Department of Health

Report on Health and Social Subjects

41

Dietary Reference Values for Food Energy and Nutrients for the United Kingdom

Report of the Panel on Dietary Reference Values
of the Committee on Medical Aspects of Food Policy

London: TSO

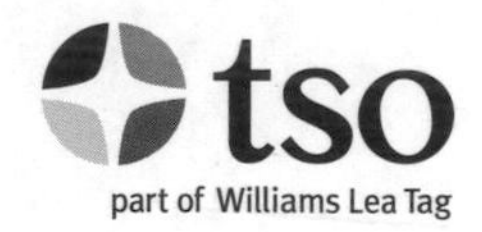

Published by TSO (The Stationery Office), part of Williams Lea Tag,
and available from:

Online
www.tsoshop.co.uk

Mail, Telephone, Fax & E-mail
TSO
PO Box 29, Norwich, NR3 1GN
Telephone orders/General enquiries: 0333 202 5070
Fax orders: 0333 202 5080
E-mail: customer.services@tso.co.uk
Textphone 0333 202 5077

TSO@Blackwell and other Accredited Agents

First published 1991

Twenty Ninth impression 2016

ISBN 978-0-11-321397-9

Printed in the United Kingdom for The Stationery Office

Preface

In 1987 the Committee on Medical Aspects of Food Policy (COMA) convened a Panel to review the Recommended Daily Amounts of food energy and nutrients for groups of people in the United Kingdom (DHSS, 1979). The Panel itself met on 7 occasions, reviewed much published information and received contributions from a number of independent experts. The Panel also set up four expert Working Groups to report on energy and protein; fat and carbohydrate; vitamins; and minerals. The Working Groups carried out the majority of the work, meeting on a total of 35 occasions. Their reports to the Panel form the major part of this Report.

The Dietary Reference Values derived by the Panel differ in a number of ways from the 1969 UK Recommended Daily Intakes (RDIs) and from the 1979 UK Recommended Daily Amounts (RDAs). The most obvious change is the range of nutrients covered. Previously COMA has considered only 10 nutrients in detail; this time the number is around 40.

We have changed the nomenclature in this Report because terms such as Recommended Daily Intakes (RDIs) and Recommended Daily Amounts (RDAs) have often led to misinterpretation. The new Reference Nutrient Intake (RNI) and the traditional RDI both represent best estimates of the requirement of those few members of the community with particularly high needs. Adopting such a stringent yardstick makes strategic sense but incorporating the descriptive term 'recommended' has led many to believe it represents the minimum desirable intake for healthy life. In reality, for the great majority of the population, the RNI or RDA is substantially more than individual needs. The Panel therefore introduced two other values for many nutrients, to provide more guidance in particular for interpretation of dietary surveys.

For the first time we have also amalgamated figures for food constituents such as fats and carbohydrates with those for micronutrients. This is because the average consumer sees no obvious distinction between 'nutrient requirements' and 'dietary recommendations for health'.

A final, but important, innovation was the decision to invite four non-UK European scientists to join our deliberations. By doing so we have been able to draw upon a wider range of experience and hope the UK Dietary Reference Values (DRVs) will be of particular help to the European Community as well as to nutritional science as a whole.

SIR DONALD ACHESON
Chairman of Committee on Medical Aspects of Food Policy

Glossary of Terms and Abbreviations

Terms relating to weight measurement

g gram

mg milligram or 10^{-3} g or one-thousandth of 1 g

μg microgram or 10^{-6} g or one-millionth of 1 g

ng nanogram or 10^{-9} g or one-thousand-millionth of 1 g

kg kilogram or 10^{3} g or 1000 g

mmol millimol = Atomic or molecular weight of element or compound in $g \times 10^{-3}$.

Terms relating to energy

kcal kilocalorie = 10^{3} or 1000 calories. A unit used to measure the energy value of food

kJ kilojoule = 10^{3} or 1000 joules. A unit used to measure the energy value of food

1kcal = 4.18 kJ

MJ megajoule = 10^{6} J or 1 million joules

BMR Basal Metabolic Rate. Rate at which the body uses energy when the body is at complete rest. Values depend on age, sex, body weight. For a 65 kg man, BMR is about 7.56 MJ/d. For a 55 kg woman, BMR is about 5.98 MJ/d

PAL Physical Activity Level. A multiple of BMR; the ratio of overall daily energy expenditure to BMR. Values range from 1.4 (for a person with light energy expenditure in work who has non-active leisure pursuits) to 1.9 (for a man in energy-demanding work whose leisure time pursuits are also energy demanding.)

Terms relating to energy and nutrient intakes

RDI Recommended Daily Intakes of Nutrients for the United Kingdom, 1969.

RDA Recommended Daily Amounts of Food Energy and Nutrients for Groups of People in the United Kingdom, 1979.

DRV Dietary Reference Value. A term used to cover LRNI, EAR, RNI and safe intake.

EAR Estimated Average Requirement of a group of people for energy or protein or a vitamin or mineral. About half will usually need more than the EAR, and half less.

LRNI Lower Reference Nutrient Intake for protein or a vitamin or mineral. An amount of the nutrient that is enough for only the few people in a group who have low needs.

RNI Reference Nutrient Intake for protein or a vitamin or mineral. An amount of the nutrient that is enough, or more than enough, for about 97% of people in a group. If average intake of a group is at RNI, then the risk of deficiency in the group is very small.

Safe intake A term used to indicate intake or range of intakes of a nutrient for which there is not enough information to estimate RNI, EAR or LRNI. It is an amount that is enough for almost everyone but not so large as to cause undesirable effects.

Terms relating to fat

Fat Dietary fat—usually triglycerides ie 3 fatty acid molecules joined to 1 molecule of glycerol.

Fatty acid A molecule of variable length consisting mainly of a carbon chain to which hydrogen atoms are attached.

Essential fatty acid (EFA) One which cannot be made in the body and which must be supplied by food.

Saturated fatty acid (SFA) One which contains the maximum possible number of hydrogen atoms.

Monounsaturated fatty acid One in which each molecule has 2 hydrogen atoms missing.

Polyunsaturated fatty acid (PUFA) A fatty acid in which each molecule has more than 2 hydrogen atoms missing.

cis and *trans* isomers Terms which relate to the spatial arrangement of atoms in molecules such as monounsaturated or polyunsaturated fatty acids. Most fatty acids which occur naturally in foods are *cis*.

Cholesterol It may be ingested in foods such as egg yolk, offal but most is made in the body. An essential component of every living cell wall. May be converted to vitamin D, and is transported around the body in blood.

LDL Low Density Lipoprotein. One of several proteins in the blood which transport cholesterol around the body. LDL is thought to be the form in which cholesterol is deposited in artery walls.

Terms relating to carbohydrates

Monosaccharides Single-molecule sugars which include glucose and fructose.

Disaccharides Sugars whose molecules consist of 2 monosaccharides joined together. Examples are sucrose (consisting of 1 glucose and 1 fructose molecule) and lactose (consisting of 1 glucose and 1 galactose molecule).

Polysaccharides Carbohydrates whose molecules consist of many monosaccharides eg starch which is many glucose molecules joined together.

NSP Non-starch polysaccharides. A precisely measurable component of foods. The best measure of 'dietary fibre'.

Simple sugars Monosaccharides and disaccharides.

Intrinsic sugars Any sugar which is contained within the cell wall of the food.

Extrinsic sugars Any sugar which is not contained within cell walls. Examples are the sugars in honey, table sugar and lactose in milk and milk products.

Non-milk extrinsic sugars Extrinsic sugars except lactose in milk and milk products.

Terms relating to proteins

Amino acid One of 20 molecules which, when joined together, make up proteins. There are many different types of proteins in food and the human body, the nature of each depending on the types of amino acids present, the proportions and the order in which they occur.

Indispensible amino acid (IAA) An amino acid which cannot be made in the body—either at all or not fast enough for the body's need—and which must be taken in food. There are 8 for adults and 10 for infants.

Contents

Committee on Medical Aspects of Food Policy
Panel on Dietary Reference Values

Chairman

Dr R G Whitehead	Director, MRC Dunn Nutrition Unit, Cambridge.

Members

Professor J V G A Durnin (Vice-Chairman)	Institute of Physiology, University of Glasgow.
Dr P J Aggett	Department of Child Health, University of Aberdeen.
Dr C J Bates	MRC Dunn Nutrition Unit, Cambridge.
Professor Dame Barbara Clayton	Geriatric Medicine Group, University of Southampton.
Dr J H Cummings	MRC Dunn Clinical Nutrition Centre, Cambridge.
Dr S Fairweather-Tait	AFRC Institute of Food Research, Norwich.
Dr G A J Pitt	Department of Biochemistry, University of Liverpool.
Dr A M Prentice	MRC Dunn Clinical Nutrition Centre, Cambridge.

Observers representing the Scientific Committee for Food of the European Commission

Dr M Gibney	Department of Clinical Medicine, Trinity College, Dublin, Eire.
Professor A P Trichopoulou	Department of Nutrition and Biochemistry, Athens School of Public Health, Athens, Greece.

Observers

Dr J G Ablett	Department of Health, London.
Dr P C Clarke	Department of Health, London.
Dr G I Forbes (until 1989)	Scottish Home and Health Department, Edinburgh.
Professor L Garby	Institute of Physiology, Odense University, Odense, Denmark.
Professor J G A J Hautvast	Department of Human Nutrition, Wageningen Agricultural University, Wageningen, Netherlands.
Dr D J Hine	Welsh Office, Cardiff.
Dr H Kilgore	Department of Health and Social Services (Northern Ireland), Belfast.
Dr R Skinner (from 1989)	Scottish Office Home and Health Department, Edinburgh.

Secretariat

Dr M J Wiseman (Medical)	Department of Health, London.
Mr R W Wenlock (Scientific)	Department of Health, London.
Dr D H Buss (Scientific)	Ministry of Agriculture, Fisheries and Food, London.
Mr K L G Follin (Administrative until 1989)	Department of Health, London.
Mrs J Caro (Administrative from 1989)	Department of Health, London.
Mrs E Lohani (Administrative)	Department of Health, London.
Mr D Roberts (Administrative until 1989)	Department of Health, London.

Panel on Dietary Reference Values Working Group on Energy and Protein

Members

Professor J V G A Durnin (Chairman)	Institute of Physiology, University of Glasgow.
Dr A M Prentice (Vice-Chairman)	MRC Dunn Clinical Nutrition Centre, Cambridge.
Professor A A Jackson	Department of Human Nutrition, University of Southampton.
Professor W P T James	Rowett Research Institute, Aberdeen.
Dr D J Millward	Department of Nutrition, London School of Hygiene and Tropical Medicine, University of London.
Dr N G Norgan	Department of Human Sciences, Loughborough University.

Observers

Dr J G Ablett	Department of Health, London.
Dr D H Buss	Ministry of Agriculture, Fisheries and Food, London.
Dr P C Clarke	Department of Health, London.
Dr R G Whitehead (Chairman of the Panel on DRV)	MRC Dunn Nutrition Unit, Cambridge.

Secretariat

Dr M J Wiseman (Medical)	Department of Health, London.
Mr R W Wenlock (Scientific)	Department of Health, London.
Mr K L G Follin (Administrative until 1989)	Department of Health, London.
Mrs J Caro (Administrative from 1989)	Department of Health, London.
Mrs E Lohani (Administrative)	Department of Health, London.
Mr D Roberts (Administrative until 1989)	Department of Health, London.

Panel on Dietary Reference Values Working Group on Fat and Carbohydrates

Members

Dr J H Cummings (Chairman)	MRC Dunn Clinical Nutrition Centre, Cambridge.
Professor Dame Barbara Clayton (Vice-Chairman)	Geriatric Medicine Group, University of Southampton.
Professor K G M M Alberti	Department of Medicine, University of Newcastle-upon-Tyne.
Dr S A Bingham	MRC Dunn Clinical Nutrition Centre, Cambridge.
Professor M G Marmot	Department of Community Medicine, University College and Middlesex School of Medicine, London.
Professor J Shepherd (from 1988)	Department of Pathological Biochemistry, University of Glasgow.
Professor D A T Southgate	AFRC Institute of Food Research, Norwich.
Professor O M Wrong (until 1988)	Department of Medicine, University College and Middlesex Hospital School of Medicine, London.

Observers

Dr J G Ablett	Department of Health, London.
Dr D H Buss	Ministry of Agriculture, Fisheries and Food, London.
Dr P C Clarke	Department of Health, London.
Mr R W Wenlock	Department of Health, London.
Dr R G Whitehead (Chairman of the Panel on DRV)	MRC Dunn Nutrition Unit, Cambridge.

Secretariat

Dr M J Wiseman (Medical)	Department of Health, London.
Mr K L G Follin (Administrative until 1989)	Department of Health, London.
Mrs J Caro (Administrative from 1989)	Department of Health, London.
Mrs E Lohani (Administrative)	Department of Health, London.
Mr D Roberts (Administrative)	Department of Health, London.

Panel on Dietary Reference Values Working Group on Vitamins

Members

Dr G A J Pitt (Chairman)	Department of Biochemistry, University of Liverpool.
Dr C J Bates (Vice-Chairman)	MRC Dunn Nutrition Unit, Cambridge.
Dr D A Bender	Department of Biochemistry, University College, London.
Dr D E M Lawson	AFRC Institute of Animal Physiology and Genetics Research, Cambridge.
Dr D P R Muller	Department of Child Health, Institute of Child Health, London.
Dr E M E Poskitt	Institute of Child Health, Royal Liverpool Children's Hospital, Alder Hey, Liverpool.
Dr M J Shearer	Clinical Science Laboratories, United Medical and Dental Schools of Guy's and St. Thomas' Hospitals Guy's Campus, London.
Dr D I Thurnham	MRC Dunn Nutrition Unit, Cambridge.

Observers

Dr J G Ablett	Department of Health, London.
Dr P C Clarke	Department of Health, London.
Dr H A Tyler	Ministry of Agriculture, Fisheries and Food, London.
Mr R W Wenlock	Department of Health, London.
Dr R G Whitehead (Chairman of the Panel on DRV)	MRC Dunn Nutrition Unit, Cambridge.
Dr M J Wiseman	Department of Health, London.

Secretariat

Dr D H Buss (Scientific)	Ministry of Agriculture, Fisheries and Food, London.
Ms A M E Mills (Scientific)	Ministry of Agriculture, Fisheries and Food, London.

Panel on Dietary Reference Values Working Group on Minerals

Members

Dr P J Aggett (Chairman)	Department of Child Health, University of Aberdeen.
Dr S Fairweather-Tait (Vice-chairman)	AFRC Institute of Food Research, Norwich.
Professor M I Gurr	Lately, Nutrition Consultant, Milk Marketing Board, Thames Ditton.
Dr M Lawson	Department of Child Health, Institute of Child Health, London.
Professor C F Mills	Rowett Research Institute, Aberdeen.

Observers

Dr J G Ablett	Department of Health, London.
Dr D H Buss	Ministry of Agriculture, Fisheries and Food, London.
Dr P C Clarke	Department of Health, London.
Dr R G Whitehead (Chairman of the Panel on DRV)	MRC Dunn Nutrition Unit, Cambridge.

Secretariat

Mr R W Wenlock (Scientific)	Department of Health, London.
Dr M J Wiseman (Medical)	Department of Health, London.
Mr K L G Follin (Administrative until 1989)	Department of Health, London.
Mrs J Caro (Administrative from 1989)	Department of Health, London.
Mrs E Lohani (Administrative)	Department of Health, London.
Mr D Roberts (Administrative)	Department of Health, London.

Acknowledgements

Written contributions were submitted from the following organisations and experts.

Dr S M Barlow
International Association of Fish Meal Manufacturers, Potters Bar, Hertfordshire.

Miss A E Black
British Dietetic Association, Birmingham.

Professor J A Blair
University of Aston, Birmingham.

Dr J T Brocklebank
Department of Paediatrics and Child Health, St James's University Hospital, Leeds.

Professor D Bryce-Smith
Department of Chemistry, University of Reading.

Dr C E Casey
Department of Medicine and Therapeutics, University of Aberdeen.

Miss S Chinn
Department of Community Medicine, United Medical and Dental Schools of Guy's and St. Thomas's Hospitals, London.

Professor M A Crawford
Nuffield Laboratory of Comparative Medicine, Institute of Zoology, London.

Dr R B Fraser
Department of Obstetrics and Gynaecology, University of Sheffield.

Professor M I Gurr
Lately, Milk Marketing Board, Thames Ditton, Surrey.

Mr W D B Hamilton
Kellogg Company of Great Britain, Ltd.

Mr J C Hammond
Food and Drink Federation, London.

Dr K Heaton
University Department of Medicine, University of Bristol.

Mrs E Hoinville
London School of Hygiene and Tropical Medicine, London.

Dr J A Kanis	Department of Human Metabolism and Clinical Biochemistry, Medical School, University of Sheffield.
Dr A B Lehmann	Department of Health Care of the Elderly, Medical School, University of Nottingham.
Professor J Lennard-Jones	St Marks's Hospital, London.
Dr A F Lever	MRC Blood Pressure Unit, Western Infirmary, Glasgow.
Professor M F Oliver	Department of Medicine, University of Edinburgh.
The National Association for Premenstrual Syndrome	Sevenoaks, Kent.
The National Osteoporosis Society	London.
Miss H Paine	Infant and Dietetic Foods Association, London.
Professor R Passmore	Edinburgh.
Mr D J Roberton	Hoffman-LaRoche, Welwyn Garden City.
Professor G Rose	Department of Medical Statistics and Epidemiology, London School of Hygiene and Tropical Medicine, University of London.
Dr C J Schorah	Department of Medical Pathology, University of Leeds.
Dr D H Shrimpton	Committee for Responsible Nutrition.
The Sugar Bureau	London
Professor J D Swales	Department of Medicine, University of Leicester.

Professor Dame Barbara Clayton of the University of Southampton, Dr C Cooper of Bristol Royal Infirmary, Professor J Grimley Evans of the Radcliffe Infirmary, Oxford, Dr J Gutteridge, National Institute of Biological Standards, Stanmore, Dr D E M Lawson of the Institute of Animal Physiology, Cambridge, and Professor B A Wharton of Glasgow University attended special meetings of the Working Groups.

The Working Groups are very grateful for the very valuable assistance given freely by all these contributors, without whom Dietary Reference Values for key nutrients could not have been formulated.

Summary tables

THE FOLLOWING TABLES SET OUT IN SUMMARY FORM THE FINDINGS OF THE PANEL:

Table 1.1 *Estimated Average Requirements (EARs) for Energy*

Age	EARs MJ/d (kcal/d)	
	males	females
0–3 months	2.28 (545)	2.16 (515)
4–6 months	2.89 (690)	2.69 (645)
7–9 months	3.44 (825)	3.20 (765)
10–12 months	3.85 (920)	3.61 (865)
1–3 years	5.15 (1,230)	4.86 (1,165)
4–6 years	7.16 (1,715)	6.46 (1,545)
7–10 years	8.24 (1,970)	7.28 (1,740)
11–14 years	9.27 (2,220)	7.72 (1,845)
15–18 years	11.51 (2,755)	8.83 (2,110)
19–50 years	10.60 (2,550)	8.10 (1,940)
51–59 years	10.60 (2,550)	8.00 (1,900)
60–64 years	9.93 (2,380)	7.99 (1,900)
65–74 years	9.71 (2,330)	7.96 (1,900)
75+ years	8.77 (2,100)	7.61 (1,810)
Pregnancy		+0.80*(200)
Lactation:		
1 month		+1.90 (450)
2 months		+2.20 (530)
3 months		+2.40 (570)
4–6 months (Group 1)**		+2.00 (480)
4–6 months (Group 2)		+2.40 (570)
>6 months (Group 1)		+1.00 (240)
>6 months (Group 2)		+2.30 (550)

*last trimester only
**See para 2.5.2

Table 1.2 *Dietary Reference Values for fat and carbohydrate for adults as a percentage of daily total energy intake (percentage of food energy)*

	Individual minimum	Population average	Individual maximum
Saturated fatty acids		10 (11)	
Cis-polyunsaturated fatty acids		6 (6.5)	10
	n−3 0.2		
	n−6 1.0		
Cis-monounsaturated fatty acids		12 (13)	
Trans fatty acids		2 (2)	
Total fatty acids		30 (32.5)	
TOTAL FAT		33 (35)	
Non-milk extrinsic sugars	0	10 (11)	
Intrinsic and milk sugars and starch		37 (39)	
TOTAL CARBOHYDRATE		47 (50)	
NON-STARCH POLYSACCHARIDE (g/d)	12	18	24

The average percentage contribution to total energy does not total 100% because figures for protein and alcohol are excluded. Protein intakes average 15 per cent of total energy which is above the RNI. It is recognised that many individuals will derive some energy from alcohol, and this has been assumed to average 5 per cent approximating to current intakes. However the Panel allowed that some groups might not drink alcohol and that for some purposes nutrient intakes as a proportion of food energy (without alcohol) might be useful. Therefore average figures are given as percentages both of total energy and, in parenthesis, of food energy.

Table 1.3 *Reference Nutrient Intakes for Protein*

Age	Reference Nutrient Intake[a] g/d
0–3 months	12.5[b]
4–6 months	12.7
7–9 months	13.7
10–12 months	14.9
1–3 years	14.5
4–6 years	19.7
7–10 years	28.3
Males:	
11–14 years	42.1
15–18 years	55.2
19–50 years	55.5
50+ years	53.3
Females:	
11–14 years	41.2
15–18 years	45.0
19–50 years	45.0
50+ years	46.5
Pregnancy[c]	+ 6
Lactation[c]:	
0–4 months	+11
4+ months	+ 8

[a] These figures, based on egg and milk protein, assume complete digestibility.

[b] No values for infants 0–3 months are given by WHO. The RNI is calculated from the recommendations of COMA. (See Table 7.1)

[c] To be added to adult requirement through all stages of pregnancy and lactation.

Table 1.4 *Reference Nutrient Intakes for Vitamins*

Age	Thiamin	Riboflavin	Niacin (nicotinic acid equivalent)	Vitamin B6	Vitamin B12	Folate	Vitamin C	Vitamin A	Vitamin D
	mg/d	mg/d	mg/d	mg/d†	μg/d	μg/d	mg/d	μg/d	μg/d
0–3 months	0.2	0.4	3	0.2	0.3	50	25	350	8.5
4–6 months	0.2	0.4	3	0.2	0.3	50	25	350	8.5
7–9 months	0.2	0.4	4	0.3	0.4	50	25	350	7
10–12 months	0.3	0.4	5	0.4	0.4	50	25	350	7
1–3 years	0.5	0.6	8	0.7	0.5	70	30	400	7
4–6 years	0.7	0.8	11	0.9	0.8	100	30	400	—
7–10 years	0.7	1.0	12	1.0	1.0	150	30	500	—
Males									
11–14 years	0.9	1.2	15	1.2	1.2	200	35	600	—
15–18 years	1.1	1.3	18	1.5	1.5	200	40	700	—
19–50 years	1.0	1.3	17	1.4	1.5	200	40	700	—
50+ years	0.9	1.3	16	1.4	1.5	200	40	700	**
Females									
11–14 years	0.7	1.1	12	1.0	1.2	200	35	600	—
15–18 years	0.8	1.1	14	1.2	1.5	200	40	600	—
19–50 years	0.8	1.1	13	1.2	1.5	200	40	600	—
50+ years	0.8	1.1	12	1.2	1.5	200	40	600	**
Pregnancy	+0.1***	+0.3	*	*	*	+100	+10***	+100	10
Lactation:									
0–4 months	+0.2	+0.5	+2	*	+0.5	+ 60	+30	+350	10
4+ months	+0.2	+0.5	+2	*	+0.5	+ 60	+30	+350	10

*No increment **After age 65 the RNI is 10 μg/d for men and women ***For last trimester only †Based on protein providing 14.7 per cent of EAR for energy

Table 1.5 *Reference Nutrient Intakes for Minerals* (SI Units)

Age	Calcium	Phosphorus[1]	Magnesium	Sodium	Potassium	Chloride[4]	Iron	Zinc	Copper	Selenium	Iodine
	mmol/d	mmol/d	mmol/d	mmol/d	mmol/d	mmol/d	µmol/d	µmol/d	µmol/d	µmol/d	µmol/d
0–3 months	13.1	13.1	2.2	9	20	9	30	60	5	0.1	0.4
4–6 months	13.1	13.1	2.5	12	22	12	80	60	5	0.2	0.5
7–9 months	13.1	13.1	3.2	14	18	14	140	75	5	0.1	0.5
10–12 months	13.1	13.1	3.3	15	18	15	140	75	5	0.1	0.5
1–3 years	8.8	8.8	3.5	22	20	22	120	75	6	0.2	0.6
4–6 years	11.3	11.3	4.8	30	28	30	110	100	9	0.3	0.8
7–10 years	13.8	13.8	8.0	50	50	50	160	110	11	0.4	0.9
Males											
11–14 years	25.0	25.0	11.5	70	80	70	200	140	13	0.6	1.0
15–18 years	25.0	25.0	12.3	70	90	70	200	145	16	0.9	1.0
19–50 years	17.5	17.5	12.3	70	90	70	160	145	19	0.9	1.0
50+ years	17.5	17.5	12.3	70	90	70	160	145	19	0.9	1.0
Females											
11–14 years	20.0	20.0	11.5	70	80	70	260[5]	140	13	0.6	1.0
15–18 years	20.0	20.0	12.3	70	90	70	260[5]	110	16	0.8	1.1
19–50 years	17.5	17.5	10.9	70	90	70	260[5]	110	19	0.8	1.1
50+ years	17.5	17.5	10.9	70	90	70	160	110	19	0.8	1.1
Pregnancy	*	*	*	*	*	*	*	*	*	*	*
Lactation:											
0–4 months	+14.3	+14.3	+2.1	*	*	*	*	+90	+5	+0.2	*
4+ months	+14.3	+14.3	+2.1	*	*	*	*	+40	+5	+0.2	*

*No increment

[1] Phosphorus RNI is set equal to calcium in molar terms

[2] 1 mmol sodium = 23 mg

[3] 1 mmol potassium = 39 mg

[4] Corresponds to sodium 1 mmol = 35.5 mg

[5] Insufficient for women with high menstrual losses where the most practical way of meeting iron requirements is to take iron supplements (see table 28.2)

Table 1.5 *Reference Nutrient Intakes for Minerals* (continued)

Age	Calcium	Phosphorus[1]	Magnesium	Sodium	Potassium	Chloride[4]	Iron	Zinc	Copper	Selenium	Iodine
	mg/d	mg/d	mg/d	mg/d[2]	mg/d[3]	mg/d	mg/d	mg/d	mg/d	µg/d	µg/d
0–3 months	525	400	55	210	800	320	1.7	4.0	0.2	10	50
4–6 months	525	400	60	280	850	400	4.3	4.0	0.3	13	60
7–9 months	525	400	75	320	700	500	7.8	5.0	0.3	10	60
10–12 months	525	400	80	350	700	500	7.8	5.0	0.3	10	60
1–3 years	350	270	85	500	800	800	6.9	5.0	0.4	15	70
4–6 years	450	350	120	700	1,100	1,100	6.1	6.5	0.6	20	100
7–10 years	550	450	200	1,200	2,000	1,800	8.7	7.0	0.7	30	110
Males											
11–14 years	1,000	775	280	1,600	3,100	2,500	11.3	9.0	0.8	45	130
15–18 years	1,000	775	300	1,600	3,500	2,500	11.3	9.5	1.0	70	140
19–50 years	700	550	300	1,600	3,500	2,500	8.7	9.5	1.2	75	140
50+ years	700	550	300	1,600	3,500	2,500	8.7	9.5	1.2	75	140
Females											
11–14 years	800	625	280	1,600	3,100	2,500	14.8[5]	9.0	0.8	45	130
15–18 years	800	625	300	1,600	3,500	2,500	14.8[5]	7.0	1.0	60	140
19–50 years	700	550	270	1,600	3,500	2,500	14.8[5]	7.0	1.2	60	140
50+ years	700	550	270	1,600	3,500	2,500	8.7	7.0	1.2	60	140
Pregnancy	*	*	*	*	*	*	*	*	*	*	*
Lactation:											
0–4 months	+550	+440	+ 50	*	*	*	*	+6.0	+0.3	+15	*
4+ months	+550	+440	+ 50	*	*	*	*	+2.5	+0.3	+15	*

*No increment

[1]Phosphorus RNI is set equal to calcium in molar terms

[2]1 mmol sodium = 23 mg

[3]1 mmol potassium = 39 mg

[4]Corresponds to sodium 1 mmol = 35.5 mg

[5]Insufficient for women with high menstrual losses where the most practical way of meeting iron requirements is to take iron supplements (see table 28.2)

Table 1.6 *Safe intakes*

Nutrient	Safe intake*
Vitamins:	
Pantothenic acid	
adults	3–7 mg/d
infants	1.7 mg/d
Biotin	10–200 μg/d
Vitamin E	
men	above 4 mg/d
women	above 3 mg/d
infants	0.4 mg/g polyunsaturated fatty acids
Vitamin K	
adults	1 μg/kg/d
infants	10 μg/d
Minerals:	
Manganese	
adults	above 1.4 mg (26 μmol)/d
infants and children	above 16 μg (0.3 μmol)/kg/d
Molybdenum	
adults	50–400μg/d
infants, children and adolescents	0.5–1.5 μg/kg/d
Chromium	
adults	above 25 μg (0.5 μmol)/d
children and adolescents	0.1–1.0 μg (2–20 nmol)/kg/d
Fluoride	
children over 6 years and adults	0.5 mg/kg/d (3 μmol/kg/day)
children over 6 months	0.12 mg/kg/d (6 μmol/kg/day)
infants under 6 months	0.22 mg/kg/d (12 μmol/kg/day)

*See para 1.3.18

1. Introduction

1.1 **Background to the Panel** The Panel on Dietary Reference Values was set up in 1987 by the Committee on Medical Aspects of Food Policy (COMA) to review the Recommended Daily Amounts (RDAs) of food energy and nutrients for groups of people in the United Kingdom which had been set in 1979. The Panel recognised from the outset that this was such a major task that it could be completed only by the creation of expert Working Groups to consider various classes of nutrients and to report their considerations and conclusions to the Panel. Four Working Groups were convened to review requirements for energy and protein; for fat and carbohydrate; for vitamins; and for minerals.

1.2 Terms of Reference of the Panel

'To review the Recommended Daily Amounts (RDAs) for food energy and nutrients for groups of people in the United Kingdom.'

1.3 Interpretation of the Terms of Reference

1.3.1 The definition of the Recommended Daily Amount (RDA) for a nutrient which was used in the previous Report of the Committee on Medical Aspects of Food Policy[1] is 'the average amount of the nutrient which should be provided per head in a group of people if the needs of practically all members of the group are to be met'. This was framed in an attempt to make it clear that the amounts referred to are averages for a group of people and not amounts which individuals must consume. In the earlier report published by COMA[2] the definition of Recommended Intakes was 'the amounts sufficient, or more than sufficient, for the nutritional needs of practically all healthy persons in a population'. The word 'Intakes' was used to emphasise that the recommendations related to foods as actually eaten.

1.3.2 In considering the options available this Panel was conscious not only of these differences in UK definitions but also of the variety of different definitions in other countries. The Panel was however aware of the continuing potential for misuse and misinterpretation of any single figure, however defined. To minimise this and to help users to interpret dietary information on both groups and individuals the Panel decided to try to set a range of intakes based as far as possible on its assessment of the distribution of requirements for each nutrient. The Panel called these various figures Dietary Reference Values (DRVs) and the Panel adopted the title of the Panel on Dietary Reference Values.

1.3.3 The Panel considered that this change in approach and nomenclature would reduce the chance of misunderstanding the true nature of its figures as estimates of reference values *and not as recommendations* for intakes by individuals or groups. These reference values can be deployed in a variety of ways, for instance as yardsticks for the assessment of dietary surveys and food supply statistics; to provide guidance on appropriate dietary composition and meal provision; or for food labelling purposes. The appropriate DRV varies with the purpose for which it is intended. The Panel was strongly of the opinion that all the values should be closely related to the biological parameters used to derive the figures, irrespective of the intended use. These values can be used as the basis for recommendations in a number of areas in which the Panel had no specific expertise, eg agriculture, economics and sociology, which require the use not only of the reference values but of other sets of knowledge and judgements as well.

1.3.4 *Criteria of adequacy* Requirements for a nutrient differ from one individual to another and may also change with alterations in the composition and nature of the diet as a whole, because such alterations may affect the efficiency with which nutrients are absorbed and/or utilized (Annex 8). Classically the requirement of an individual for a nutrient has been the amount of that nutrient required to prevent clinical signs of deficiency. While this must always be an important element in defining a requirement, it can be argued that societies should expect more than the basic need to avoid deficiency, and that some allowance should be made, where appropriate, for a degree of storage of the nutrient to allow for periods of low intake or high demand without detriment to health. Claims have also been made that at very high levels of intake some nutrients have especially beneficial or therapeutic effects but the Panel decided that these effects did not fall within their definition of requirement. The Panel did, however, try to give some guidance on possible effects of very high intakes (see also para 1.3.9).

1.3.5 Because, apart from essential fatty acids (EFA), there is no absolute requirement for fats, sugars or starches, it is not possible to derive useful reference figures for them based on a range of requirements. Rather, the Panel has made pragmatic judgements based on the *changes* from current intakes which would be expected to result in certain changes in physiological and or health outcomes. These judgements have been made bearing in mind the likely changes which might occur in the prevailing socio-cultural environment in the UK, and should not be taken to represent 'ideal' figures.

1.3.6 The information from which estimates of requirements have been made can be categorised as follows:

a. the intakes of a nutrient needed to maintain a given circulating level or degree of enzyme saturation or tissue concentration;

b. the intakes of a nutrient by individuals and by groups which are associated with the absence of any signs of deficiency diseases;

c. the intakes of a nutrient needed to maintain balance noting that the period over which such balance needs to be measured differs for different nutrients, and between individuals;

d. the intakes of a nutrient needed to cure clinical signs of deficiency;

e. the intakes of a nutrient associated with an appropriate biological marker of nutritional adequacy.

1.3.7 The Panel found no single criterion to define requirements for all nutrients. Some nutrients may have a variety of physiological effects at different levels of intake. Which of these effects should form the parameter of adequacy is therefore to some extent arbitrary. For each nutrient the particular parameter or parameters which were used to define adequacy are given in the text. None of these criteria is perfect, but they were judged to be the best available on which to base DRV so that they were relevant to prevailing circumstances. In some cases the evidence on which they are based is reliable experimental data, in others it is from associations, often epidemiological, and in others evidence may be limited to anecdotal data of variable persuasiveness.

1.3.8 *Definition of Dietary Reference Values* Although information is usually inadequate to calculate the precise distribution of requirements in a group of individuals for a nutrient, it has been assumed to be normally distributed (Figure 1.1). This gives a notional mean requirement or Estimated Average Requirement (EAR) with the inter-individual variability in requirements illustrated in figure 1.1. The Panel has defined the Reference Nutrient Intake (RNI) as point c in the distribution, that is two notional standard deviations (2sd) above the (EAR) (point b). Intakes above this amount will almost certainly be adequate. A further value at point a, two notional standard deviations (2sd) below the mean, the Lower Reference Nutrient Intake (LNRI), represents the lowest intakes which will meet the needs of some individuals in the group. Intakes below this level are almost certainly inadequate for most individuals. For some nutrients the derivation of DRVs was not possible from these principles, and this is stated in the text. In particular, for those nutrients where no requirement could be defined (starches, sugars, fat and fatty acids), the DRVs are not derived on these principles, although analogous figures based on pragmatic judgements have been proposed (see para 1.6.6).

1.3.9 At higher levels of consumption there may be evidence of undesirable effects. Guidance on such high levels of consumption is given in the text. The RNI remains equivalent to the 1969 RDI—that is the amount sufficient or more than sufficient to meet the nutritional needs of practically all healthy persons in a population[2], and therefore exceeds the requirements of most.

1.3.10 By setting the RNI at a notional 2 sd above the EAR the Panel was aware that this might, in theory, be perceived as leaving up to 2.5 per cent of the population inadequately provided for, but considered that this was unlikely to be so in practice In any population choosing spontaneous diets it is likely that, while the distribution stays roughly the same, the individuals comprising the extremes will vary, so that consistent intakes at the extremes are unlikely. Information is not usually available to determine the mean and sd with such precision and in such circumstances the Panel has chosen an intake that, as far as can be ascertained, is adequate for everyone. The risk of 2.5 per cent of the

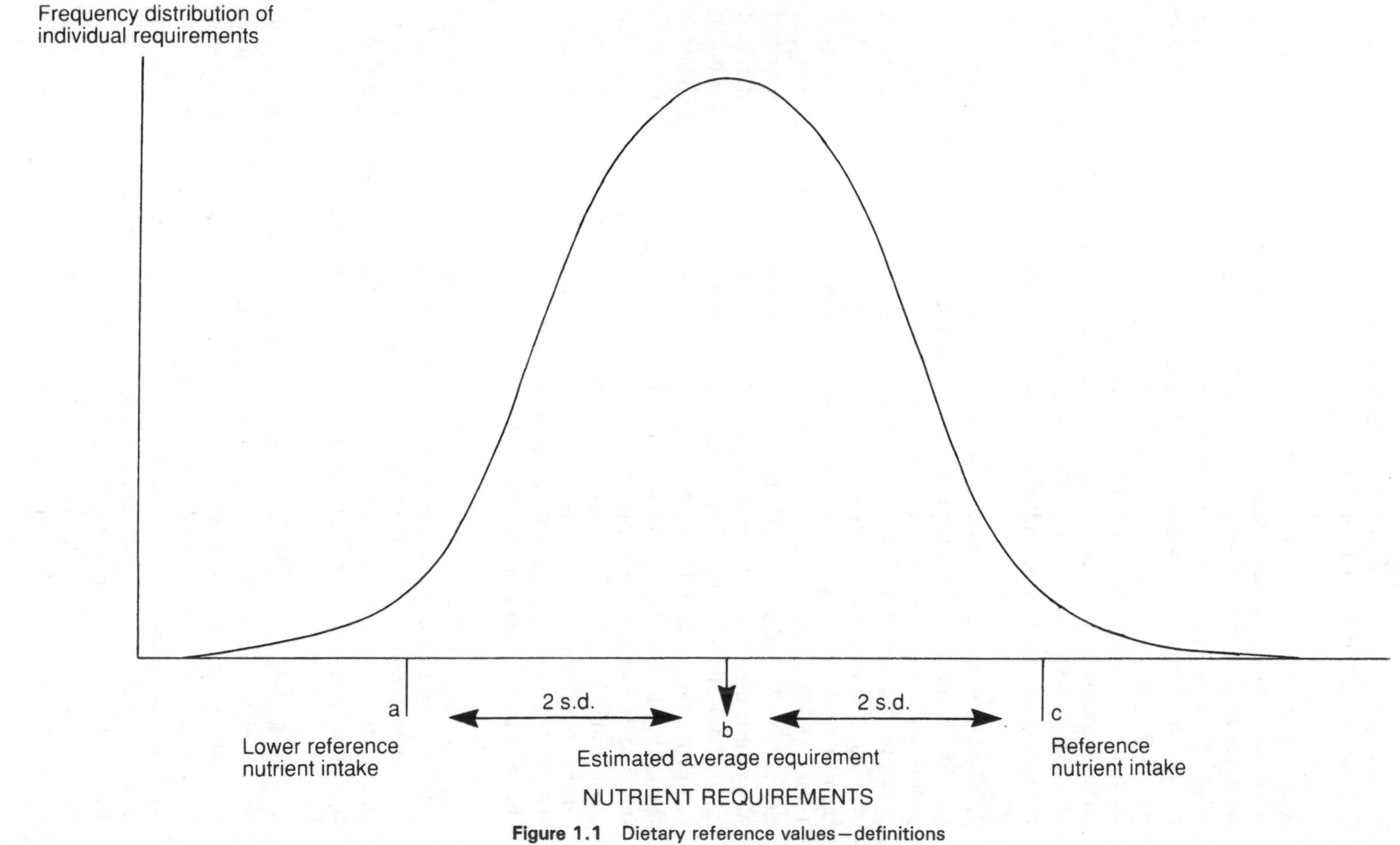

Figure 1.1 Dietary reference values—definitions

population not being adequately supplied by the RNI is therefore considered very remote.

1.3.11 *Interpretation of Dietary Reference Values* For most nutrients the Panel found insufficient data to establish any of these DRVs with great confidence. There are inherent errors in some of the data, for instance in individuals' reports of their food intake, and the day-to-day variation in nutrient intakes also complicates interpretation. Even given complete accuracy of a dietary record, its relation to habitual intake remains uncertain, however long the recording period. The food composition tables normally used to determine nutrient intake from dietary records contain a number of assumptions and imperfections. Furthermore, there is uncertainty about the relevance of many biological markers, such as serum concentrations of a nutrient, as evidence of an individual's 'status' for that nutrient. Thus uncertainties relating to the appropriate parameter by which to assess the requirement, to the completeness of the database for any nutrient, and to the precision and accuracy of dietary intake data lead to the need to make judgements.

1.3.12 Equally, when nutrient intakes are measured there is demonstrable inter-individual variation, which is not necessarily related to the variation in requirements. Figure 1.2 demonstrates a distribution of intakes identical to the distribution of requirements but where any individual's intake is not necessarily the same as his own requirement. An individual whose intake is at point a—the LRNI—*may* be meeting his requirements for a nutrient, but it is highly probable that he is not. Similarly it is just possible, but very improbable, that an individual consuming a nutrient at point c—the RNI—will be consuming insufficient amounts of that nutrient. Whatever parameter is used the risk of deficiency in an individual at a given intake will vary from virtually zero at point c to virtually 100 per cent at point a. It should be recognised that the time course of the relationship between intake and status varies between different nutrients. For instance daily energy intakes should approximate requirements while assessment of intakes of some micronutrients needs to be integrated over days, weeks, or even longer. Furthermore not only may nutrients have effects on health at the time they are eaten, but there is growing evidence that diet may be one of the factors in early, even intrauterine, life which has an influence on later health in adult life.

1.3.13 If the distribution of intakes in a group of individuals is identical to that of their requirements for a nutrient it is probable that some with lower intakes will have higher requirements and *vice versa*. If there is no correlation between intakes and requirements in a group, then an average intake equal to the EAR carries a substantial risk of deficiency in the group represented by the upper dotted line depicting risk (Figure 1.2). In order to avoid this risk completely, the distribution of intakes of the group would have to be such that the lowest intakes exceeded the highest requirements. If, as is likely, there is some correlation between intakes and requirements, then the higher that correlation the lower the risk. In fact, there may be relationships between intake and requirements on the basis of body size, which in part determines energy

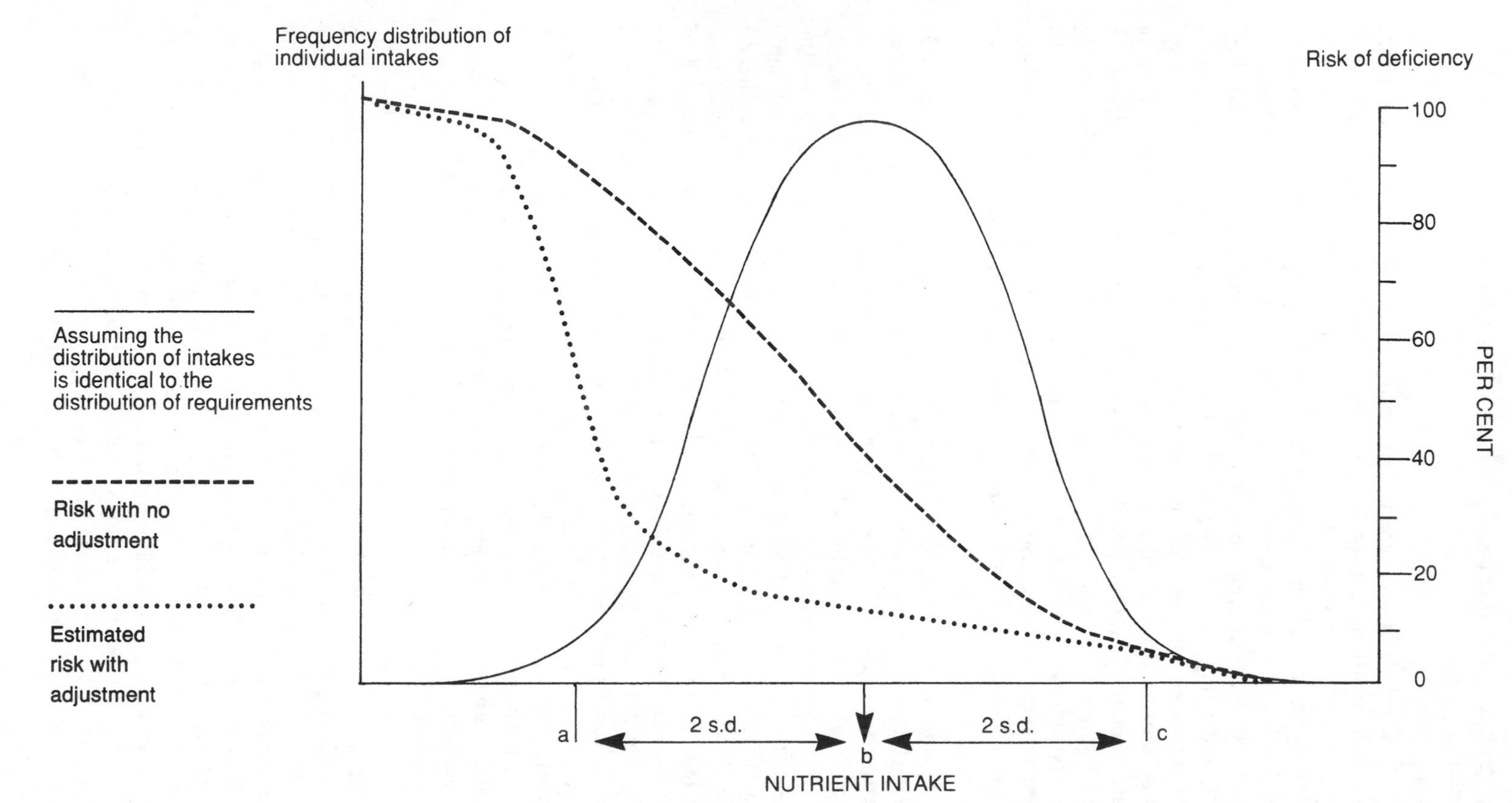

Figure 1.2 Dietary intakes and risk of deficiency

requirements and therefore energy (and food) intakes. The degree to which this occurs is not known. The lower dotted line in Figure 1.2 represents the Panel's assessment of the actual risk of deficiency in a group, taking account of this. Furthermore, apparent requirements of individuals at prevailing intake levels may not represent basal requirements. If intake by an individual falls below the usual intake, there may be adaptive mechanisms which reduce the risk of deficiency but which may not be fully effective until a period of time has elapsed. This effect varies between different nutrients.

1.3.14 *Weights and standard age ranges* As requirements for most nutrients vary with both age and sex, the Panel has attempted to set DRVs for all such groups of the population. In theory at least DRVs could be set for each sex at every age but in practice the evidence is insufficient and the population has been assigned to broad groups divided by age and sex. The 'standard age groups' adopted by the Panel are given below. Some DRVs are also related to body weight and in the past the standard weights used for calculations in respect of British children have been those of Tanner *et al*[3]. The Panel has sought new weight data for use in calculating DRVs for people of all ages in the UK. These are described in Annex 1 to this Report with descriptions of source studies. These weights are given below for each of the standard age groups.

Children		Males		Females	
Age	Weight (kg)	Age	Weight (kg)	Age	Weight (kg)
0–3 months	5.9	11–14 years	43.1	11–14 years	43.8
(formula-fed)		15–18 years	64.5	15–18 years	55.5
4–6 months	7.7	19–50 years	74.0	19–50 years	60.0
7–9 months	8.9	50+ years	71.0	50+ years	62.0
10–12 months	9.8				
1–3 years	12.6			Pregnancy	
4–6 years	17.8			Lactation: 0–4 months	
7–10 years	28.3			4+ months	

The Panel considered the elderly as a separate group but found few data on their particular nutrient requirements. Wherever possible the separate requirements of the elderly for specific nutrients are addressed in the text. The Panel recommended that more investigations be carried out into nutrient requirements of the UK population, their nutritional status and methods for its measurement, particularly for the elderly and for children.

1.3.15 *Pregnancy* DRVs reflecting any additional estimated requirement for pregnancy are given as a single incremental figure. For most nutrients, however, no increment for pregnancy is given. This does not necessarily imply no increase in metabolic demand during pregnancy, but rather that such extra demands should be met by normal adaptation or increased efficiency of utilisation, or from stores of the nutrient. Indeed, in women, it is partly for such a purpose that stores are required, so removing the need for an increase in dietary intake, which in practice does not occur. These incremental DRVs therefore depend at least in part on the adequacy of the prepregnancy stores, which would be expected if the prepregnant requirements were met. The Panel recognised that there may be subgroups or individuals in whom this is not necessarily the case, and endorsed the easy availability of cheap adequately formulated vitamin tablets for pregnant and lactating women, which are available free to those in receipt of income support. Woman are advised that in order to avoid risk of undesirable effects from vitamin A, any supplementation should only be on the advice of a doctor or ante-natal clinic.

1.3.16 *Breast-fed and infant formula-fed infants* The Panel endorsed human (breast) milk as best for babies and saw no value in setting DRVs for breast-fed infants. The Panel therefore decided that DRVs would be set only for infants fed with artificial feeds (formulas) whose nutrient intakes are dependent on the composition of the artificial feeds being offered. For most nutrients the DRV of infants who are not wholly breast-fed represents *at least* the same amount of each nutrient from formulas and other foods as the wholly breast-fed infant of the same age would receive. The amount of any nutrient consumed by a wholly breast-fed infant can be calculated from the concentration in breast milk and the volume consumed, but the efficiency of absorption of energy and some nutrients from formulas is less than from breast milk and some adjustment may be needed. Thus, in some cases the DRVs for infants aged 0–3 months who are formula-fed are in excess of those which might be expected to be derived from breast milk. This should not be taken to mean that provision of these nutrients from breast milk is unsatisfactory. In addition, the DRVs for some nutrients such as calcium and phosphorus may be higher than the levels obtained from some proprietary brands of infant formulas. However, the Panel did not see its role as reviewing the compositional criteria for infant formulas, and noted these discrepancies which are within the ranges currently permitted in the UK[4], although some fall outside the ranges permitted by the draft European Commission Directive on Infant Formulae and Follow-on Milks.

1.3.17 The RNIs are summarised in tables 1.1 to 1.5 but in each section dealing with a nutrient all the DRVs, that is the RNIs and wherever possible the LRNIs and the EARs, are provided in tables. Mass units are still generally better understood by most nutritionists and dietitians, but the RNI for minerals are given first in SI units in table 1.5.

1.3.18 *Safe intakes* For some nutrients, which are known to have important functions in humans, the Panel found insufficient reliable data on human requirements and were unable to set any DRVs for these. However, they decided on grounds of prudence to set a safe intake, particularly for infants and children, and these are given in table 1.6. The safe intake was judged to be a level or range of intake at which there is no risk of deficiency, and below a level where there is a risk of undesirable effects. They are not therefore intended as a 'toxic level', and although exceeding these safe intakes would not necessarily result in undesirable effects, equally there is no evidence for any benefits. The Panel agreed that the safe range of intakes set for the nutrients in table 1.6 need not be exceeded.

1.4 **Uses of Dietary Reference Values** These DRVs apply to groups of healthy people and are not necessarily appropriate for those with different needs arising from disease, such as infections, disorders of the gastro-intestinal tract or metabolic abnormalities. **The DRVs for any one nutrient presuppose that requirements for energy and all other nutrients are met.** There are a number of potential uses of Dietary Reference Values. For any particular use, one or other DRV may be appropriate, as discussed in more detail in the following sections.

1.4.1 *For assessing diets of individuals*

1.4.1.1 The imprecision of most estimates both of individuals' nutrient intakes and of nutritional status, and thus of the estimation of the DRVs themselves, means that utmost caution should be used in applying the figures to the interpretation (or assessment) of individual diets. Even with a perfect measure of an individual's habitual intake of a nutrient (a difficult goal), the DRVs can give no more than a guide to the adequacy of diet for that individual.

1.4.1.2 If the habitual intake is below the LRNI it is likely that the individual will not be consuming sufficient of the nutrient to maintain the function selected by the Panel as an appropriate parameter of nutritional status for that nutrient, and further investigation, including biological measures, may be appropriate.

1.4.1.3 If the intake is above the RNI, then it is extremely unlikely that the individual will not be consuming sufficient.

1.4.1.4 If the intake lies between the two, then the chances of the diet being inadequate (in respect of the chosen functional parameter for any nutrient) fall as the intake approaches the RNI (para 1.3.13; Figure 1.2). It is impossible to say with any certainty whether an individual's nutrient intake, if it lies between the LRNI and the RNI, is or is not adequate, without some biological measure in that individual.

1.4.2 *For assessing diets of groups of individuals*

1.4.2.1 When measures of individual diets are aggregated, one of the sources of imprecision is attenuated—that is intraindividual day to day variability. Assuming that the interindividual variability is random, then in a sufficiently large group, this source of imprecision is also diminished. Thus the group mean intake will more precisely represent the habitual group mean intake than any of the individual measures will represent habitual individual intakes.

1.4.2.2 If the dietary data are robust enough, some information on percentiles of intake may be available. Thus it may be possible (see Fig 1.2; para 1.3) to say 'X per cent of the group had intakes below the RNI'. If X is zero then the risk of deficiency in the whole group is extremely small. As X increases further so the risk of deficiency in the group increases. If the data allow only the calculation of a mean or median intake for a group, then, because of the nature of the relationship between intake and the risk of deficiency (Figure 1.2), an average (or median) intake equal to the RNI can be taken to represent a very small risk of deficiency within the group.

1.4.3 *For prescribing diets or provision of food supplies* When prescribing diets, the intention is to ensure adequacy of the diet. In this situation it is prudent to prescribe diets containing nutrients at the RNI—so that, if eaten, the risk of deficiency would be very small in any individual. In this circumstance, almost all individuals receiving such diets will consume in excess (sometimes considerably so) of their requirements. The same principles can be applied to provision of food supplies to institutions, nations etc.

1.4.4 *For labelling purposes*

1.4.4.1 National RDAs or RDIs have been used as a basis for providing information on nutrient contents of foods on their labels. This has the advantage of giving a useful denominator, which would seem to be easily understood by individuals who might otherwise be unable to interpret the information on nutrient content of food. For instance, the public may find it more valuable to know that a food contains X per cent of the RDA/RDI than Y mg in 100 g of the food.

1.4.4.2 However, as RDAs and RDIs have usually been set at the upper end of the range of requirements, individuals might misinterpret information given in this form to imply that the RDA or RDI was equal to their requirement or to the average requirement for a nutrient, when in fact it is, with the exception of energy (which is not given on food labels in this form), always in excess of that.

1.4.4.3 The range of DRVs presented here offers an opportunity to escape from this dilemma at least for some nutrients. The advantages of a system based on labelling with the EAR would be to maintain comparability between foods and provide a standard presentation. EARs for different ages and sexes might be used on different foods according to the likely consumers—at least for baby foods. In addition consumers would interpret the EAR as just that, and would not therefore be provoked into unnecessary attempts to reach consumption levels virtually certain to be in excess of requirements.

1.5 DRV for energy

1.5.1 Classically RDAs have been set for energy and for nutrients whose deficiency in the diet results in recognisable and specific syndromes. RDAs have been set at levels well above those estimated to minimise the occurrence of these syndromes. RNIs for all nutrients, but not energy, can be set at the upper end of the range of requirements because an intake moderately in excess of requirements has no adverse effects, but reduces the risk of deficiency. For energy, however, this is not the case. Recommendations for energy have therefore always been set as the average of energy requirements for any population group. The Panel has therefore calculated EARs for energy, but not LRNIs or RNIs.

1.5.2 There is a variety of methods for estimating energy requirements. The greatest amount of data comes from dietary surveys that measure energy consumption over a variable length of time. This requires the assumption that on average the population is in energy balance at the time of measurement. Until recently measurements of energy expenditure (eg direct or indirect calorimetry) were less applicable to large scale studies over periods of several days. The newer and increasing use of doubly labelled water ($^2H_2{}^{18}O$) to provide an indirect measure of energy expenditure in free living individuals integrated over days and weeks has led to a useful developing database.

1.5.3 Current surveys in the UK, both of dietary and household purchase data, indicate energy intakes by the population below the prevailing RDAs[1]. This discrepancy may be because these data represent true requirements, or are less accurate measures than those on which the RDAs were based, even though the methodology is the same, or because previous recommendations may have included an amount to cover a particular level of activity which may not be achieved. The conjunction of more traditional methods with the still relatively small database emerging from newer technology has nevertheless allowed the Panel greater confidence in setting the EARs for energy given in table 1.1.

1.5.4 *Obesity* As in most developed countries, problems relating to insufficient energy intakes are uncommon in the UK, and do not arise from insufficient food supplies but generally from accompanying physical or psychological diseases. In contrast, however, many of the diseases which are characteristic of developed countries are related to overweight and obesity in the population which result from a chronic excess of dietary energy intake over energy expenditure. The Panel has not attempted to prescribe levels of energy expenditure, but has set DRVs for energy on the basis of current estimates of energy expenditure. In doing so the Panel was aware of evidence that overweight and obesity are increasing in the British population. In 1980 39 per cent of adult males and 32 per cent of adult females were overweight, defined as a Body Mass Index (BMI) in excess of 25.0 (see section 5.6). However, by 1987 these figures had risen to 45 and 36 per cent respectively. In 1980 obesity, defined as a BMI in excess of 30, was present in 6 per cent of adult men and 8 per cent of adult women and had risen to 8 and 12 per cent respectively by 1987[5].

1.6 DRVs for fat and carbohydrates

1.6.1 Setting DRVs for fat and carbohydrates (including 'fibre'), represents a major departure from previous exercises. Each of them comprises a varied group of nutrients and, with the exception of the essential fatty acids, their removal from the diet is not necessarily associated with recognised syndromes. The health consequences of eating diets containing different amounts of, or proportions of dietary energy as, fat, and of different fatty acid types, go beyond the avoidance of classical essential fatty acid (EFA) deficiency. Both coronary heart disease (CHD) and some forms of cancer have been associated with high intakes of fat, but their occurrence is not related to dietary fat alone. The Panel has endeavoured to define specific roles for fatty acids in terms of optimal health, taking account of the prevailing diet (Table 1.7) and changes which it considered practicable and likely (Table 1.2).

1.6.2 The discussion of various components of 'fibre' is made difficult both by lack of data and by inconsistences in what is considered to be 'fibre'. A number of hypotheses has been proposed linking low 'fibre' intake with a variety of diseases, although none can unequivocally be described as a specific 'fibre' deficiency disease. There is no agreed and universally applicable definition which embraces the variety of compounds with different physiological effects, a fact which has frequently gone unrecognised in the literature. The Panel has proposed that non-starch polysaccharides (NSP), which can be analysed accurately, reproducibly and specifically, and form the main component of 'fibre', should form the basis for recommendations even though the Panel recognised that this group of compounds also has a variety of different effects.

1.6.3 Dietary carbohydrate comprises a variety of sugars, oligosaccharides and starches as well as NSP, and, to a lesser extent other complex carbohydrates. Consideration was restricted to the broad groups, NSP, sugars and starches. There is an increasing realisation that there is substantial overlap between NSP and starches in their chemical, physical and physiological properties. Many of the physiological effects attributed traditionally to 'fibre' can be reproduced by certain forms of starch (eg 'resistant starch').

1.6.4 It is not clear from the data whether correlations between these dietary components and health outcomes are best seen when their intakes are expressed

Table 1.7 *Intake of fat, fatty acids and carbohydrates by the British population (g/d)*

Nutrient	Adults[5]			NFS 1989[6]
	total sample	male (n = 1,087)	female (n = 1,110)	
total fat	87.8	102.3	73.5	90.2
fatty acids:				
total *cis*-polys	13.3	15.7	10.9	13.6
n-3	1.7	1.9	1.3	—
n-6	11.7	13.8	9.6	—
total *cis*-monos	26.7	31.4	22.1	33.1
total sats	36.5	42.0	31.1	36.8
total *trans*	4.8	5.6	4.0	—
total:				
carbohydrate	232	272	193	230
sugars	100	115	86	95
starch	130	156	106	136
NSP[6]	11.6	11.2	12.5	12.4
Energy (kcal/d)	2,061	2,450	1,680	1,940
(MJ/d)	8.6	10.3	7.0	8.1

as absolute amounts or when related to dietary energy. Intakes vary with age, weight, sex and other parameters, and it is not clear how best to standardise the data for comparisons between different groups. Furthermore, data are virtually confined to situations of constant energy intake. In this Report the Panel has attempted to draw conclusions from reliable data, but has also had to make judgements based on complex and often inconsistent information. In some instances insufficient data were available to draw firm conclusions, and this is made clear in the text. The Panel has tried to identify those areas where further research would help understanding of the impact of these dietary components on health. More than for many other nutrients, the figures proposed for fat and carbohydrate represent judgements. The figures should not be taken as firm recommendations, but rather as guidelines which if achieved, would be expected to result in the relevant arbitrary end points.

1.6.5 Because the recommendation for energy is given as an average of requirements for the population, this section gives an estimate of the desirable contributions of fat and carbohydrate to dietary energy (Table 1.2). Except for special reasons, therefore, only a single average figure is given. In those cases where tentative individual maxima or minima can be given, these are stated. The figures in Table 1.2 are given in mass units only for non-starch polysaccharide.

1.6.6 The DRVs in this section are therefore not defined in the same way as those in the other sections of this Report. Apart from the essential fatty acids, none of the other nutrients in this section has been shown to be essential, so there can be no Estimated Average Requirement (EAR). The average figures presented in Table 1.2 are therefore proposals for population average intakes, and not for individuals, that are consistent with good health, given the prevailing socio-cultural environment. They can nevertheless be used for many of the same purposes and in the same ways as other uses of DRVs given in Section 1.3. In some cases suggesting a population average is not appropriate—for instance when data refer only to a necessary threshold minimum (or maximum) intake below (or above) which *individuals* might expect to be at higher risk of specific problems. These tentative individual minima and maxima are analogous, but not identical, to the LRNIs and the RNIs for other nutrients (see Table 1.2).

1.7 **DRVs for protein** Conventionally there have been two bases for setting protein requirements. The first, based on observations made in free living populations, has relied on the apparent adequacy of those intakes, and estimated requirements have been expressed as g/d or as a percentage of dietary energy. The Panel recognised this as a pragmatic solution, but without a sound biological basis. The second approach, derived from estimates of basic nitrogen requirements with additions for specific situations such as growth and pregnancy, which was adopted by joint FAO/WHO/UNU Expert Consultation in 1985[8], has formed the basis of the Panel's deliberations and enabled calculations of DRVs including EARs shown in Table 1.3.

1.8 **Meetings of the Panel**

1.8.1 The Panel was convened in 1987 at the recommendation of the Committee on Medical Aspects of Food Policy (COMA). The various Working Groups convened by the Panel met for a total of 35 times. The Panel itself met 7 times. The values put forward were agreed by all members of the Panel.

1.8.2 We are grateful to all members of the Working Groups and to those who have prepared working papers or have made documents available.

1.9 **References**

[1] Department of Health and Social Security. *Recommended Daily Amounts of Food Energy and Nutrients for Groups of People in the United Kingdom*. London: HMSO, 1979. (Reports on health and social subjects; 15).

[2] Department of Health and Social Security. *Recommended Intakes of Nutrients for the United Kingdom*. London: HMSO, 1969. (Reports on public health and medical subjects; 120).

[3] Tanner J M, Whitehouse R H, Takaishi M. Standards from birth to maturity for height, weight, height velocity and weight velocity: British children, 1965. *Arch Dis Child* 1966; **41**: 454–471, 613–635.

[4] Department of Health and Social Security. *Artificial Feeds for the Young Infant*. London: HMSO, 1980. (Reports on health and social subjects; 18).

[5] Gregory J, Foster K, Tyler H, Wiseman M. *The Dietary and Nutritional Survey of British Adults*. London: HMSO, 1990.

[6] Ministry of Agriculture, Fisheries and Food. *Household Food Consumption and Expenditure 1989*. London: HMSO, 1990.

[7] Bingham S A, Pett S, Day K C. Non-Starch Polysaccharide intake of a representative sample of British adults. *J Hum Nutr Diet* 1990; **3**: 333–337.

[8] World Health Organization. *Energy and Protein Requirements. Report of a Joint FAO/WHO/ UNU Meeting*. Geneva: World Health Organization, 1985. (WHO Technical Report Series; 724).

2. Energy

2.1 Energy requirements of children aged 0–3 years

2.1.1 *Introduction* Previous considerations of the energy requirements of pre-school children in the UK have been based on energy intakes reported from dietary surveys of healthy, well-nourished children[1,2]. Many of the studies used by the DHSS and FAO/WHO/UNU[3] committees were common to both reports and the resultant recommendations were therefore very similar (Figure 2.1). The derivation of the new recommendations differs from the previous approach in a number of ways because of greater availability of a variety of measurements of energy expenditure.

2.1.2 *Energy Expenditure*

2.1.2.1 The development during the early 1980s of the doubly-labelled water (DLW) method for use in humans has provided additional data on which to base recommendations for energy intake. The method provides a measure of total energy expenditure (TEE) in free-living individuals without constraining their patterns of activity or food intake. TEE includes the energy costs of basal metabolism, physical activity, thermogenesis and the costs of synthesising new tissue. Children's total energy requirements can be calculated by adding estimates of the energy value of new tissue deposited during normal growth to the estimates of TEE obtained by the DLW method. Nevertheless, the Panel was mindful of the need to rely on a number of assumptions in calculating TEE from DLW data, as well as the considerable technical difficulties encountered by most workers in making the determination. The Panel considered the DLW data to be a valuable additional resource, but emphasised the need for caution in interpretating data derived using this relatively new technique.

2.1.2.2 Figure 2.1 summarises published data on TEE in 355 healthy infants in 5 separate studies[4–8]. The uniformity in the group mean values obtained by several different research groups in diverse populations suggests that they can be interpreted with some confidence[9]. Potential sources of error do exist and the possibility of a unidirectional error cannot be excluded. In Figure 2.2 estimates of the energy value of new tissue deposited during normal growth (hatched area) have been added to a smoothed curve derived from the weighted means of the energy expenditure values shown in Figure 2.1. The stored energy was calculated by applying an assumed growth rate equivalent to the 50th centile given in Annex 1 to data on the body composition of infants[10].

2.1.2.3 Whitehead and Paul have reanalysed the original energy intake data used by FAO/WHO/UNU[3] according to the mode of feeding[11]. The results, shown in Figure 2.3, demonstrate that infants fed old-style formulas consumed significantly more energy than those on modern, adapted formulas or breast-

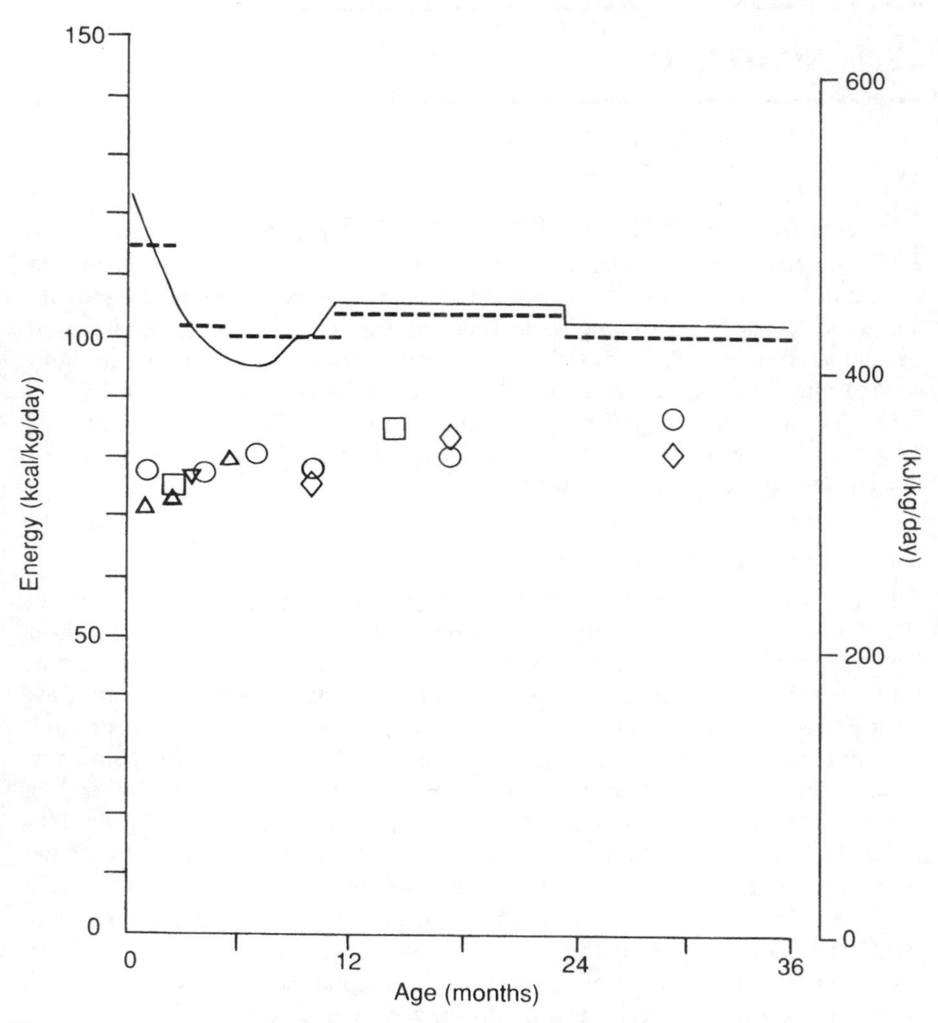

Figure 2.1 *Energy Requirements 0–36 months* Group mean estimates of total energy expenditure compared with DHSS[2] (- - -) and FAO/WHO/UNU[3] recommended dietary allowances (—). Data from references 4–8. Circles = Vasquez-Velasquez 1988[7]; Prentice *et al* 1988[5]; triangles = Lucas *et al* 1987[8]; inverted triangles = Roberts *et al* 1988[6]; diamonds = Vasquez-Velasquez, 1988[7]; Prentice *et al* 1988[5]; Squares = Fjeld *et al* 1988[4].

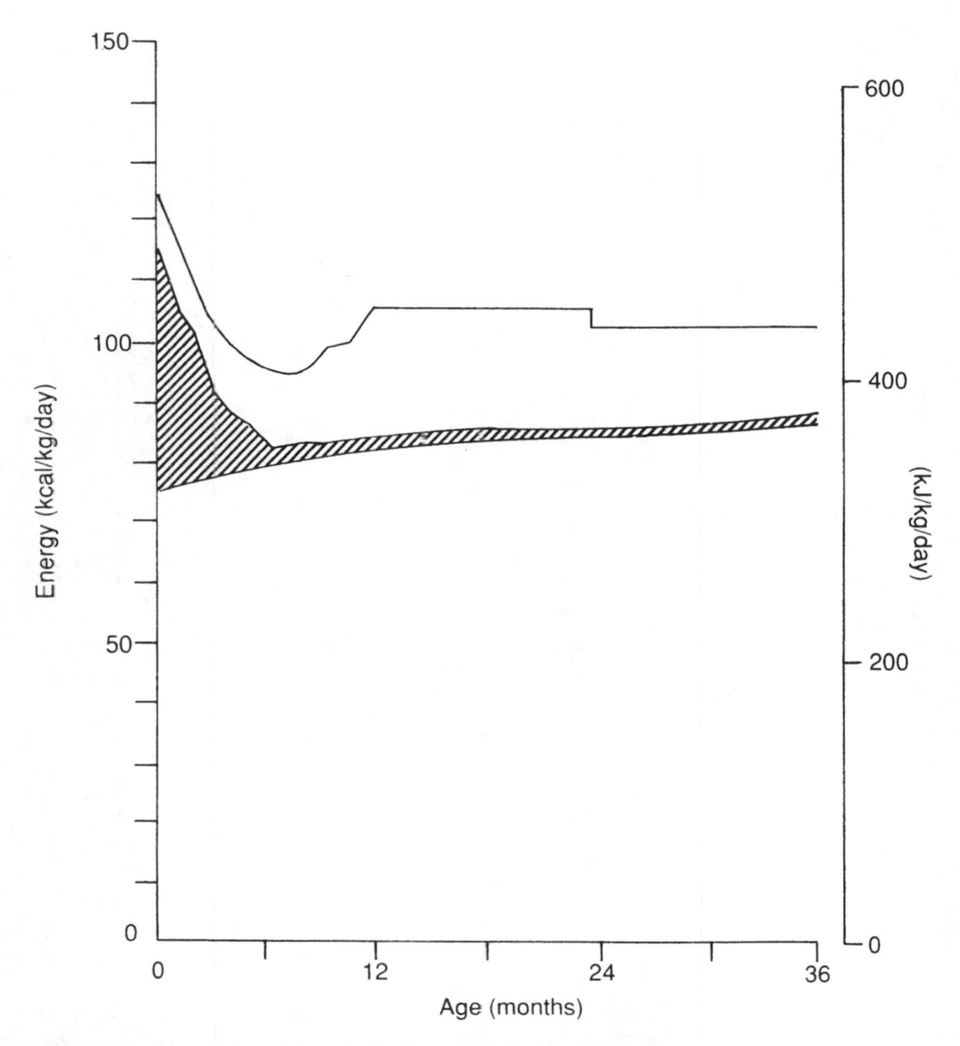

Figure 2.2 *Energy Requirements 0–36 months* Revised estimations of energy requirements (middle line) derived by adding the energy deposited during growth (hatched area) to a smoothed mean curve for energy expenditure computed from the data in Figure 2.1.

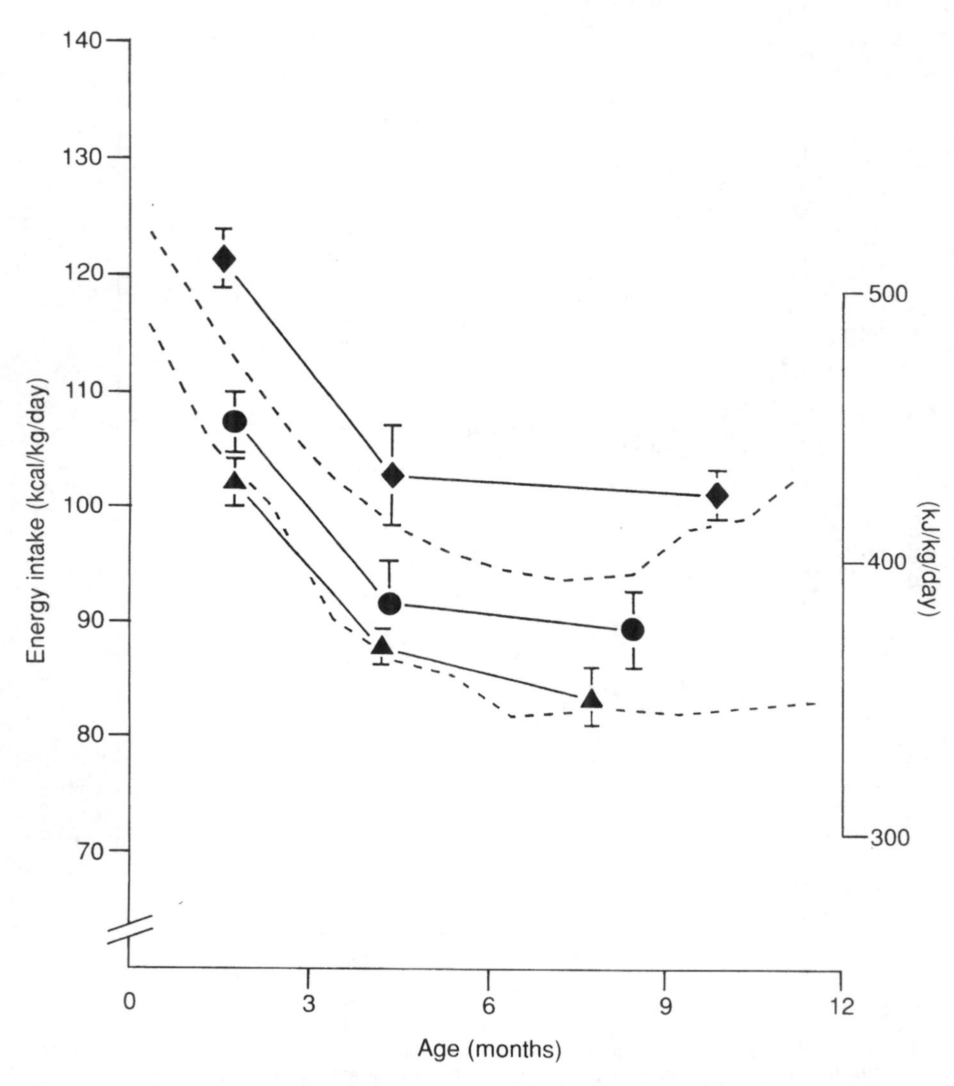

Figure 2.3 *Energy Requirements 0–36 months* Subdivision according to mode of feeding of the energy intake data from 0–12 months used as the basis of the FAO/WHO/UNU report[3].

Diamonds = old high-energy formulas; circles = modern formulas; triangles = wholly or partly breast-fed. Upper broken line = FAO/WHO/UNU[3] recommendations; lower broken line = new estimates of requirements from Figure 2.2. Intake data from Whitehead and Paul[11].

milk. There is evidence that suggests that infants fed pre-1975 infant formulas may have raised their energy expenditure to dissipate excess energy as heat[12].

2.1.3 *Observed dietary intakes*

2.1.3.1 Problems of interpretation are inherent not only in measures of energy expenditure, but also in the use of observed intakes as a sole basis for determining requirements. Firstly the latter are dependent on accurate dietary data. Recent studies using doubly-labelled water as a measure of energy expenditure at the same time as 7-day weighed food intakes in adolescents and adults have shown some discrepancies from observed intakes[13,14]. The interpretation of these data remains controversial[15,16]. These studies need to be replicated and do not necessarily apply to infants. Nevertheless, they emphasise the need for caution in reliance on any single method of measurement although the information available from dietary studies is much greater than that currently available from studies of energy expenditure. Secondly, the approach is dependent on a reliable conversion from gross energy to metabolisable energy which is usually achieved by applying Southgate and Durnin's modified Atwater factors which were derived experimentally in adults[18] and are not necessarily applicable to young children.

2.1.3.2 However, among infants and young children the Panel was unable to find evidence of a discrepancy between the two methods as shown among adolescents and adults. Data from 9 recent studies of food intake in infancy were considered by the Panel. These were from Australia, Canada, France, Netherlands, Sweden and UK and covered over 1500 infants. The results have been summarised and reviewed elsewhere[19]. On average the new results were slightly lower than DHSS and FAO/WHO/UNU recommendations[2,3], and were consistent with the energy intakes of breast-fed infants and those fed on modern formulas (figure 2.3).

2.1.4 *Basis of estimation of requirements*

2.1.4.1 The Panel endorsed breast feeding as the optimum mode of feeding during the first 4 to 6 months of life for healthy term babies. In view of the differences between estimates of energy requirements between breast and formula-fed infants (see para 2.1.2.3) and the fact that DRVs for breastfed infants have no value in practice, the Panel agreed that it was not necessarily appropriate to base estimates for all children on data derived from breastfed infants. The current estimates are therefore *only* for formula-fed infants.

2.1.4.2 The Panel noted that recommendations of FAO/WHO/UNU had included a 5 per cent increment for a perceived underestimate of intakes of energy from breastmilk in the first year of life, and for an appropriate level of physical activity in the second and third years[3]. The Panel was not convinced that this approach was relevant to the UK population, and has used the FAO/WHO/UNU values without this increment. This is consistent with the Panel's view that it was not prudent to include a prescriptive component in estimates of energy requirements. However, separate prescriptive advice might well be given

Table 2.1 *Estimated Average Requirements of energy for children aged 0–36 months*

Age	Average weight[a]		Intake per kg of body weight	Estimated Average Requirements	
months	kg		kJ(kcal)/kg/d	kJ(kcal)/d	
	Boys	Girls		Boys	Girls
1	4.15	4.00	480 (115)	1,990 (480)	1,920 (460)
3	6.12	5.70	420 (100)	2,570 (610)	2,390 (570)
6	8.00	7.44	400 (95)	3,200 (760)	2,980 (710)
9	9.20	8.55	400 (95)	3,680 (880)	3,420 (820)
12	10.04	9.50	400 (95)	4,020 (960)	3,800 (910)
18	11.30	10.65	400 (95)	4,520 (1,080)	4,260 (1,020)
24	12.39	11.80	400 (95)	4,960 (1,190)	4,720 (1,130)
30	13.42	12.84	400 (95)	5,370 (1,280)	5,140 (1,230)
36	14.40	13.85	400 (95)	5,760 (1,380)	5,540 (1,320)

[a] NCHS weights[17] for 1 month. All other weights from Annex 1.

to increase energy expenditures and thus counter the possible current downward trend in physical activity.

2.1.5 *Estimated Average Requirements* The Panel found that the measurements of total energy expenditure using DLW were on average in agreement with observed dietary energy intakes from modern infant formulas and with FAO/WHO/UNU values without the 5 per cent increment. The EARs for energy for infants are summarised in Table 2.1 and were derived by combining the evidence from different sources outlined above. The figures are intended only for formula-fed infants and assume that the Southgate and Durnin factors[18] are used to estimate the metabolisable energy content of foods. In the absence of contradictory evidence the EARs for boys and girls are assumed to be identical when expressed on a body weight basis.

2.1.6 *Research needs* The Panel noted the recent reports which link slower growth during the first year of life to higher risk of ill health during adulthood, and recognised the need for more detailed information on the effects of nutrition and growth during fetal development, infancy and childhood on later well-being[20].

2.2 Energy requirements of children aged 3–10 years

2.2.1 The Panel found insufficient data to calculate EARs based on measurements of energy expenditure in children aged 3 to 10 years. Therefore, the Panel accepted that EARs should be based on intakes.

2.2.2 There are a number of studies which provide data for the UK on energy intakes in this age group[21–25]. These are consistent with the values quoted as 'Intakes' by FAO/WHO/UNU[3]. The Panel therefore accepted these values as

Table 2.2 *Estimated Average Requirements for children aged 3–10 years* [a]

Age Years	Average Weight		Intake per kg of body weight		Estimated Average Requirements	
	kg[b]		kJ(kcal)/kg/d		MJ(kcal)/d	
	Boys	Girls	Boys	Girls	Boys	Girls
3	15.3	14.9	405 (97)	385 (92)	6.23 (1,490)	5.73 (1,370)
4	17.0	16.8	395 (94)	365 (87)	6.73 (1,600)	6.12 (1,460)
5	19.3	18.9	370 (88)	345 (82)	7.19 (1,720)	6.48 (1,550)
6	21.7	21.3	350 (84)	320 (76)	7.57 (1,810)	6.77 (1,620)
7	24.2	23.8	325 (78)	295 (71)	7.92 (1,890)	7.05 (1,680)
8	26.8	26.6	305 (73)	275 (66)	8.24 (1,970)	7.28 (1,740)
9	29.7	29.7	290 (69)	255 (61)	8.55 (2,040)	7.51 (1,790)

[a] Values are derived from the intake figures in Table 23 of FAO/WHO/UNU[3].
[b] From Annex 1

pertinent to the UK population for children aged 3–10 years. FAO/WHO/UNU suggested that these measured intakes should be increased by 5 per cent to allow for 'a desirable level of physical activity'[3]. However, such an addition would not necessarily lead to any increase in activity and so might be conducive to the unwelcome development of obesity. The Panel's EARs for energy are summarised in table 2.2.

2.3 Energy requirements for children and adolescents aged 10–18 years and for adults aged 19–59 years

2.3.1 *Introduction*

2.3.1.1 EARs for dietary energy for older children and adults have been calculated following the approach of FAO/WHO/UNU. That is, wherever possible, energy expenditure data have been used rather than data on energy intake, with energy expenditure expressed as multiples of the basal metabolic rate (BMR)[3]. The Panel agreed that measurements of energy expenditure provided a more direct basis for estimating energy requirements than energy intake data.

2.3.1.2 The use of BMR as the basis for calculating energy expenditure is a different approach from that of previous UK Reports[1,2]. The reasons for the present approach are that (1) a substantial proportion of daily energy expenditure is accounted for by the BMR, (2) there are formulae available, derived from a large amount of data, to calculate BMR of groups of either sex using only age and body weight, (3) if greater precision is required BMR can actually be measured on an individual with relative ease, and (4) the other important variable affecting total energy expenditure—physical activity—can also be usefully expressed as a multiple of BMR.

2.3.1.3 Total daily energy expenditure is the sum of the BMR, the thermic effect of the food eaten ('dietary induced thermogenesis') and the energy expended in physical activity. The thermic effect of the food eaten is normally included in any measurement or estimation of energy expenditure and is not assessed separately. Total energy expenditure (TEE), expressed as a multiple of BMR, is affected by the physical activity level (PAL; see para 2.3.9.). In consequence, to estimate total energy expenditure, and therefore dietary energy requirements, for a group of individuals, it is necessary to have information on the sex, age, and body weight to calculate BMR and on the energy expended in the various activities of work and leisure. While this estimation would normally be done for groups of individuals, if actual measurements of BMR are made on an individual, together with the energy cost of physical activity, then the energy requirement for that individual can also be estimated. Hence the same basic approach can be used for groups of older children, adolescents, adults and the elderly, and for individuals.

2.3.2 *Basal metabolic rate* BMR is determined principally by body mass and composition, whch vary with sex and age, and an estimation of BMR from body weight can be made in separate age and sex groups. The recommended equations for estimating BMR are those of Schofield *et al*[26] given in Annex 2. They differ slightly from those of FAO/WHO/UNU for children and adults by being based on additional data and are derived from measurements on over 1300 10–17 year olds, 3500 men and 1200 women. Although few data from the United Kingdom were included, these equations are regarded as providing adequate estimates. Neither the inclusion of alternative variables such as height or surface area, nor more complex transformations of body weight such as logarithmic or quadratic, improved the estimation significantly.

2.3.3 *The energy expended in physical activity* The energy expenditure in physical activity has traditionally been calculated from the duration of the various work and leisure activities and assigning an energy cost to each of them. This energy cost can be expressed as a multiple of BMR—eg 1.2 × BMR for sitting if no physical activity takes place, 4 × BMR for walking on the level at an average pace, 1.7 × BMR for standing activities at work, etc. PAR (physical activity ratio) is used as an abbreviation for 'multiple of BMR for an activity'. The energy costs of activities performed over short periods of time (half to one hour) as PAR are given in Annex 3.

2.3.4 *Duration and intensity of physical activity* When PAR is used to provide an energy cost for specific activity, such as 'sitting doing office work', 'standing cooking', or 'walking', it is important to be aware of whether or not it represents a duration of the activity where normal variants are included—such as occasionally getting up and moving around for a few seconds while sitting doing office work, sitting down briefly or standing relatively still for part of the time while cooking, or stopping briefly while walking. Values given in the literature for the energy cost of 'activities' do not usually include these variants and refer only to the actual activity as performed continuously. On the whole, for purposes of calculating EAR, a value for the way in which any activity would normally be done during a moderately prolonged period of time—eg cooking for 1½ hours, or walking for half an hour—is the one which is usually most helpful, and these are the values given in Annex 3. When performed over longer periods of time PAR are lower due to rest periods, etc.

2.3.5 *The influence of occupation* Previous reports have attempted to provide estimates of daily energy ependiture on the basis of the occupations of the groups of people involved eg 'sedentary', 'moderately active', 'very active'[1,2]. By itself this is of limited use for several reasons. There are probably fewer occupations now which could be classified as 'very active' compared to one or two decades ago and very few data are available from experimental evidence which can be related to almost any contemporary occupational situation. Various occupations are categorised in Annex 4 according to PAR integrated over the working day. Nowadays the influence of non-occupational activities may have an even greater influence than the actual work. Unless separate allowances are made for work and leisure, and unless specific information is available for the actual work situation, the general use of 'occupation' by itelf to indicate energy requirements will allow only very rough estimates.

2.3.6 *Non-occupational activities* It is difficult to calculate the energy expended in non-occupational activities in any simple, precise way for groups of people. FAO/WHO/UNU attempted to solve this difficulty by adopting a philosophy which may not be appropriate for the UK population. That philosophy was based on an assumption that independently of any other leisure activities, everyone should expend energy in the three categories of (a) 'household tasks', (b) 'community activities', and (c) activity of benefit for cardiovascular and general health[3]. The Panel concluded that, desirable though these 'social' activities might be, unless there is evidence that they already exist in any population, making an allowance for energy expended in such activities might be a prescription in excess of the energy requirement.

2.3.7 *Intensity of activity* An estimate of the contribution to total energy expenditure from activity can be derived from calculations of time spent in various activities at specified PAR. The assumption is made that 'bed' accounts for 8 in every 24 hours. An average working day in the UK lasts for 7.5 hours and the working week consists of 5 days, giving an average of about 5.5 hours over the 7-day week. The remaining 'non-occupational' time (10.5 hours) can be divided into one of 3 categories based on 2 hours of activity at different PAR levels and 8.5 hours at an arbitary PAR of 1.4. 'Non-active' individuals would spend 2 hours of the 10.5 of non-occupational activity at a level of BMR × 2, giving an overall value of BMR × 1.5 for the 10.5 hours of non-occupational activity. 'Moderately active' people who spend 2 out of the 10.5 hours at an energy expenditure of BMR × 3 would have an overall value of BMR × 1.7 for the 10.5 hours non-occupational activity. 'Very active' people who spend 2 hours of the 10.5 at BMR × 4 would have a non-occupational overall energy cost of BMR × 1.9. An example of how this can be used to estimate energy expenditure for men and women in 'light' occupations is given in Annex 5.

2.3.8 *Estimation of daily energy expenditure of groups* Daily energy expenditure of groups of individuals can be estimated from several levels of data with consequent different levels of accuracy. Three levels of estimates are described below in order of increasing accuracy and precision. Other combinations of measured and estimated data are possible.

2.3.9 *Physical Activity Level (PAL)* PAL is the ratio of overall daily energy expenditure to BMR and is characterised by a description of lifestyle. When based *only* on occupation, this level may produce unreliable estimates, as described earlier, but it has been a common method of estimating energy requirements and recommended energy intakes. An adjustment for non-occupational activity can be made as described in para 2.3.7 above. Combining estimates of PAR for occupational and non-occupational acitivity (see paras 2.3.5–2.3.7), a matrix of PAL for 3 categories of both occupational and non-occupational activity can be derived. Such a matrix for adults is given in table 2.3. In the absence of further information, UK population groups should be assumed to have light occupations and non-active non-occupational activity, and PAL of 1.4.

2.3.10 *More precise time use and activity at work and in non-occupational activity* With some information on time use at work, in bed and the remainder and on the type of occupational and non-occupational activities, physical activity ratios (PAR) can be ascribed to these components and daily energy expenditure estimated.

Daily energy expenditure = BMR × [time in bed + (time at work × PAR) + (non-occupational time × PAR)].

PAR can be assigned to occupations using the provisional classification shown in Annex 4. An example of this approach is given in Annex 5 for a light occupation and the three categories of non-occupational activity described earlier.

2.3.11 *Detailed time use and activity description* With more detailed, representative information on typical time use and measured energy costs of activities, daily energy expenditure can be estimated more accurately.

Daily energy expenditure = BMR[time in bed + sum of (time in each activity × PAR)].

Table 2.3 *Calculated Physical Activity Level (PAL) of adults at 3 levels each of occupational and non-occupational activity**

Non-occupational activity	Occupational Activity					
	Light		Moderate		Moderate/Heavy	
	M	F	M	F	M	F
Non-active	1.4	1.4	1.6	1.5	1.7	1.5
Moderately active	1.5	1.5	1.7	1.6	1.8	1.6
Very active	1.6	1.6	1.8	1.7	1.9	1.7

*Based on assumptions of PAR and time use as detailed in paragraphs 2.3.5–2.3.7 and in Annexes 4 and 5 and rounded to 2 significant figures

If the energy costs of activities cannot be measured, the energy costs of activities as PAR can be taken from Annexes 3 and 4. Annex 6 illustrates this approach for a group of women office workers.

2.3.12 *Estimating the daily energy expenditure of individuals* In order to estimate daily energy expenditure of individuals it is necessary to have a measurement of BMR, detailed time use data and activity description as in para

2.3.11 above and wherever possible measurements of the energy cost of activities. This is the classical approach of diary record of activities and indirect calorimetry. BMR must be measured as even when allowances are made for age, sex and weight, the precision of the estimate in any individual is insufficient. Once BMR has been measured the same procedures as outlined for groups of individuals in paras 2.3.9 to 2.3.11 above can be followed.

2.3.13 *Estimated Average Requirements of energy* Depending on the data available one of the three methods illustrated in paras 2.3.9 to 2.3.11 can be employed to ascertain the EAR of a group.

2.3.14 *Older children and adolescents* In contrast to younger children, there is sufficient provisional information on time use and energy cost of activities in the school day to allow estimates of daily energy expenditure and recommended energy intakes for children and adolescents aged 10–17 years. Typical time use and energy costs of activities are given in Table 2.4. The same time use pattern has been taken for boys and girls but the intensity of activities (PAR) is lower in girls. The EARs for energy for 10–17 year olds are shown in Table 2.5, and the calculations underlying them are given in Annex 7. The EARs for children in the standard age ranges from birth to 18 years are given in table 2.6.

2.3.15 *Adults* The EARs for dietary energy for groups of men and women of various ages, body weights and physical activity levels are shown in Table 2.7. Owing to the inactive life style of much of the population, a PAL of 1.4 should be assumed in the absence of other information on activity. EARs based

Table 2.4 *Estimated time use and energy cost of activities (PAR) in older children and adolescents aged 10–18 years*

Activity		Energy cost (PAR)	
	hours	Boys	Girls
Bed	8	1.0	1.0
School	6	1.6	1.5
Light	7	1.6	1.5
Moderate	2.5	2.5	2.2
High	0.5	5.0	5.0
PAL	24	1.56	1.48

Table 2.5 *Estimated Average Requirements (MJ/d) of children and adolescents (10–18 years) according to body weight and physical activity level (PAL)*

Body Weight kg	BMR* MJ/d	PAL 1.4	1.5	1.6	1.8	2.0
males						
30	4.97	7.0	7.5	8.0	9.0	9.9
35	5.34	7.5	8.0	8.6	9.6	10.7
40	5.71	8.0	8.6	9.1	10.3	11.4
45	6.08	8.5	9.1	9.7	11.0	12.2
50	6.45	9.0	9.7	10.3	11.6	12.9
55	6.82	9.6	10.2	10.9	12.3	13.6
60	7.19	10.1	10.8	11.5	12.9	14.4
65	7.56	10.6	11.3	12.1	13.6	15.1
females						
30	4.58	6.4	6.9	7.3	8.2	9.2
35	4.86	6.8	7.3	7.8	8.7	9.7
40	5.14	7.2	7.7	8.2	9.2	10.3
45	5.42	7.6	8.1	8.7	9.8	10.8
50	5.70	8.0	8.5	9.1	10.3	11.4
55	5.98	8.4	9.0	9.6	10.8	12.0
60	6.26	8.8	9.4	10.0	11.3	12.5

BMR* = Basal metabolic rate calculated from data in Annex 1 and Annex 2.

Table 2.6 *Estimated Average Requirements (EARs) for energy of children 0–18 years**

Age	EAR MJ/d (kcal/d) Boys	Girls
0–3 months	2.28 (545)	2.16 (515)
4–6 months	2.89 (690)	2.69 (645)
7–9 months	3.44 (825)	3.20 (765)
10–12 months	3.85 (920)	3.61 (865)
1–3 years	5.15 (1,230)	4.86 (1,165)
4–6 years	7.16 (1,715)	6.46 (1,545)
7–10 years	8.24 (1,970)	7.28 (1,740)
11–14 years	9.27 (2,220)	7.72 (1,845)
15–18 years	11.51 (2,755)	8.83 (2,110)

*Calculated by interpolation from tables 2.1, 2.2, 2.4 and 2.5 and weights from Annex 1.

Table 2.7 *Estimated Average Requirements (EARs) for energy (MJ/d) for groups of men and women at various ages, weights and activity levels*

Body Weight kg	BMR MJ/d	Physical Activity Level (PAL)								
		1.4	1.5	1.6	1.7	1.8	1.9	2.0	2.1	2.2
Men 19–29 yr										
60	6.7	9.3	10.0	10.7	11.4	12.0	12.7	13.4	14.1	14.7
65	7.0	9.8	10.5	11.2	11.9	12.6	13.3	14.0	14.7	15.4
70	7.3	10.2	11.0	11.7	12.5	13.2	13.9	14.6	15.4	16.1
75	7.6	10.7	11.5	12.2	13.0	13.7	14.5	15.2	16.0	16.8
80	7.9	11.1	11.9	12.7	13.5	14.3	15.1	15.9	16.7	17.5
Men 30–59 yr										
65	6.8	9.5	10.2	10.8	11.5	12.2	12.9	13.5	14.2	14.9
70	7.0	9.8	10.5	11.2	11.9	12.6	13.3	14.0	14.7	15.4
75	7.3	10.2	10.9	11.6	12.4	13.1	13.8	14.5	15.3	16.0
80	7.5	10.5	11.3	12.0	12.8	13.5	14.3	15.0	15.8	16.5
85	7.7	10.8	11.6	12.4	13.2	13.9	14.7	15.5	16.3	17.0
Women 18–29 yr										
45	4.8	6.8	7.2	7.7	8.2	8.7	9.2	9.7	10.2	10.6
50	5.1	7.2	7.7	8.2	8.7	9.2	9.7	10.3	10.8	11.3
55	5.4	7.6	8.2	8.7	9.3	9.8	10.4	10.9	11.5	12.0
60	5.8	8.1	8.7	9.2	9.8	10.4	11.0	11.5	12.1	12.7
65	6.1	8.5	9.1	9.7	10.3	10.9	11.5	12.1	12.7	13.3
70	6.4	8.9	9.6	10.2	10.8	11.5	12.2	12.8	13.4	14.0
Women 30–59 yr										
50	5.2	7.3	7.9	8.4	8.9	9.4	9.9	10.5	11.0	11.5
55	5.4	7.6	8.2	8.7	9.2	9.7	10.3	10.8	11.3	11.9
60	5.6	7.8	8.4	8.9	9.5	10.0	10.6	11.2	11.7	12.3
65	5.7	8.0	8.6	9.2	9.8	10.3	10.9	11.5	12.0	12.6
70	5.9	8.3	8.9	9.5	10.1	10.7	11.3	11.8	12.4	13.0

Table 2.8 *Estimated Average Requirements (EARs) for energy for groups of men and women with physical activity level of 1.4*

	Weight* kg	EAR	
		MJ/d	kcal/d
Men			
19–49 years	74	10.6	2,550
50–59 years	74	10.6	2,550
Women			
19–49 years	60	8.1	1,940
50–59 years	63	8.0	1,900

*From Annex 1

on this assumption in men and women are given in Table 2.8. Further information on activity is required to identify other PALs correctly (see Annexes 3–6).

2.3.16 *Differences from previous values* The calculated values for light activity occupational groups who are relatively inactive in their non-occupational time are lower than those of previous reports[1,2]. This is mostly because of an apparent overestimate of daily working time in these reports (an average day was taken as having 8 hours of work and no allowance was made for the non-working weekend). However, this effect is countered by using median body weights which are higher than those used previously. The estimated energy expenditure in the light activity group with PAL = 1.4 reflects the inactive life style of much of the population, but is supported by recent energy expenditure data using the doubly labelled water method and energy intake data[27]. The Panel considered that a higher level of activity and energy expenditure would be desirable.

2.3.17 *Validation* As in the 3–10 year age group, there have been few data to allow simultaneous comparisons of energy intake with expenditure among 11 to 18 year olds. In view of the shortage of information in this age group and in adolescents the Panel commissioned a special study of energy expenditure measured by the doubly-labelled water method[9] in about 12 boys and 12 girls at each age of 3, 5, 7, 9, 12, 15 and 18 years. The final data set contained 177 measurements. The results are plotted in figure 2.4 against the new EAR for 3–10 year olds (Table 2.2) and against the food intake figures collated by FAO/WHO/UNU for the 10–18 year olds[3]. In general there is excellent agreement, but unlike the data for 3–10 year olds, the estimates of total energy expenditure in the older children exceeded those of dietary energy intake. There are a number of possible reasons for this discrepancy, which may coexist. Firstly, there may be methodoligical problems associated with either measurement. There is evidence that in some instances dietary records may underestimate habitual energy intake[14]. Equally it is possible that the assumptions used in calculating energy expenditure using $^{2}H_2{}^{18}O$ may not always be appropriate. Secondly, the measurements of energy expenditure may have been unrepresentative of the population. The small sample sizes and the high levels of the estimates of energy expenditure are consistent with this. In contrast, there are data on energy intake derived from a substantial number of individuals. Nationally representative samples of 10–11 year old and 14–15 year old children provided robust data for those ages[25]. The Panel considered it prudent to rely on the larger data set, but agreed that the discrepancy with the newer method gave grounds for caution.

2.3.18 *Ethnic differences* The existence of ethnic differences in BMR after allowing for body size, composition, sex, age, nutritional status and climate remains controversial. There is little evidence for differences between ethnic groups resident in the UK. It is proposed that the same approaches to the EAR for energy can be used for all ethnic groups in the United Kingdom.

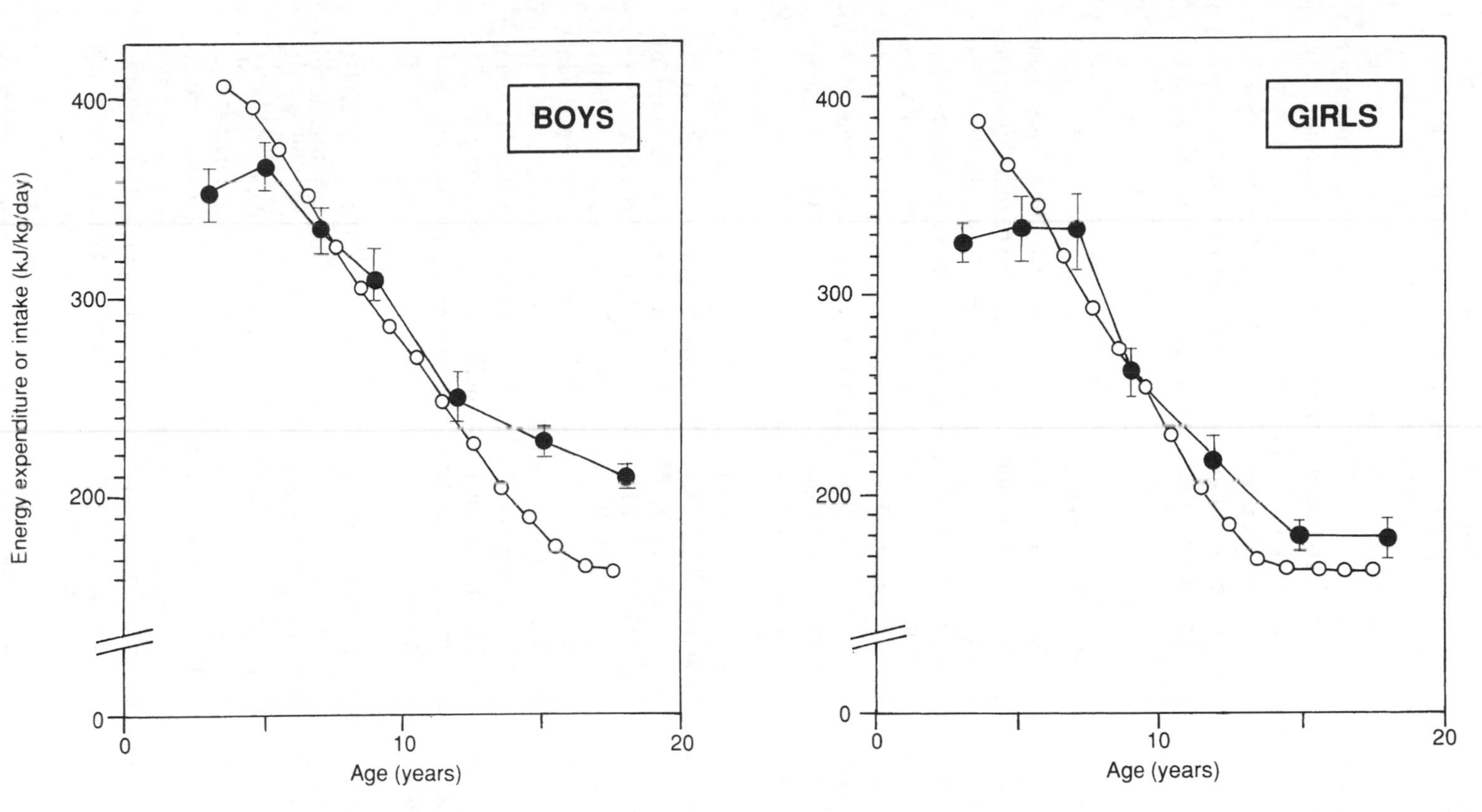

Figure 2.4 *Comparison of new estimates of energy expenditure measured by doubly-labelled water with estimates of intake summarised by FAO/WHO/UNU*[3]

Closed Circles = energy intake figures from FAO/WHO/UNU[3]

Open Circles = New EARs for 3–10 years and energy intake figures from FAO/WHO/UNU for 10–18 years.[3]

2.3.19 *Exercise and health* A separate and additional allowance for physical activity to maintain cardiovascular function and health, strength or flexibility has been considered carefully. Evidence for benefit from this physical activity is impressive[28]. For some exercise programmes the energy cost may be significant. A programme of 3 sessions per week, 30 minutes per session at an average intensity of 50 per cent of the VO_2 max would involve net energy expenditure of 2.5 MJ (600 kcal) over the week or 0.4 MJ (96 kcal)/d. This would increase PAL from 1.4 in a previously non-active group to 1.5. However, there is evidence that much shorter periods of more moderate exercise would also offer improved health benefits without requiring a significant addition to total energy expenditure[29].

2.4 **Energy requirements for pregnancy**

2.4.1 Maintenance of a normal pregnancy requires energy. This arises from the increases in tissue mass and in metabolic activity and can be quantified. The changes in tissue mass comprise the increased mass of the uterus, the formation of the fetus and placenta, the expanded blood volume, and the deposition of an extra 2 to 2.4 kg of adipose tissue which provides an energy reserve for lactation. Mothers who do not intend to breastfeed their child do not require this latter energy reserve. The costs resulting from the extra energy metabolism are occasioned by the larger tissue mass of the mother, so that both basal metabolic rate (BMR) and the energy cost of movement become greater.

2.4.2 It can be calculated that the energy cost of the changes in tissue mass is on average about 40,000 kcal (167 MJ) in women of about 60 kg non-pregnant body weight. The total increase in BMR integrated over the duration of pregnancy is about 30,000 kcal (126 MJ), giving an overall total of about 70,000 kcal (293 MJ)[30]. However, the costs could be modified in two ways. Firstly, there might be reduction in BMR as a result of endocrine change in the pregnant woman, but the evidence does not support this. Secondly, physical activity in the mother might be reduced especially in the latter part of pregnancy. It might be difficult to detect the diminution in physical activity and compensation would be shown up by food energy intakes during pregnancy which were lower than might otherwise be expected.

2.4.3 The apparent extra energy requirement of about 70,000 kcal (293 MJ) is seldom matched by an equivalent increase in food intake. Many cross-sectional, a few semi-longitudinal surveys and one large longitudinal survey in the UK have failed to demonstrate substantial alteration in energy intake until the last few weeks of pregnancy. This evidence shows an average increase in intake of energy of less than 0.42 MJ/d (100 kcal/d) in the third trimester and virtually no change before then[31-39]. Similar results have been found by another longitudinal study in Holland[40]. Outcomes of these pregnancies were satisfactory. Therefore there is no apparent risk to the mother or the fetus with only a modest increase in energy intake in the last trimester of pregnancy.

2.4.4 Thus the true additional energy requirements of pregnancy, under the conditions prevailing in Western societies such as the UK, are probably modest.

However in view of the disparity between the calculations and the experimental findings caution must be exercised. The Panel therefore agreed that the increment in EAR for pregnancy should be 0.8 MJ/d (200 kcal/d) above the pre-pregnant EAR only during the last trimester. Women who are underweight at the beginning of pregnancy, and women who do not reduce activity, may need more.

2.5 Energy requirements for lactation

2.5.1 The energy requirements for lactation are calculated as increments to be added to the mother's EAR. The derivation of these increments is summarised in Table 2.9.

2.5.2 The values for milk output were derived by combining data from British[19] and Swedish mothers[41], and include a 4 per cent correction to allow for insensible water losses by the infant during test-weighing. These values are representative of the norm for well nourished women[42] and differ from those in the FAO/WHO/UNU[3] by less than 10 per cent in the early months. The EARs recognise two distinctive groups of breastfeeding mothers. Firstly, women who practise exclusive or almost exclusive breastfeeding until the baby is 3–4 months old and then progressively introduce weaning foods as part of an active weaning process which often lasts only a few months (Group 1). Secondly, women who introduce only limited complementary feeds after 3–4 months and whose intention is that breast milk should provide the primary source of nourishment for 6 months or more (Group 2).

2.5.3 The gross energy content of breast milk was taken to be 280 kJ/100 g (67 kcal/100 g) representing an average between the value assumed by DHSS[2]

Table 2.9 *Additional energy requirements for lactation*

Month	Milk volume[a] ml/d	Energy cost[b] MJ(kcal)/d	Allowance for weight loss[c] MJ(kcal)/d	Total additional requirement MJ(kcal)/d
All breastfeeding women				
0–1	680	2.38 (570)	−0.5 (120)	1.9 (450)
1–2	780	2.73 (650)	−0.5 (120)	2.2 (530)
2–3	820	2.87 (690)	−0.5 (120)	2.4 (570)
Group 1[d]				
3–6	700	2.45 (590)	−0.5 (120)	2.0 (480)
6 onwards	300	1.05 (250)	Nil	1.0 (240)
Group 2[d]				
3–6	750	2.63 (630)	−0.25 (60)	2.4 (570)
6 onwards	650	2.28 (540)	Nil	2.3 (550)

[a] Based on studies from Cambridge[19] and Sweden[45].

[b] Gross energy density of the milk assumed to be 280 kJ/100 g (67 kcal/100 g). Dietary to milk energy conversion efficiency assumed to be 80 per cent.

[c] Assuming an average weight loss of 500 g/month with an energy equivalence of 29 MJ/kg (6900 kcal/kg).

[d] see para 2.5.2

and a more recent lower estimate claimed to be more representative of the true energy density of milk as suckled by the infant[8]. The Panel accepted many of the arguments in support of the lower estimate, but this has yet to be independently confirmed.

2.5.4 Previous reports have erroneously used the metabolisable energy content of milk rather than the gross energy which must be supplied by the mother. This has led to an underestimate by about 5 per cent. Correcting for this error partly offsets the effect of assuming a lower energy density in breast milk and the resultant EAR is only slightly lower than that previously used by DHSS[2].

2.5.5 The efficiency of conversion from maternal dietary to gross milk energy has previously been assumed to be 80 per cent. This estimate was derived from the 95 per cent confidence limits of a very indirect estimate using milk volumes calculated from infant growth rates and measures of energy intake in different groups of lactating and non-lactating women[43]. However, recent estimates support the 80 per cent assumption[44].

2.5.6 There is conflicting evidence in support of the assumption that lactation necessarily induces maternal weight loss[44,45]. A value for weight loss of 500g/month has been assumed which would allow for the gradual mobilisation of fat deposited during pregnancy. This allowance is halved for Group 2 mothers over the second 3 months in order to simulate a gradual transition to a state where the entire costs of lactation are met from the diet. It should be noted that there is a wide variation in post-partum weight changes between individuals and hence in individual energy requirements. The Panel found no evidence that gradual weight loss during lactation is detrimental to milk production, but did not advise intentional dieting until after weaning.

2.5.7 The maternal EAR, to which the incremental needs for lactation are to be added, should be calculated in the same way as for non pregnant women. The only way by which a lactating mother would require a smaller addition to her non-pregnant non-lactating energy intake than the energy required to produce the normal volume of breast milk would be by some energy-saving mechanism. The most probable one is by an obligatory reduction in physical activity. However, it seems likely that for many women the enforced rest periods associated with breastfeeding will be offset by the additional work involved in caring for a new baby. The estimates in table 2.9 for these incremental requirements closely match increments in food intake observed among lactating women in affluent societies[46].

2.6 Energy requirements for the elderly

2.6.1 There are few data on energy requirements of the elderly in the UK. Although some were obtained 20 to 30 years ago, the data are still valid. Durnin measured the intakes and expenditures of elderly peiple living alone at home[47], and Jerham *et al* measured energy intakes and expenditures of elderly male crofters in North West Scotland[48]: the results are shown in Table 2.10.

Table 2.10 *Daily energy intakes in groups of elderly people*[47,48,54–57]

	McGandy *et al* (1966) USA		Borgstrom *et al* (1979) Sweden		Uauy *et al* (1978) USA		Calloway & Zanni (1980) USA	Durnin *et al* (1961) Scotland		Jerham *et al* (1969)
Sex	M	M	M	F	M	F	M	F	M	M
N	50	37	17	20	6	6	6	17	9	6
Age (y)	67–74	77–79	67–73	67–73	68–74	70–84	63–77	60–69	64–77	58–78
Height (mean) (m)	1.74	1.72	1.68	1.60	1.70	1.59	1.74	1.55	1.74	1.74
Weight (mean) (kg)	77.7	70.9	76.4	68.8	73.7	68.9	82.2	60.7	70.0	77.0
Energy intake MJ (kcal)	9.6 (2297)	8.8 (2093)	8.6 (2050)	6.7 (1600)	9.7 (2325)	8.0 (1904)	10.7 (2554)	7.9 (1894)	8.6 (2055)[1]	12.2 (2905)[2]
Energy intake MJ (kcal)/kg	0.12 (29.6)	0.12 (29.5)	0.11 (26.8)	0.10 (23.3)	0.13 (31.5)	0.12 (27.6)	0.13 (31.2)	0.13 (31.2)	0.12 (29.4)	0.16 (37.7)
Intake/estimated BMR	1.53	1.47	1.38	1.25	1.62	1.49	1.58	1.57	1.34	1.80

1. Energy expenditure was 9.5 MJ(2,325 kcal)/d
2. Energy expenditure was 12.2 MJ (2,420 kcal)/d

Recently, unpublished data have been acquired on randomly sampled groups of elderly living at home and in residential accommodation, mainly in Italy: comparisons with the smaller body of information on the elderly in the UK show a similar pattern. The energy expenditure of the elderly is reduced for two principal reasons. On average the level of physical activity falls, particularly among those who become sick, infirm or disabled although there is a large variation between individuals. There is also a decline in the basal metabolic rate which relates particularly to the fall in the fat free mass. Thus in the elderly there may be an accentuation of the process apparent in middle age when weight may remain steady but fat replaces lean tissue.

2.6.2 *The old and very old* The retirement age of men and women varies but the effects of retirement on physical activity do not necessarily lead to a fall in energy expenditure. A longitudinal study in Nottingham showed that healthy steel workers may actually increase their activity levels after retirement[49,50]. Over the age of 75 years, however, sickness and disability are increasingly likely with evidence of a fall in body weight as well as in the mass of lean tissue. In a large representative study of the elderly living in their own homes, on average significantly less activity was recorded in those aged over 75 years compared with those aged 66 to 75 years. However, this was not always so for men, who were also significantly more active than women. Distributions were skewed with a few very active people but most very inactive[51].

2.6.3 *Basal metabolic rate* The widely used equations of Schofield *et al* incorporate only 50 men and 38 women over the age of 60 years and include data on groups in the tropics or in unusual circumstances[26]. These limited data are therefore not reliable for predictive purposes. Individual unpublished data on 101 Glaswegian men aged 60–70 years and on 170 Italian men and 180 Italian women have been made available to the Panel for inclusion with data from Schofield *et al*[26]. Annex 2 shows the equations for the two sexes in the two age groups. There are appreciable changes above 75 years of age and the Schofield equations appear particularly inappropriate for the older group of men. BMR/kg fat free mass may not be different in young and older adults and the fall in the total mass of lean tissue with age may be the dominant effect in accounting for the decline in BMR.

2.6.4 *Physical activity patterns* With age all activities show a decline, so in general there is a progressive fall in energy expenditure[52]. However, there is considerable variation in activity levels in all age groups and an active 70-year-old may have as high an energy expenditure as a sedentary 40-year-old (see para 2.6.2). In addition the cost of physical activity may be increased in the elderly due to reduced efficiency of movement. For instance Bassey and Terry found that for women the energy cost of walking was substantially greater in the eighth decade compared with the third[53]. More information on the variation of energy expenditure in the elderly in the UK is required.

2.6.5 *Energy Intakes* Table 2.10 gives some data on selected groups of a variety of countries. With one exception, they are fairly sedentary populations, but not more so than many younger groups. However, when elderly people are

Table 2.11 *Estimated Average Requirements (EARs) for energy in groups of men and women aged 60 years and over*

	Weight	EAR	
	(kg)	MJ/d	kcal/d
Men			
60–64y	74.0	9.93	2,380
65–74y	71.0	9.71	2,330
75+y	69.0	8.77	2,100
Women			
60–64y	63.5	7.99	1,900
65–74y	63.0	7.96	1,900
75+y	60.0	7.61	1,810

inactive, their total energy expenditure and intake may be so low as to result in an inadequate intake of some nutrients. If calculated energy requirements for some groups of elderly people suggest that such a risk exists, encouragement is needed to achieve a higher intake of energy preferably by stimulating physical activity and thus greater energy expenditure. Such advice and encouragement may be especially necessary in institutionalised elderly people, in whom energy intake may not even be sufficient to meet the low energy expenditure, so that weight loss may be a particular problem. In this case, encouragement of higher intakes of energy is appropriate.

2.6.6 *Estimated Average Requirements* In view of these considerations the Panel agreed *a standard value for PAL in the elderly of 1.5 × BMR should be used* for ages 60 years onwards, irrespective of sex or of whether the groups were housebound or institutionalised or living at home. The Panel recognised that energy expenditure was likely to be greater in free-living than institutionalised elderly people, and that the bed-ridden would have markedly reduced energy expenditure. The Panel considered that the paucity of the data did not allow further valid sub-division, and that the prescriptive use of this value of 1.5 × BMR would be unlikely to lead to harm, in particular from provision of insufficient food energy. EARs for energy in the elderly were calculated from data in Annexes 1 and 2 and are given in Table 2.11.

2.7 References

1 Department of Health and Social Security. *Recommended Intakes of Nutrients for the United Kingdom*. London: HMSO, 1969. (Reports on public health and medical subjects; 120).

2 Department of Health and Social Security. *Recommended Daily Amounts of Food Energy and Nutrients for Groups of People in the United Kingdom*. London: HMSO, 1979. (Reports on health and social subjects; 15).

3 World Health Organization. *Energy and Protein Requirements. Report of a Joint FAO/WHO/UNU Meeting*. Geneva: World Health Organization, 1985. (WHO Technical Report Series; 724).

4 Fjeld C R, Schoeller D A, Brown K H. Energy expenditure of malnourished children during catch-up growth. *Proc Nutr Soc* 1988; **47**: 227–231.

[5] Prentice A M, Lucas A, Vasquez-Velasquez L, Davies P S W, Whitehead R G. Are current guidelines for young children a prescription for overfeeding? *Lancet* 1988; **ii**: 1066–1069.

[6] Roberts S B, Savage J, Coward W A, Chew B, Lucas A. Energy expenditure and intake in infants born to lean and overweight mothers. *New Engl J Med* 1988; **318**: 461–466.

[7] Vasquez-Velasquez L V. Energy expenditure and physical activity of malnourished Gambian infants. *Proc Nutr Soc* 1988; **47**: 233–239.

[8] Lucas A, Ewing G, Roberts S B, Coward W A. How much energy does a breast-fed infant consume and expend? *Br Med J* 1987; **295**: 75–77.

[9] International Dietary Energy Consultative Group. Prentice A, ed. *The Doubly-Labelled Water Method for Measuring Energy Expenditure: Technical Recommendations for Human Applications*. Vienna: IAEA/IDECG NAHRES4, 1990.

[10] Fomon S J, Haschke F, Ziegler E E, Nelson S E. Body composition of reference children from birth to age 10 years. *Am J Clin Nutr* 1982; **35**: 1169–1175.

[11] Whitehead R G, Paul A A. Diet and growth in healthy infants. *Hong Kong J Paediatr* 1988; **5**: 1–20.

[12] Davies P S W, Ewing G, Coward W A, Lucas A. Energy metabolism in breast and formula fed infants. In: Atkinson S *et al*, eds. *Breastfeeding, Nutrition, Infection and Infant Growth in Developed and Emerging Countries*. St John's Newfoundland: ARTS Biomedical Publishers, 1990; P521 (Abstract).

[13] Livingstone M B E, Davies P S W, Prentice A M, *et al*. Comparisons of simultaneous measures of energy intake and expenditure in children and adolescents. *Proc Nut Soc* 1991; **50**: 15A).

[14] Livingstone M B E, Prentice A M, Strain J J, *et al*. Accuracy of weighed dietary records in studies of diet and health. *Br Med J* 1990; **300**: 708–712.

[15] Day N E, Roberts S J. Accuracy of weighed dietary records. *Br Med J* 1990; **300**: 1398.

[16] Jackson A A, Wootton S. Accuracy of weighed dietary records. *Br Med J* 1990; **300**: 1138–1139.

[17] Hamill P V, Drizd T A, Johnson C L, Reed R B, Roche A F. *NCHS Growth Curves for Children, Birth to 18 years*. Hyattsville MD: National Center for Health Statistics, 1977. (Vital and Health Statistical Series; 11).

[18] Southgate D A T, Durnin J V G A. Calorie conversion factors: an experimental reassessment of the factors used in the calculation of the energy value of human diets. *Br J Nutr* 1970; **24**: 517–535.

[19] Paul A A, Black A E, Evans J, Cole T J, Whitehead R G. Breast-milk intake and growth in infants from 2 to 10 months. *J Hum Nutr Dietet* 1988; **1**: 437–450.

[20] Barker D J P. The fetal and infant origins of adult disease. *Br Med J* 1990; **301**: 1111.

[21] Cook J, Altman D G, Moore D M C *et al*., A survey of the nutritional status of schoolchildren. *Br J Prev Soc Med* 1973; **27**: 91–99.

[22] Black A E, Billewicz W Z, Thomson A. The diets of preschool children in Newcastle-upon-Tyne, 1968–1971. *Br J Nutr* 1976; **35**: 105–113.

[23] Durnin J G V A. Energy balance in childhood and adolescence. *Proc Nutr Soc* 1984; **43**: 271–279.

[24] Griffiths M, Rivers J P W, Payne P R. Energy intake in children at high and low risk of obesity. *Hum Nutr: Clin Nutr* 1987; **41**: 425–430.

[25] Department of Health. *The Diets of British Schoolchildren*. London: HMSO, 1989. (Reports on health and social subjects; 36).

[26] Schofield W N, Schofield C, James W P T. Basal metabolic rate—review and prediction. *Hum Nutr: Clin Nutr* 1985; **39** (suppl): 1–96.

[27] Gregory J, Foster K, Tyler H, Wiseman M. *The Dietary and Nutritional Survey of British Adults*. London: HMSO, 1990.

[28] Fentem P H, Turnbull N B, Bassey E J. *Benefits of Exercise: the Evidence*. Manchester: Manchester University Press, 1990.

[29] Blair S N. How much fitness is needed to decrease all cause mortality in men and women. *Proceedings of the Annual Meeting of the American College of Sports Medicine* 1991 (in press).

[30] Hytten F E, Leitch I. *The Physiology of Human Pregnancy*. 2nd Ed. Oxford: Blackwell Scientific Publications, 1971.

[31] English R M, Hitchcock N F. Nutrient intakes during pregnancy, lactation and after the cessation of lactation in a group of Australian women. *Br J Nutr* 1968; **22**: 615–624.

[32] Emerson K, Saxena B N, Poindexter E L Caloric cost of normal pregnancy. *Obstets Gynaecol* 1972; **40**: 786–794.

[33] Smithells R W, Ankers C, Lennon D *et al*. Maternal nutrition in early pregnancy. *Br J Nutr* 1977; **38**: 497–506.

[34] Darke S J, Disselduff M M, Try G P. Frequency distributions of mean daily intakes of food energy and selected nutrients obtained during nutrition surveys of different groups of people in Great Britain between 1968 and 1971. *Br J Nutr* 1980; **44**: 243–252.

[35] Doyle W, Crawford M A, Laurence M *et al*. Dietary survey during pregnancy in a low socio-economic group. *Hum Nutr: Appl Nutr* 1982; **36A**: 95–106.

[36] Eaton P M, Wharton F A, Wharton B A. Nutrient intake of pregnant Asian women at Sorrento Maternity Hospital, Birmingham. *Br J Nutr* 1984; **52**: 457–468.

[37] Anderson A S, Lean M E J. Dietary intake in pregnancy. A comparison between 49 Cambridgeshire women and current recommended intake. *Hum Nutr: Appl Nutr* 1986; **40A**: 40–48.

[38] Black A E, Wiles S J, Paul A A. The nutrient intakes of pregnant and lactating mothers of good socio-economic status in Cambridge, UK: some implications for recommended daily allowances of minor nutrients. *Br J Nutr* 1986; **56**: 59–72.

[39] Durnin J V G A. Energy requirements of pregnancy: an integration of the longitudinal data from the five-country study. *Lancet* 1987; **ii**: 1131–1133.

[40] van Raaij J A T M, Vermatt-Miedema S H, Schonk C M, Peck P E M, Hautvast J G A J. Energy requirements of pregnancy in the Netherlands. *Lancet* 1987; **ii**: 953–954.

[41] World Health Organization. *The Quantity and Quality of Breast-milk: Report on the WHO Collaborative Study on Breast-feeding*. Geneva: World Health Organization, 1985.

[42] Prentice A M, Paul A A, Prentice A, Black A E, Cole T J, Whitehead R G. Cross-cultural differences in lactational performance. In: Hamosh P, ed. *Human Lactation 2: Maternal and Environmental Factors*. New York: Plenum Press, 1986; 13–44.

[43] Thomson A M, Hytten F E, Billewicz W Z. The energy cost of human lactation. *Br J Nutr* 1970; **24**: 565–574.

[44] Prentice A M, Prentice A. Energy costs of lactation. *Ann Rev Nutr* 1988; **8**: 63–79.

[45] Sadurskis A, Kabir N, Wager J, Forsum E. Energy metabolism, body composition and milk production during lactation in healthy Swedish women. *Am J Clin Nutr* 1988; **48**: 44–49.

[46] Prentice A M, Whitehead R G. The energetics of human reproduction. *Symp Zool Soc Lond* 1987; **57**: 275–304.

[47] Durnin J V G A. Food intake and energy expenditure of elderly people. *Geront Clin* 1961; **4**: 128–133.

[48] Jerham, V J, Lavides V C, Durnin J V G A. A nutrition survey on crofters in North-West Scotland. *Nutrition* 1969; **23**: 159–164.

[49] Patrick J M, Bassey E J, Fentem P H. Changes in body fat and muscle in manual workers at and after retirement. *Eur J Appl Physiol* 1982; **49**: 187–196.

[50] Patrick J M, Bassey E J, Irving J M, Blecher A, Fentem P H. Objective measurements of customary physical activity in elderly men and women before and after retirement. *Q J Exptl Physiol* 1986; **71**: 47–58.

[51] Dallosso H M, Morgan K, Bassey E J, Ebrahim S B J, Fentem P H, Arie T H D. Levels of customary physical activity among the old and very old living at home. *J Epidemiol Community Hlth* 1988; **42**: 121–127.

[52] Patrick J M. Customary physical activity in the elderly. *Proc symp Biol Human Aging* Cambridge: Cambridge University Press, 1984.

[53] Bassey E J, Terry A M. The oxygen cost of walking in the elderly. *J Physiol* 1986; **373**: 42P.

[54] McGandy R B, Barrows C H, Spadias A, Meredith A, Stone J L, Norris A H. Nutrient intakes and energy expenditure in men of different ages. *J Geront* 1966; **21**: 581–587.

[55] Borgstrom B, Norden A, Akesson B, Abdulla M, Jagerstad M. Nutrition in old age. Chemical analyses of what old people eat and their states of health during a 6 year follow-up. *Scand J Gastro-ent* 1979; **52** (suppl): 1–299.

[56] Uauy R B, Scrimshaw N S, Young V. Human protein requirements: Nitrogen balance response to graded levels of egg protein in elderly men and women. *Am J Clin Nutr* 1978; **31**: 779–785.

[57] Calloway D H, Zanni E. Energy requirements and energy expenditure of elderly men. *Am J Clin Nutr* 1980; **33**: 2088–2892.

3. Fat

3.1 Essential fatty acids

3.1.1 *Definition* The essential fatty acids (EFAs) are linoleic acid (C18:2, n-6), and alpha linolenic acid (C18:3, n-3). There are several longer chain fatty acids, of which arachidonic acid (C20:4, n-6), eicosapentaenoic acid (C20:5, n-3) and docosahexaenoic acid (C22:6, n-3) are physiologically important, which can be made to a limited extent in the tissues from linoleic and alpha linolenic acids. They are not strictly essential fatty acids but in EFA deficiency, intakes of these longer chain fatty acids may become critical.

3.1.2 *Functions of EFAs* EFAs in phospholipids are important for maintaining the function and integrity of cellular and sub-cellular membranes. They also participate in the regulation of cholesterol metabolism, being involved in its transport, breakdown and ultimate excretion. They are precursors of prostaglandins, thromboxane, leukotrienes and of arachidonic, eicosapentaenoic and docosahexaenoic acids. It has been postulated that in infants there may be a specific dietary requirement for these longer chain fatty acids during rapid brain development[1]. In contrast to breastmilk, infant formulas do not contain longer chain fatty acids. Premature infants have been shown to have a specific requirement for these fatty acids[2] but there is no evidence for this in full-term infants.

3.1.3 *Sources of EFAs* EFAs are present in all natural lipid structures but are relatively more common in the storage lipids of plants and of marine animals than of land animals. Most vegetable oils and some fish are therefore good dietary sources. Intakes in Great Britain, estimated from the Dietary and Nutritional Survey of British Adults, were 11.7 g/d of n-6 fatty acids and 1.6 g/d of n-3 fatty acids[3]. The main sources of n-6 fatty acids were vegetables, fruit and nuts (3.0 g), cereal products (2.6 g) and fat spreads (2.4 g). The main sources of n-3 fatty acids were vegetables (0.4 g), meat and meat products (0.3 g), cereal products (0.3 g) and fat spreads (0.3 g).

3.1.4 *Deficiency* A deficiency state arising from an inadequate intake of linoleic acid has been demonstrated in children[4]. Although a specific deficiency state arising from inadequate dietary alphalinolenic acid has not been demonstrated in healthy humans, it is regarded as a dietary essential. Long chain fatty acids of the n-3 series are needed for the development and function of the brain and retina.

3.1.5 *Dietary Reference Values* DRVs for EFAs have been derived only on the basis of prevention of EFA deficiency, although it has been proposed that levels of EFA intake above those required to prevent deficiency may be important in modulating the risk of cardiovascular disease. This aspect of EFA intake is discussed in section 3.4. Most adult Western diets provide 8 to 15 g/d of EFAs and healthy people have a body reserve of 500 to 1000 g in adipose tissue. Overt evidence of EFA deficiency in adults is seen only in clinical situations when they provide less than 1 to 2 per cent of total dietary energy or less than 2 to 5 g/d of linoleic acid. The total EFA concentration in human milk represents about 6 per cent of its energy. the lower level recommended in *Artificial Feeds for Young Infants*[5] of linoleic and alpha linolenic acids in a feed for normal infants was that together they should constitute at least 1 per cent of the total energy (the amount required to cure deficiency). This does not match the concentrations usually found in human milk and there have been suggestions that the lower level be 3 per cent of total energy[6], or 4.5 per cent for linoleic acid and 0.5 per cent for alpha linolenic acid[2]. There is no evidence that these higher levels offer advantages over the lower ones. The Panel therefore recommended that for infants, children and adults linoleic acid should provide at least 1 per cent of total energy and alpha linolenic acid at least 0.2 per cent of total energy.

3.2 **Free radicals and lipid peroxidation**

3.2.1 *Introduction* In the last decade there has been a substantial increase in information on the biological importance of oxygen-derived species, such as hydrogen peroxide and free radicals (eg hydroxyl or superoxide). These highly active species have the capacity to damage cellular components by oxidation at any site where the species are produced[7]. The extent of damage is dependent both on the activity and on the biological half life of the radical, although the body has a substantial capacity to repair such damage. Nevertheless, radicals produced intracellularly can damage DNA and lead to mutations[8]. It is thought that the hydroxyl radical is important in natural killer T-lymphocyte activity[9]. Structural integrity is an important factor in preventing tissue oxidation[7]. However, all membrane lipids, particularly polyunsaturated fatty acids, are vulnerable to peroxidation, and once established, lipid perodixation is auto-catalytic. Transitional metal ions, such as iron and copper are particularly important catalysts of peroxidation in biological systems. Although largely bound in organic complexes, there is evidence, particularly for iron, that in a number of tissues they may be bound loosely enough to act as a catalyst for these reactions[8,10]. These effects have led to claims that lipid peroxidation may be a pathogenetic factor in conditions such as ageing, and in the development of cancer and atherosclerosis[11]. Such claims have in turn led to concern that an increase in dietary polyunsaturated fatty acids (PUFAs) may increase risk of these conditions, although there is no evidence for such a relationship.

3.2.2 *Biology*

3.2.2.1 Free radicals are produced *in vivo* in the course of normal oxidative metabolism, as a result of cytochrome P_{450} activity and as part of the respiratory burst of activated phagocytes in cell mediated immunity. To counteract the oxidative process, there are two main groups of natural antioxidants: preventive substances which are mainly iron chelators or binding compounds[1] and radical scavengers which include superoxide dismutase, vitamins E and C, urate and carotenes[12]. Selenium is essential for glutathione peroxidase which can also metabolise lipid peroxides to fatty acids. A disproportion in the balance between these two arms of the process might result in tissue damage. Although a number of the components involved in these reactions (substrates, catalysts, antioxidants) can be derived from the diet, it is not established how their dietary intake modulates their activity in the body.

3.2.2.2 There are a few conditions in which lipid peroxidation and free radicals have an established pathogenetic role in reperfusion injury and in tissue rejection following transplant surgery[10,13]. Peroxidised lipids have also been found in a number of disease states[7], but it is likely that this is a result of pre-existing disease rather than a primary causal factor, as damaged tissues are more prone to peroxidation than healthy ones. Under these circumstances peroxidation is likely to lead to a continuation of damage rather than initiate it. Only in few of the clinical situations where oxygen radicals are accepted contributors to their pathogenesis, such as Keshan Disease, is antioxidant therapy effective[14]. This may be related, at least in part, to the failure of the antioxidant to reach the site of radical activity and cellular damage (see also Section 19).

3.2.2.3 There is no direct evidence bearing on the role of dietary fat in this area. Populations with high ratios of dietary polyunsaturated to saturated fatty acids (P:S ratio) are not characterised by high rates of cardiovascular disease or bowel or breast cancer. Such populations usually do not derive a large proportion of dietary energy from total fat. Initial reports that diets high in PUFAs, used to lower blood cholesterol and modify cardiovascular disease risk, were associated with an increase in gallstones and pancreatic cancer have not subsequently been substantiated.

3.2.3 *Conclusions*

i. It is likely that peroxidation of tissue polyunsaturated fatty acids (PUFAs) is a response to pre-existing tissue damage, although this may contribute to continuation of disease processes;

ii. Balance within tissues between free radical activity and antioxidant status is important for the maintenance of cellular integrity;

iii. Intake of antioxidants is the major dietary contributor to that balance;

iv. No evidence exists that high dietary intakes of PUFAs have been associated with any human disease.

3.2.4 *Guidance on high intakes* The Panel noted that despite the paucity of evidence, recommendations have been made by other expert committees that dietary PUFA should not contribute more than 10 per cent to dietary energy. The Panel found insufficient evidence either to support or contradict these recommendations, but accepted that existing evidence justified a cautious approach. The Panel therefore proposed that the dietary intake of polyunsaturated fatty acids by individuals should not exceed 10 per cent of total food energy.

3.3 **Positional and trans isomers of fatty acids**

3.3.1 *Introduction* The introduction in most molecules of a double bond gives rise to the possibility of geometric (*cis-trans*) isomerism. Fatty acids containing more than one double bond are common in nature. Unsaturated fatty acids from all vegetable, and most animal, sources adopt the *cis* configuration. In addition, a fatty acid may have similar numbers of double bonds at different positions in the chain (positional isomerism). Interest in the metabolic effects of *trans*-fatty acids has grown recently because of suggestions that their consumption may be linked to the development of human disease, particularly cardiovascular disease. Trends to increased consumption of hydrogenated vegetable and fish oils in margarines and other spreads has led to an increased *trans*-fatty acid consumption as these fats are a rich dietary source of *trans* and positional isomers of fatty acids[15-17]. Consumption of these products is, however, now declining[18].

3.3.2 *Dietary sources of isomeric fatty acids* Industrial hydrogenation is the chief but not the only source of dietary *trans* fatty acids. Ruminal bacteria of domestic cattle and sheep generate *trans* isomers. There is a significant accumulation of these *trans* fatty acids in the milk and therefore other dairy products, and in beef and lamb[19]. In the United States, margarines and shortenings are almost entirely produced from vegetable oils, while the UK makes substantial use of fish oils. These may contain up to 18 per cent of fatty acids with 20 or more carbon units compared to less than 1 per cent in vegetable oils. The variety of unnatural positional or geometric isomers which results from their hydrogenation is therefore wider. It also varies with the source (deep water *versus* inshore) and variety of the fish used. Hydrogenation is used not only to process foodstuffs for direct human consumption, but also to a lesser extent to prepare animal feed. Small amounts of *trans* fatty acids therefore find their way into the human food chain via poultry and pork. The high temperature to which vegetable oils are subjected during deep frying renders them susceptible to direct isomerisation in the frying process, particularly where the fat is used repeatedly. Many deep-fried foods do, as a result, contain variable quantities of *trans* or *cis* fatty acid isomers which are not encountered in nature.

3.3.3 *Dietary consumption of trans fatty acids* The National Food Survey[18] gives information based on household food purchases in Great Britain which indicates that average consumption of *trans* fatty acids is about 5 g/d, although the range is wide, depending on diet and the sources of dietary fat, and intakes up to 25 or 30 g/d are possible[17]. The Dietary and Nutritional Survey of British Adults showed that intakes of *trans* fatty acids in 1986/87 averaged 5.6 and 4.0 g/d for men and women respectively[3]. The intakes of other isomeric fatty acids have not been estimated. *Trans* fatty acids consumed by mothers will be transmitted to suckling infants via breastmilk. The reported quantities of *trans* isomers in human milk vary from 2–18 per cent of the total fatty acids, corresponding approximately to the quantities in the diet[20,21] and change rapidly in response to diet modification. One study has shown that adolescents consume the same proportion of *trans* fatty acids, mostly *trans*, 18:1 as adults. No *trans* 18:2 isomers were detectable in significant amounts in the diet[22].

3.3.4 *Digestion, absorption and metabolism of trans fatty acid isomers* In general *trans* unsaturated fats are digested, absorbed and metabolised in a manner and at a rate which is indistinguishable from their *cis*-unsaturated counterparts[21].

3.3.5 *Isomeric fatty acids and health* Enrichment of the diet with *trans* fatty acids, following the previous widespread use of partially hydrogenated vegetable and fish oils has raised concerns regarding the health risks of this development. The structural similarities between *cis, cis* linoleate and its all *trans* counterpart raised the possibility that the *trans* isomer might exhibit essential fatty acid activity or, alternatively, might affect linoleate metabolism and aggravate essential fatty acid deficiency, but this theory has not been confirmed. No data are available on other (positional) isomers of fatty acids. Toxicological effects have not been ascribed to any of the *trans* isomers, with the exception of *trans* 9, *trans* 12 octadecadienoic acid which at high levels in the diet was found to impair delta 6 desaturase activity and decrease prostaglandin synthesis in experimental animals[23]. However, insignificant amounts of this isomer are found in hydrogenated fats and it is barely detectable in human tissues.

3.3.6 *Atherosclerosis* Extensive studies have failed to confirm a relationship between *trans* and positional isomers and atherogenesis. Investigations of the influence of *trans* fatty acids on plasma cholesterol level have shown both elevating and neutral effects. Many studies were flawed, and reliable data on the effects of *trans* fatty acids at the levels likely in any conventional UK diet are scarce. Diets containing high levels of *trans* fatty acids (about 11 per cent of energy) raise LDL-cholesterol concentrations when compared with C18:1 *cis* fatty acids (oleic acid), although not to the same extent as a diet high in C12 and C16 saturated fatty acids. In the same study HDL cholesterol fell when *trans*, but not saturated, fatty acids were exchanged with oleic acid[24].

3.3.7 *Cancer* An association between the incidence of cancer of the colon, breast and prostate and the use of industrially hydrogenated vegetable fats has been reported[25], but other known risk factors, or socioeconomic factors, might have accounted for the association.

3.3.8 *Conclusions*

i. The biological effects of dietary isomeric fatty acids in the UK remain to be fully elucidated and knowledge of the range of intakes and trends is incomplete. A number of areas have been inadequately studied (eg hydrogenated fish oils, positional isomers). The properties of *trans* fatty acids so far studied are such that they cannot generally be regarded as equivalent either to their *cis* counterparts or to saturated fatty acids. The Panel concluded that the data did not adequately refute or support the allegations of potential long term adverse effects on health of isomeric fatty acid intake in the UK.

ii. The average and extremes of intakes of isomeric (including *trans*) fatty acids should be monitored in the UK. More research is needed on biological effects of different isomeric fatty acids, particularly those resulting from hydrogenation of fish oils. In the meantime *trans* fatty acid intake in the population should not increase further than the current estimated average of 5 g/d or 2 per cent of dietary energy.

3.4 Cardiovascular disease

3.4.1 *Death from cardiovascular disease* Mortality from coronary heart disease (CHD) in the UK is amongst the highest in the world[15], and has been related to fat intakes. Although these rates have been declining for more than 15 years, CHD accounts for more deaths in men than any other single cause, and is particularly important in men under the age of 55. CHD deaths in women equal those from all causes of cancer combined. CHD is a major cause of morbidity as well as mortality, encompassing a spectrum of severity from asymptomatic atherosclerosis through symptomatic disease, eg angina pectoris, acute myocardial infarction, heart failure, to sudden death. Death from CHD usually follows a myocardial infarction, following an interruption of the blood supply to heart muscle via the coronary arteries. Coronary occlusion usually takes the form of a thrombosis in a main coronary artery which has previously been considerably narrowed by atheroma. It is the concurrence of atherosclerosis and thrombosis which results in infarction. The pathogenesis of each, however, may be different. Cardiovascular disease also includes cerebrovascular and peripheral vascular disease. Although fewer deaths are attributable to the latter conditions, they are nevertheless considerable causes of morbidity.

3.4.2 *Atherosclerosis* This is characterised by the accumulation of cholesterol-rich lipid deposits within the arterial wall, eventually leading to endothelial damage, plaque formation and narrowing of the arterial lumen. The major arteries of the heart (coronary arteries), of the brain and of the legs are particularly prone to develop atherosclerosis. The pathogenesis of this condition is not clear, but it appears to involve cholesterol in low density lipoproteins (LDL) being taken up by macrophages within the arterial wall. The relationship of fatty streaks, which may be found in the arteries of children and young adults, to later atherosclerosis is not known.

3.4.3 *Thrombosis* This is usually the final event in coronary occlusion, and is the result of intravascular platelet aggregation, with an associated fibrin matrix. The formation of a thrombus requires an adequate supply of clotting factors, particularly of Factor VII and fibrinogen. Increased concentrations of these precursors have been linked to increased risk of CHD. Smoking has been associated with an increase in plasma fibrinogen.

3.4.4 *Risk factors for atherosclerosis* The development of atherosclerosis depends on numerous risk factors both genetic and environmental. Smoking, high blood pressure and raised serum cholesterol are the major ones, while before the menopause women are relatively protected. Familial CHD risk is often unassociated with the major risk factors. Smoking is associated with a dose related increase in risk of death from CHD, independently of other risk factors. Risk of death from CHD is strongly correlated with blood pressure. About 50 per cent of the variation in CHD risk can be attributed to these known environmental risk factors. Other modulators of risk may include dietary components such as antioxidant vitamins, which influence macrophage uptake of LDL, and long-chain fatty acids which may affect blood clotting.

3.4.5 *Serum cholesterol* There is a continuous increase in risk of death from CHD with increasing serum cholesterol. This is a consistent finding which has been demonstrated both within and between populations. In Western societies risk of death from CHD is 4 fold greater in the top 10 per cent than in the bottom 10 per cent of the distribution of serum cholesterol. It has been calculated that, allowing for measurement error, a 10 per cent difference in serum cholesterol is associated with a 30 per cent difference in CHD rates. Cholesterol is transported in the plasma in association with specific proteins which direct its metabolism. Four major lipid-protein complexes (lipoproteins) are recognized (chylomicrons, very low density (VLDL), low density (LDL) and high density lipoproteins (HDL)). Coronary heart disease risk has been linked primarily with LDL which carries 70 per cent of plasma cholesterol. LDL in modified form is thought to be avidly assimilated by macrophages in the arterial wall and has been identified as a component of atherosclerotic lesions. Conversely, plasma concentrations of HDL are inversely associated with CHD mortality. There are specific inherited abnormalities of LDL cholesterol metabolism which result in markedly increased risk of CHD and premature death.

3.4.6 *Dietary saturated fatty acids and serum cholesterol* The major non-genetic determinant of serum cholesterol levels is diet, and death rates from CHD in different countries are associated with national fat consumption[26]. The association between CHD mortality is closest with saturated fatty acid (SFA) supplies, which has been demonstrated in both international and national studies. Similarly, national average SFA supplies correlated closely with national average serum cholesterol concentration[27]. As the amount of dietary SFA increases, the serum levels both of LDL cholesterol and of total cholesterol rise[26,28]. Not all SFA have the same effects. The major effect on serum cholesterol is due to myristic acid (C14) which accounts for 67 per cent of the explained variance. Palmitic acid (C16) has a lesser effect, and there is no evidence that SFA of longer (stearic, C18) or shorter (C10, C12) chain lengths have any effect on serum cholesterol[26,28]. However, despite these differences, it is usual to consider total saturated fatty acids as a class for practical purposes.

3.4.7 *Dietary polyunsaturated fatty acids and serum cholesterol* Increasing dietary n-6 polyunsaturated fatty acid (PUFA) intake decreases both total and LDL cholesterol, independently of any change in SFA. However, n-3 PUFA, such as docosahexaenoic and eicosapentaenoic acids in fish oils, and alpha linolenic acid, do not appear to have any effect on serum total cholesterol levels, but may be involved with clotting pathways. Increased n-3 PUFA intake may inhibit thrombus formation, and has been shown to reduce the risk of further myocardial infarction in men with at least one previous episode. n-3 PUFA also lower serum triglyceride concentrations.

3.4.8 *Dietary monounsaturated fatty acids and serum cholesterol* Low CHD rates have been described in countries following a so-called "Mediterranean diet". Although some of these countries, eg Greece and Southern Italy, have relatively high intakes of *cis*-monounsaturated fatty acids[26,29], the Mediterranean diet is characterised more by low saturates and low total fat intakes as well as a number of other factors including high intakes of fruit, vegetables and wine. Most Mediterranean countries have much lower total fat and SFA intakes than the UK whilst having similar or slightly greater *cis*-monounsaturated fatty acid intakes. Experimental studies in man show that *cis*-monounsaturated fats are neutral with regard to changes in total cholesterol in blood[26,28]. There is insufficient evidence at present that a specific increase in *cis*-monounsaturated fatty acid intake would help to prevent coronary heart disease.

3.4.9 *Total fat and serum cholesterol* Although in international studies total fat supplies are associated both with average cholesterol concentration and with CHD mortality[30], an effect of total fat intake on cholesterol metabolism or CHD risk independent of SFA or PUFA intakes has not been demonstrated. Although there is some evidence from small clinical studies that levels of Factor VII may be determined at least in part by total dietary fat intake, irrespective of its composition[31], these data are preliminary. Nevertheless, they provide support for the view that it may be important not to allow an unrestricted intake of fat, irrespective of its composition. Therefore the Panel concluded that DRV for fat should be calculated from the summation of the reference values for individual classes of fatty acids.

3.4.10 *Dietary cholesterol* Dietary cholesterol intake has a small effect on serum cholesterol levels. The effect of dietary cholesterol in raising serum cholesterol is minimised when SFA intake represents a small proportion of energy.

3.4.11 *Serum cholesterol reduction and risk of CHD* A number of long-term prospective studies has been carried out to assess the effect on CHD of reducing serum cholesterol, either by diet alone or with drugs, or with other interventions. These studies uniformly demonstrate a fall in CHD events when serum cholesterol is decreased[32,33]. These long-term studies have all been performed on men, and most on men who might be considered at relatively high risk for CHD. A reduction of CHD in women or in the population at average risk has not been demonstrated. However, there seems no reason to suppose that the effect of the interventions would not be qualitatively similar, as the relationship between CHD risk and serum cholesterol is continuous, and reduction in risk is proportional to reduction in serum cholesterol. In intervention trials overall mortality was not altered. Although these trials were not designed with the power to demonstrate such a difference, this has been a matter of concern. Studies to assess an effect on all cause mortality would need to be even larger and/or longer than those already carried out.

3.4.12 *Serum cholesterol and risk of other diseases* It has been suggested that a low serum cholesterol may increase the risk of cancer. However, in populations with low average serum cholesterol concentrations, spontaneous cancer rates are no higher than in those with higher cholesterol levels. Furthermore cancer rates in Western population groups with low cholesterol concentrations fall if those developing cancer soon after sampling are excluded, suggesting that the low cholesterol may be a result of pre-existing undiagnosed cancer. Some cancer cells have been shown to have receptors for LDL cholesterol which might explain such an effect, and LDL catabolism has been shown to be increased in metastatic prostatic cancer[34]. Dietary intervention studies show that where coronary heart disease risk is lowered in association with a fall in blood cholesterol, there is no specific rise in cancer deaths which is out of proportion to the change in other death rates[35]. The balance of the evidence therefore is against a specific predisposing effect of low blood cholesterol to cancer. If low blood cholesterol is causally associated with cancer development it is likely that the effect is small and limited only to those with very low cholesterol levels. The possible disadvantages of a low blood cholesterol are outweighed by the benefits to the population as a whole in terms of coronary disease prevention (see also 3.5.4.3). A meta-analysis of a number of primary prevention intervention studies has suggested that lowering of blood cholesterol may increase deaths not related to illness[36]. The potentially different adverse effects of various methods of cholesterol reduction deserve further investigation.

3.4.13 *Dietary change and serum cholesterol* Based on the results of a large series of human metabolic studies (para 3.4.6), the relationship between dietary intakes of SFA, PUFA and cholesterol on the one hand, and serum cholesterol on the other, have been described in equations[26,28]. These equations can be used to predict in groups of people the effect on serum cholesterol concentrations of changes in dietary intakes of these nutrients assuming energy intakes remain constant. The Panel concluded that a reduction in serum LDL concentration would be expected to result in a fall in risk of cardiovascular disease in the population[32,33]. It further recognized that further substantial data applicable to the general population were unlikely to be forthcoming in the foreseeable future. A reduction in serum LDL cholesterol levels in the general population could most effectively be achieved by a reduction in SFA consumption. Low SFA intake is not known to have any adverse effects. Increased PUFA intake might have some undesirable sequelae (see para 3.2.3). Although an increased intake of monounsaturated fatty acids might reduce LDL cholesterol, the weight of evidence in support of this is much less than that pertaining to SFA and PUFA, but an increased intake does not necessarily increase serum cholesterol. Any effects of total fat on serum cholesterol appear to be mediated mainly through the sum of the effects of its component fatty acids. It is not known to what extent changes in energy balance may affect these predictions.

3.4.14 *Relationship of serum cholesterol to CHD risk* The evidence relating serum cholesterol to CHD risk does not suggest a threshold effect—that is a particular level of serum cholesterol above which the risk is high, and below which the risk is low. Rather, the risk appears to increase continuously with serum cholesterol[37]. The Panel accepted that here, even more than for many other areas, any reference value would be based on a judgement involving practical and cultural considerations, as well as the scientific evidence.

3.4.15 *Method of expression of fat intakes* Conventionally, fat intakes have been expressed as a proportion of dietary energy to control for dietary energy intake, and so to some extent for energy expenditure and body size. However, while the composition of the diet is important, it is possible that the absolute amount of fat consumed is also relevant. There is no reason to suppose that reducing the *proportion* of dietary energy from fat by increasing *total* energy intake from greater consumption of low-fat foods would lead to decreased CHD risk, particularly in the absence of increased energy expenditure. Furthermore, energy from alcohol may contribute to total energy intake. Conventionally, recommendations for fat intake have been made as a proportion of food energy (ie excluding alcohol), to avoid the possibility of achieving the targets by increasing alcohol intake rather than reducing SFA intake.

3.4.16 *Alcohol and energy intakes* The Panel endorsed the recommendations of the Royal College of Physicians that men should not drink more than 21 units (168 g) and women 14 units (112 g) of alcohol weekly (representing about 7 per cent of dietary energy)[38]. However 21 per cent of adult men and 35 per cent of adult women are not regular consumers of alcohol[3]. In order to facilitate the flexible use of reference values for fat and carbohydrate, the Panel agreed to present them as percentages both of total dietary energy, and of food energy. If the recommendations for limiting alcohol intake were achieved, the differences between the two sets of figures would be less.

3.4.17 *Derivation of Dietary Reference Values* Expert groups both in Europe and in the USA have accepted conventional categories of serum cholesterol such that less than 5.2 mmol/l represents a desirable level, 5.2-6.4 mmol/l is mildly elevated, 6.5-7.8 mmol/l is moderately elevated, and more than 7.8 mmol/l is severely elevated[39,40]. In Great Britain average serum cholesterol in adults is about 5.8 mmol/l and average daily SFA intake is 36.5 g/day, representing 16 per cent of dietary energy[3]. Data from the NFS are consistent with this figure (see table 1.7). Based on the Keys equation[26] it is possible to calculate that a reduction in average SFA intake to 10 per cent of total energy would be expected to result in a decrease in serum cholesterol concentration of about 0.4 mmol/l. If this reduction were confined to SFA of 14 or 16 carbon atoms, then the reduction in serum cholesterol would be expected to be greater. This in turn would be expected to reduce the risk of CHD in the UK substantially. Only about 5 per cent of adults in the UK currently derive 10 per cent of energy or less from SFA. These calculations have been based on the assumption that the distribution of national fatty acid intakes around the mean remains similar, although the mean intakes might change. The evidence relating to this assumption is very scanty, and the Panel agreed that such an assumption might not prove accurate. The Panel recommended that research be done into the changes in population distributions of intakes of nutrients in response to efforts to change them.

3.4.18 *Dietary Reference Values* The Panel therefore proposed that:

i. Saturated fatty acids should provide an average for the population of 10 per cent of total dietary energy;

ii. *Cis*-polyunsaturated fatty acids should continue to provide an average of 6 per cent of total dietary energy for the population and be derived from a mixture of n-6 and n-3 PUFAs;

iii. *Cis*-monounsatured fatty acids (principally oleic acid) should continue to provide on average 12 per cent of dietary energy for the population;

iv. Total fatty acid intake can be calculated as the sum of the component fatty acids (see 3.8) to average 33 per cent of total dietary energy for the population. The Panel stressed that the DRVs for fat and fatty acids were closely interdependent and interrelated, and could not be taken in isolation.

3.5 **Cancer**

3.5.1 *Introduction* Cancer accounts for 23 per cent of all deaths in Britain. With few exceptions, the risk of cancer increases with age (Fig 3.1). Of the most common cancers, rates in Britain are declining for stomach cancer, but increasing for cancer of the skin and bladder. In women, the incidence of breast and lung cancer is increasing. In men, rates for cancer of the prostate are increasing[41].

3.5.2 *Geographical variations in cancer incidence* There is a marked geographical variation worldwide in age standardised incidence of different types of cancer[42]. Incidence rates in migrants change to match those of the host population within one or two generations, suggesting a strong environmental component. An association has been described between dietary factors and the occurrence of most common cancers in the UK. Fat intake has been particularly associated with cancer of the breast, large bowel, pancreas and prostate[43]. Evidence linking fat with these cancers is derived from animal studies and human epidemiological data[44].

3.5.3 *Animal Studies* In animal studies cancers are initiated using large doses of known carcinogens, such as polycyclic hydrocarbons, but at a dose several orders of magnitude greater than encountered in human food or other environmental sources. For this and other reasons the relevance of experimental cancers to human cancer remains in doubt. Breast tumour incidence is approximately doubled in the animals fed 40 per cent energy as fat compared with those fed 20 per cent[45]. Present levels of fat in the British diet are 38 per cent of total energy (Table 1.7). Diets high in fat are generally high in energy so the effect of fat on tumour promotion may be related to total energy intake. A 20 per cent reduction in food intake has an effect equal to a similar reduction in fat in suppressing tumour formation by 40–60 per cent[45]. In recent studies no overall effect of dietary fat on tumour promotion independent of energy has been found[46–48]. Recent experiments suggest that polyunsaturated fatty acids of the n-3, but not the n-6, series (principally eicosapentaenoic acid) tend to suppress tumour promotion, whereas there is a tumour requirement for the n-6 series of approximately 10 per cent of total energy[45].

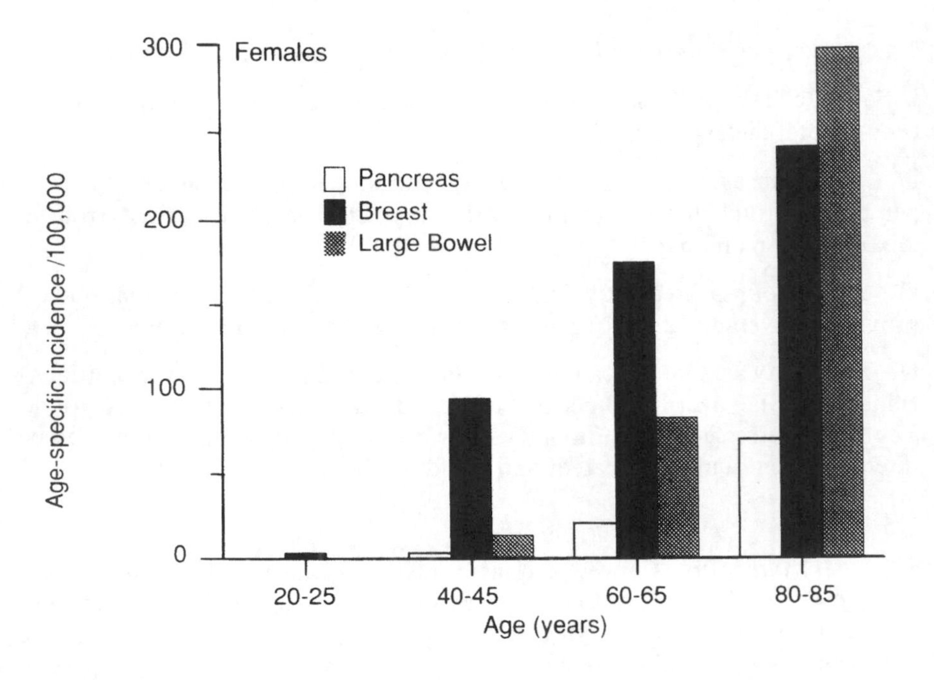

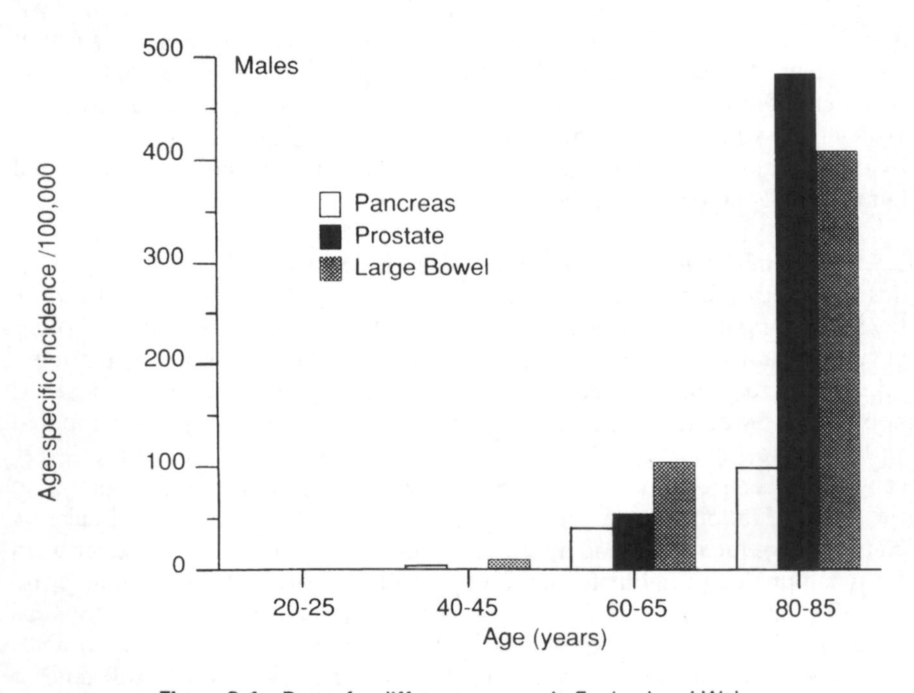

Figure 3.1 Rates for different cancers in England and Wales

3.5.4 *Epidemiology*

3.5.4.1 *Breast cancer* Total dietary fat intake is consistently related to human breast cancer mortality and incidence in cross-country studies[43]. However, most case control and prospective studies within any one country do not find a relationship between dietary fat and breast cancer incidence [48-52], although this might be expected in view of the narrow range of dietary intakes within any one population[53]. There is an increased risk of postmenopausal breast cancer with obesity[54], possibly due to increased oestrone production by adipose tissue[55]. In a prospective study by the American Cancer Society mortality from cancers both of the breast in women and of the large bowel in men were increased when weights were 40 per cent above average[56]. Risk of endometrial cancer is greatly increased with overweight. In contrast, there is probably an inverse association between premenopausal breast cancer and body weight[54].

3.5.4.2 *Colon Cancer* The incidence of human colon cancer is related to dietary fat intake in cross-country studies, although it is at least as strongly related to meat consumption[43]. However, case control studies have not shown a consistent association between dietary fat consumption and risk of colon cancer[50,51]. Recent results from the largest and best controlled prospective studies of fat and colon cancer show an increased risk with high saturates and high monounsaturated fat intakes[57]. This study also confirmed the association with high meat intake. Earlier studies found no increased risk with total fat in an Hawaiian Japanese population based on a 24 hour diet recall[51]. Preliminary studies of Seventh Day Adventists show an increased risk of colon cancer with high total fat consumption[52]. In a prospective study of colorectal adenomas in men, saturated fat was positively associated with risk (independent of energy intake) whilst dietary fibre was protective[58]. Internationally, there is a positive association between cholesterol intake and large bowel cancer incidence[59].

3.5.4.3 *Cancer and serum cholesterol* In a number of case control and prospective studies, low serum cholesterol has shown an association with increased risk of cancer. This has been attributed to the metabolic effects of pre-existing disease, because the associations are attenuated when the data were analysed to exclude individuals who were diagnosed as having cancer soon after their serum cholesterol was measured[60] (see 3.4.12). In addition, most of the studies were small so that the findings were shown only for lung cancer, which is the most common cancer, and which is primarily related to cigarette smoking, with inconsistent associations in the few patients who developed colon or breast cancer[61]. In the largest studies of more than 92,000 people in Sweden and California, serum cholesterol was either positively but weakly, or not at all related to large bowel cancer risk[62, 63].

3.5.4.4 *Prostatic cancer* shows a positive association internationally with total fat intake[43]. In addition there is a relation between fat intake and prostate cancer mortality between counties within the USA. There are some reports of higher fat intakes in patients with prostate cancer compared with controls[44].

3.5.5 *Dietary fat and aetiology of cancer* A number of mechanisms whereby fat could be involved in cancer promotion has been suggested[64]. Hormones, particularly oestrogens, are known to be important promoters of both animal and human breast cancer but there are conflicting reports on the effect of fat on circulating levels of oestrogen, other female sex hormone levels and sex hormone binding globulin[53]. Other suggested mechanisms include modulation of immune function and prostanoid synthetic pathways, and membrane lipid peroxidation[64]. In bowel cancer, it has been proposed that the concentration of faecal bile acids is increased by high fat diets and that secondary bile acids act as tumour promoters. However, individuals living in areas with a high risk of colon cancer do not have a higher faecal bile acid concentration or total faecal bile acid output compared with those living in areas with a low risk, neither do cases of large bowel cancer have higher faecal bile acid outputs or concentrations compared with controls[65]. Other factors modulating the solubility of free bile acids may be involved[66].

3.5.6 *Conclusions* The Panel concluded that there is currently insufficient evidence on which to base a recommendation for a decrease in fat intakes to prevent cancer, although an increase in consumption of any fatty acid should not be encouraged. The Panel agreed that the DRVs based on other considerations and presented in para 3.8 were consistent with a prudent view of the current data relating dietary fat and the occurrence of cancer.

3.6 **Obesity**

3.6.1 *Introduction* Obesity is a state of excess body fatness, and it is associated with an increased risk of non-insulin dependent diabetes, hypertension, atherosclerotic cardiovascular disease, endometrial cancer, gallstones and other conditions. Body fatness can be measured as the generally accepted, but imperfect, Body Mass Index (BMI: weight (kg)/height $(m)^2$), with a BMI between about 20 and 25 representing the normal range, and a BMI greater than about 30 being unequivocally recognized as obesity. A BMI between 25 and 30 may be described as overweight. The BMI takes no account of the distribution of body fat nor of muscularity. Central obesity may carry greater cardiovascular risks than peripheral obesity[67]. Obesity and the diseases related with it become more common with increasing age[68,69]. The risk of developing obesity-related diseases increases with the degree of fatness, although the relationship is not linear. Obesity tends to run in families, and both environmental and genetic factors play a part in who will become obese[69]. In Great Britain between 1980 and 1987 the proportion of adults with BMI in excess of 25 increased from 35 to 40 per cent, and of those with BMI in excess of 30 from 7 to 10 per cent[3].

3.6.2 *Energy Expenditure* On average, energy expenditure in obese subjects is greater than in non-obese controls[69,70]. Obese subjects not only have greater fat mass than non-obese subjects, but they also have a greater fat free mass (FFM). FFM is a major determinant of the resting metabolic rate, and therefore of total energy expenditure, and this explains the greater energy expenditure found in obese subjects[69]. Resting metabolic rate per unit of FFM is similar between obese subjects and non-obese controls[70]. Although much of the variance in resting metabolic rate between individuals can be accounted for by differences in FFM, there is also a significant familial component, at least in some populations[71]. In a prospective study initial resting metabolic rate per unit of FFM was lower in those individuals who subsequently gained weight than in those who did not, in spite of similar FFM between the two groups at baseline[72]. Normal levels of resting metabolic rate per unit of FFM were reached in the former group only when weight stabilised at a higher level. Control of energy expenditure is therefore a result of the interaction between genetic and environmental factors.

3.6.3 *Energy intake* Obesity can be the result of many years of daily energy imbalance accruing over time and the imbalance may only be slight. It is virtually impossible to obtain accurate data of food and nutrient intake over that time span and most data are derived from individuals or groups of individuals who have already become obese. Such data from dietary surveys have not always been accepted. Most workers have found that self-reported energy intake is lower than that which might be expected from objective measures of intake or energy expenditure[73,74]. There is evidence to support the view that obese individuals are especially likely to underrecord[75,76] although this has also not been found by all authors[74,77]. Almost all dietary surveys in Western countries find that total energy intake is highly correlated with total fat intake[77,78] and shows a negative correlation with BMI[78,79]. The explanation for this is not known, but is unlikely to be due simply to underrecording by obese individuals, as the correlation occurs throughout the whole range of BMI from lean to obese[79].

3.6.4 *Fat intake* With such uncertainty surrounding energy intake in obese individuals, it is not surprising that there are even fewer data relating the intakes of individual dietary components to obesity. There are no prospective data relating fat intake to subsequent development of obesity and no evidence that a high fat intake affects energy expenditure. In cross sectional studies total fat intake has been found to be both positively and negatively related to BMI[78,79]. There is evidence that the energy cost of fat deposition from dietary fat is less than from other dietary components, but this effect is very small[80]. However, meals containing predominantly carbohydrates stimulate carbohydrate oxidation whilst those containing mainly fat fail to promote fat oxidation, and favour fat storage [81,82]. As fat provides more calories per gram than other dietary constituents do, its addition to a food or diet necessarily increases the energy density. Low fat diets are usually bulkier than high fat diets for a given energy content, and this may have an effect in limiting energy intake. It has been shown that reducing the energy density of the diet results in a significant reduction in energy intake at least in the short term[83-85]. Whether this is related to the development of obesity remains unknown, but low fat diets are valuable in the management of established obesity[86].

3.6.5 *Conclusions* The Panel concluded that there was insufficient evidence either to establish or to exclude a special role for dietary fat in the development of obesity. Nevertheless, fat increases the energy density of diets, and is palatable. This may be conducive to increased food energy intake in some individuals with a genetic or behavioural predisposition. Dietary fat restriction is a valuable contribution to the management of established obesity.

3.7 **Diabetes mellitus**

3.7.1 *Introduction* Diabetes mellitus is a condition characterised by an elevated concentration of glucose in the blood because of inadequate secretion or impaired action of insulin. It also results in a number of other metabolic changes. There are two main types of diabetes in the UK. Insulin-dependent diabetes mellitus tends to arise in childhood or young adulthood and affects approximately 0.25–0.5 per cent of the population. Non-insulin dependent diabetes mellitus is more common and is often associated with obesity. Its prevalence increases with age and it may affect up to 30 per cent of individuals over 75 years of age. Diabetes mellitus is associated with the development of specific complications affecting the nerves, eyes and kidneys. In addition it is a powerful additional risk factor for cardiovascular disease which is the chief cause of death among diabetic subjects.

3.7.2 *Diet and diabetes* There is no suggestion that diet has any role to play in the genesis of insulin-dependent diabetes. Diet may be related to the development of non-insulin dependent diabetes insofar as obesity is a risk factor for it, but there is no evidence that dietary fat has any special role (see 3.6.5). In contrast dietary manipulation has always formed a cornerstone of the treatment of diabetes. Prior to the discovery of insulin in 1922 extreme carbohydrate restriction although largely ineffective was the only treatment available. Even 50 years after insulin treatment was introduced, carbohydrate restriction of some degree, usually to 40 per cent or less of dietary energy, was the basis of dietary recommendations for both main types of diabetes. In consequence, the energy content of the diabetic diet was maintained by increasing the proportion of fat, typically to 40–45 per cent of dietary energy. High fat diets, which in the UK are usually also high in saturated fatty acids, are associated with higher blood cholesterol concentrations, a risk factor for cardiovascular disease, to which diabetic subjects are particularly prone. For the last 15 years at least a reduction of fat, particularly of saturated fatty acids, has been recommended for the UK population to reduce the risk of cardiovascular disease[15]. More recently a diet high in complex carbohydrate and low in fat and saturated fatty acids has also been recommended for diabetic subjects[87].

3.7.3 *Metabolic aspects* Concentrations of total and low density lipoprotein (LDL) cholesterol in the blood are positively related to the development of cardiovascular disease[15]. Elevated concentrations of triglycerides may carry additional risks, particularly in diabetic subjects. Conversely, high density lipoprotein (HDL) concentration is inversely related to cardiovascular disease, and may be independently protective (see para 3.4.10). Diets high in complex carbohydrate and low in fat do not have a detrimental effect in diabetic control[88]. Nevertheless evidence that such diets are positively beneficial is less persuasive[89]. Very high carbohydrate diets (60 per cent of dietary energy or more) may increase blood triglyceride concentration and lower HDL concentration in diabetic people[90]. The qualitative effects of saturated and monounsaturated fatty acids appear to be similar in diabetic to non-diabetic subjects[91,92].

3.7.4 *Conclusions* The Panel concluded that there is no evidence for a direct effect of dietary fat on the development of either insulin-dependent or non-insulin-dependent diabetes mellitus. The Panel endorsed recent dietary recommendations that in diabetes fat should provide about 30–35 per cent of energy, with no more than about one third of that from saturated fatty acids.

3.8 **Dietary Reference Values for fat**

i. Saturated fatty acids should provide an average for the population of 10 per cent of total dietary energy (see 3.4.18).

ii. *Cis*-monounsaturated fatty acids (principally oleic acid) should continue to provide on average about 12 per cent of dietary energy for the population (see 3.4.18; 3.5.6).

iii. *Cis*-polyunsaturated fatty acids should continue to provide an average of 6 per cent of total dietary energy for the population and be derived from a mixture of n-6 and n-3 PUFA (see 3.4.18). For infants, children and adults linoleic acid should provide at least 1 per cent of total energy and alpha linolenic acid at least 0.2 per cent of total energy (see 3.1.6). Dietary intake of PUFAs by individuals should not exceed 10 per cent of total energy (see 3.2.4).

iv. *Trans* fatty acid intake in the population should not increase further than the current estimated average of 5 g/d or 2 per cent of dietary energy (see 3.3.9).

v. Total fat intake should be calculated from the sum of fatty acid intakes and glycerol (see 3.4.9) ie. Total fat = saturates + monounsaturates + polyunsaturates + *trans* + glycerol. An increase in consumption of any fatty acid should be avoided (see para 3.5.6).

vi. Total fatty acid intake should therefore average 30 per cent, and total fat intake ie including glycerol 33 per cent, of total dietary energy including alcohol or 35 per cent of energy derived from food (see Table 1.2).

3.9 **References**

[1] Crawford M A, Sinclair A J. Nutritional influences in the evolution of mammalian brain. In: Elliot T, Knight J, eds. *Lipids, Malnutrition and the Developing Brain*. Amsterdam: Elsevier, 1972; 267–292.

[2] ESPGAN Committee on Nutrition. Nutrition and feeding of preterm infants. *Acta Paed Scand* 1987; Supple 336.

[3] Gregory J, Foster K, Tyler H, Wiseman M. *The Dietary and Nutritional Survey of British Adults*. London: HMSO, 1990.

[4] Hansen A E, Knott E M, Wiese F, Shaperman E, McQuarrie I. Eczema and essential fatty acids. *Am J Dis Child* 1947; **73**: 1–18.

[5] Department of Health and Social Security. *Artificial Feeds for the Young Infant*. London: HMSO, 1988. (Reports on health and social subjects; 18).

[6] Food and Agriculture Organization. *Dietary Fats and Oils in Human Nutrition*. Rome: Food and Agriculture Organization, 1980. (FAO Food and Nutrition Series; 20).

[7] Dormandy T L. An approach to free radicals. *Lancet* 1983; **ii**: 1010–1014.

[8] Halliwell B, Gutteridge J M C. *Free Radicals in Biology and Medicine*. Oxford: Clarendon Press, 1985.

[9] Suthanthiran M, Solomon S D, Williams P S, Rubin A L, Novogrodsky A, Stenzel K H. Hydroxyl radical scavengers inhibit human natural killer cell activity. *Nature* 1984; **307**: 276–278.

[10] McBrien D C H, Slater T F. *Free Radicals, Lipid Peroxidation and Cancer*. London: Academic Press, 1982.

[11] Stringer M D, Gorog P G, Freeman A, Kakkar V V. Lipid peroxides and atherosclerosis. *Br Med J* 1989; **298**: 281–284.

[12] Thurnham D I. Antioxidants and prooxidants in malnourished populations. *Proc Nut Soc*. 1990; **45**: 247–259.

[13] Grankvist K, Marklund S, Taljedal I B. Superoxide dismutase is a prophylactic against alloxan diabetes. *Nature* 1981; **294**: 158–160.

[14] Diplock A T. Metabolic and functional defects in selenium deficiency. *Phil Trans Roy Biol Soc Lond* 1981; **294**: 105–117.

[15] Department of Health and Social Security. *Diet and Cardiovascular Disease*. London: HMSO, 1984. (Report on health and social subjects; 28).

[16] Federation of American Societies for Experimental Biology. *Health Aspects of Dietary Trans Fatty Acids*. Bethesda: FASEB, 1985.

[17] British Nutrition Foundation. *Report of the Task Force on Trans Fatty Acids*. London: British Nutrition Foundation, 1987.

[18] Ministry of Agriculture, Fisheries and Food. *Household Food Consumption and Expenditure; 1989*. London: HMSO, 1990.

[19] Christie W W. The composition, structure and function of lipids in the tissues of ruminant animals. In: Christie W, ed. *Lipid Metabolism in Ruminant Animals*. Oxford: Pergamon Press, 1981; 95–191.

[20] Lammi-Keefe C J, Jensen R G. Lipids in human milk a review: Composition and fat soluble vitamins. *J Pediatr Gastroenterol Nutr* 1984; **3**: 172–198.

[21] Emken E A. Nutrition and biochemistry of *trans* and positional fatty acid isomers in hydrogenated oils. *Ann Rev Nutr* 1984; **4**: 339–376.

[22] Van den Reek M M, Craig-Smith M C, Weete J, Clarke A J. Fat in the diets of adolescent girls with emphasis on isomeric fatty acids. *Am J Clin Nutr* 1986; **43**: 530–537.

[23] Kinsella J E, Bruchner G, Mai J, Shimp J. Metabolism of *trans* fatty acids with emphasis on the effects of *trans-trans* octadecadienoate on lipid composition, essential fatty acids and prostaglandins. An overview. *Am J Clin Nutr* 1981; **34**: 2307–2318.

[24] Mensink R P, Katan M B. Effect of dietary trans fatty acids on high-density and low-density lipoprotein cholesterol levels in healthy subjects. *New Engl J Med* 1990; **323**: 439–445.

[25] Enig M G, Munn R J, Keeney M. Dietary fat and cancer trends: a critique. *Fed Proc Am Soc Exp Biol* 1978; **37**: 2215–2220.

[26] Keys A. *Seven Countries: multivariate analysis of death and coronary heart disease*. Cambridge Mass: Harvard University Press, 1980.

[27] Shaper A G. *Coronary Heart Disease: Risks and Reasons*. London: Current Medical Literature Ltd, 1988.

[28] Hegsted D M, McGandy R B, Myers M L, Stare F J. Quantitative effects of dietary fat on serum cholesterol in man. *Am J Clin Nutr* 1965; **17**: 281–295.

[29] Ferro-Luzzi A, Sette S. The Mediterranean diet: an attempt to define its present and past composition. *Eur J Clin Nutr* 1989: 43 (suppl): 13–29.

[30] World Health Organization. *Prevention of Coronary Heart Disease*. Geneva: World Health Organisation, 1982. (WHO Technical Report Series; 678).

[31] Marckmann P, Sandstrom B, Jesperson J. Effects of total fat content and fatty acid composition in diet on factor VII coagulant activity and blood lipids. *Atherosclerosis* 1990; **80**: 227–233.

[32] Brett A S. Treating hypercholesterolemia. How should practising physicians interpret the published data for patients? *New Engl J Med* 1989; **321**: 676–680.

[33] Leaf A. Management of hypercholesterolemia. Are preventive interventions advisable? *New Engl J Med* 1989; **321**: 680–684.

[34] Henriksson P, Ericsson S, Stege R, Eriksson M, Rudling M, Berglund L, Angelin B. Hypocholesterolaemia and increased elimination of low-density lipoproteins in metastatic cancer of the prostate. *Lancet* 1989; **ii**: 1178–1180.

[35] Rose G, Shipley M. Effects of coronary risk reduction on the pattern of mortality. *Lancet* 1990, **335**: 275–277.

[36] Muldoon M F, Manuck S B, Matthews K A. Lowering cholesterol concentration and mortality: a quatitative review of primary prevention trials. *Br Med J* 1990; **301**: 309–314.

[37] Stamler J, Wentworth D, Neaton J D. Is relationship between serum cholesterol and risk of premature death from coronary heart disease continuous and graded? *J Am Med Ass* 1986; **256**: 2823–2828.

[38] Royal College of Physicians. *A Great and Growing Evil: the medical consequences of alcohol abuse*. London: Tavistock, 1987.

[39] Shepherd J, Betteridge D J, Durrington P *et al*. Strategies for reducing coronary heart disease and desirable limits for blood lipid concentrations: guidelines of the British Hyperlipidemia Association. *Br Med J* 1987; **295**: 1245–1246.

[40] National Cholesterol Education Program. *Report of the Expert Panel on Detection, Evaluation, and Treatment of High Blood Cholesterol in Adults*. Bethesda, Maryland: National Institutes of Health, 1989.

[41] Muir C, Waterhouse J, Mack T, Powell J, Whelan S. *Cancer Incidence in Five Continents*. Vol 5, Lyon: IARC, 1987 (Scientific Publication no 88).

[42] Parkin D M, Laara E, Muir C S. Estimates of the worldwide frequency of sixteen major cancers in 1980. *Int J Cancer* 1988; **41**: 184–197.

[43] Armstrong B, Doll R. Environmental factors and cancer incidence in different countries with special reference to dietary practices. *Int J Cancer* 1975; **15**: 617–631.

[44] National Research Council. *Diet, Nutrition and Cancer: National Academy of Sciences, Assembly of Life Sciences*. Washington D C: National Academy Press, 1982.

[45] Ip C. Fat and essential fatty acids in mammary carcinogenesis. *Am J Clin Nutr* 1987; **45** (suppl 1): 218–224.

[46] Albanes D. Total calories, body weight and tumor incidence in mice. *Cancer Res* 1987; **47**: 1987–1992.

[47] Beth M, Berger M R, Aksoy M, Schmähl D. Comparison between the effects of dietary fat level and of calorie intake on methylnitrosourea induced mammary carcinogenesis in female SD rats. *Int J Cancer* 1987; **39**: 737–744.

[48] Cohen L A, Choi K, Wang C. Influence of dietary fat, caloric restriction and voluntary exercise on N-Nitrosomethylurea-induced mammary tumorigenesis in rats. *Cancer Res* 1988; **48**: 4276–4283.

[49] Goodwin P J, Boyd N F. Critical appraisal of the evidence that dietary fat intakes are related to breast cancer risk in humans. *J Nat Cancer Inst* 1987; **79**: 473–485.

[50] Kinlen L J. Fat and breast cancer. *Cancer Surveys* 1987; **6**: 585–599.

[51] Kolonel L N. Fat and colon cancer: how firm is the epidemiologic evidence? *Am J Clin Nutr* 1987; **45**: 336–341.

[52] Willett W. The search for the causes of breast and colon cancer. *Nature* 1989; **338**: 389–394.

[53] Prentice R, Pepe M, Self S. Dietary fat and breast cancer. *Cancer Res* 1989; **49**: 3147–3156.

[54] Willett W C. Implications of total energy intake for epidemiology studies of breast and bowel cancer. *Am J Clin Nutr* 1987; **45** (suppl 1): 354–360.

[55] Herschopf R J, Bradlow H L. Obesity, diet, endogenous estrogens, and the risk of hormone-sensitive cancer. *Am J Clin Nutr* 1987; **45** (suppl 1): 283–298.

[56] Lew E A, Garfinkel L. Variations in mortality by weight among 750,000 men and women. *J Chron Dis* 1979; **32**: 563–576.

[57] Willett W C, Stampfer M J, Colditz G A *et al*. Relation of meat, fat and fibre intake to the risk of colon cancer in a prospective study among women. *New Engl J Med* 1990; **323**: 1664–1672.

[58] Giovannucci E, Meir J, Colditz G *et al*. Relation of diet to the risk of colorectal adenoma in men. *Am J Epidemiol* 1990; **132**: 783.

[59] Liu K, Stamler J, Moss D, Garside D, Persky V, Soltero I. Dietary cholesterol, fat and fibre and colon-cancer mortality. *Lancet* 1979; **ii**: 782–785.

[60] Broitman S A. Dietary cholesterol, serum cholesterol and colon cancer: a review. *Adv Exp Med Biol* 1988; **206**: 137–152.

[61] Isles C G, Hole J H, Gillis C R, Hawthorne V M, Lever A F. Plasma cholesterol, coronary heart disease and cancer in the Renfrew and Paisley survey. *Br Med J* 1989; **298**: 920–924.

[62] Tornberg S A, Holm L E, Cartensen J M, Eklund G. Risks of cancer of the colon and rectum in relation to serum cholesterol and beta lipoprotein. *New Engl J Med* 1986; **315**: 1629–1633.

[63] Klatsky A L, Armstrong M A, Friedman G, Hiatt R A. The relations of alcoholic beverage use to colon and rectal cancer. *Am J Epidemiol* 1988; **128**: 1007–1015.

[64] Welsch C W. Enhancement of mammary tumorigenesis by dietary fat: review of potential mechanisms. *Am J Clin Nutr* 1987; **45** (suppl 1): 192–202.

[65] Setchell K D R, Street J M, Sjovall J. Fecal bile acids. In: Setchell K *et al*, eds. *The Bile Acids: chemistry, physiology and metabolism*. New York: Plenum Press, 1987; 441–571.

[66] Bruce W R. Recent hypotheses for the origin of colon cancer. *Cancer Res* 1987; **47**: 4237–4242.

[67] Lapidus L, Bengtsson C, Larsson B, Pennert K, Rybo E, Sjostrom L. Distribution of adipose tissue and risk of cardiovascular disease and death; a 12 year follow up of participants in the population study of women in Gothenburg, Sweden. *Br Med J* 1984; **289**; 1257–1261.

[68] Knight I. *The Heights and Weights of Adults in Great Britain*. London: HMSO, 1984.

[69] Garrow J S. *Obesity and Related Diseases*. Edinburgh: Churchill Livingstone, 1988.

[70] Ravussin E, Bernard B, Schutz Y, Jecquier E. 24 hour energy expenditure and resting metabolic rate in obese, moderately obese and control subjects. *Am J Clin Nutr* 1982; **35**: 566–573.

[71] Bogardus C, Lillioja S, Ravussin E *et al*. Familial dependence of the resting metabolic rate. *New Engl J Med* 1986; **315**: 96–100.

[72] Ravussin E, Lillioja S, Knowler W C *et al.* Reduced rate of energy expenditure as a risk factor for body-weight gain. *New Engl J Med* 1988; **318**: 467–472.

[73] Livingstone M B E, Strain J J, Nevin G B, Barker M E, Hickey R J, McKenna P G. The use of weighed dietary records and the doubly-labelled ($^2H_3{}^{18}O$) water method method to compare energy intake and expenditure. *Proc Nutr Soc* 1989; **48**: 21A.

[74] Lissner L, Habicht J-P, Strupp B J, Levitsky D A, Haas J D, Roe D A. Body composition and energy intake; do overweight women overeat and underreport? *Am J Clin Nutr* 1989; **49**: 320–325.

[75] Steen B, Isaakson B, Svanborg A. Intake of energy and nutrients and meal habits in 70 year old males and females in Gothenberg, Sweden. A population study. *Acta Med Scand* 1977: **611** (Suppl): 39-86.

[76] Prentice A M, Black A E, Coward W A *et al.* High Levels of energy expenditure in obese women. *Br Med J* 1986; **292**: 983–978.

[77] Myers R J, Klesges R C, Eck L H, Hanson C L, Klem M L. Accuracy of self reports of food intake in obese and normal-weight individuals: effects of obesity on self-reports of dietary intake in adult females. *Am J Clin Nutr* 1988; **48**: 1248–1251.

[78] Romieu I, Willett W C, Stampfer M J *et al.* Energy intake and other determinants of relative weight. *Am J Clin Nutr* 1988: **47**: 406–412.

[79] Keen H, Thomas B J, Jarrett R J, Fuller J H. Nutrient intake, adiposity and diabetes. *Br Med J* 1979; **1**: 655–658.

[80] James W P T. Dietary aspects of obesity. *Postgrad Med J* 1984; **60** (Suppl 3): 50–55.

[81] Flatt J P, Ravussin E, Acheson K J, Jequier E. Effects of dietary fat on post-prandial substrate oxidation and on carbohydrate and fat balances. *J Clin Invest* 1985; **76**: 1019–1024.

[82] Shutz Y, Flatt J P, Jequier E. Failure of dietary fat to promote fat oxidation: a factor favouring the development of obesity. *Am J Clin Nutr* 1989; **50**: 307–314.

[83] Porikos K P, Hesser M F, Van Itallie T B. Caloric regulation in normal weight men maintained on a palatable diet of conventional foods. *Physiol Behav* 1982; **29**: 293–300.

[84] Porikos K P, Booth G, Van Itallie T B. Effect of covert nutritive dilution on the spontaneous food intake of obese individuals: a pilot study. *Am J Clin Nutr* 1977; **30**: 1638–1644.

[85] Lissner L, Levitsky D A, Strupp B J, Kalkwarf H J, Roe D A. Dietary fat and the regulation of energy intake in human subjects. *Am J Clin Nutr* 1987; **46**: 886–892.

[86] Royal College of Physicians. *Obesity: A Report of the Royal College of Physicians. J Roy Coll Phys* 1983, **17**.

[87] European Association for the Study of Diabetes—Diabetes and Nutrition Study Group. Nutritional recommendations for individuals with diabetes mellitus. *Diab Nutr Metab* 1988; **1**: 145–149.

[88] Simpson R W, Mann J I, Eaton J, Moore R A, Carter R, Hockaday T D R. Improved glucose control in maturity-onset diabetes treated with high-carbohydrate-modified-fat diet. *Br Med J* 1979; vol **1**: 1753–1756.

[89] Reaven G M. Dietary therapy for non-insulin-dependent diabetes mellitus. *New Engl J Med* 1988; **319**: 862–864.

[90] Coulston A M, Hollenbeck C B, Swislocki A L M, Reaven G M. Persistence of hypertriglyceridemic effect of low-fat high-carbohydrate diets in NIDDM patients. *Diabetes Care* 1989; **12**: 94–101.

[91] Garg A, Bonanome A, Grundy S M, Zhang Z, Unger R H. Comparison of a high-carbohydrate diet with a high-monounsaturated-fat diet in patients with non-insulin-dependent diabetes mellitus. *New Engl J Med* 1988; **319**: 829–834.

[92] Bierman E L, Brunzell J D. Diet low in saturated fat and cholesterol for diabetes. *Diabetes Care* 1989; **12**: 162–163.

4. Non-starch Polysaccharides

4.1 **Introduction** In considering the nutritional role of what is known as "dietary fibre" the Panel was hindered in making a sound scientific assessment of the literature because of imprecision in its terminology. Over the years a variety both of definitions and of analytical techniques has been used which are not necessarily comparable. The Panel supported the proposition by others that the term "dietary fibre" should become obsolete[1] and decided for reasons given below, that specific evidence in relation to dietary non-starch polysaccharides (NSP) would be reviewed. NSP are the major fraction of "dietary fibre" whatever definition is used, are chemically identifiable and can be measured with reasonable precision. Where possible the physical properties of NSP have also been taken into account.

4.2 **Definition and Analysis**

4.2.1 The term "dietary fibre" lacks a precise definition and has been interpreted in many ways. Trowell defined it as "the plant polysaccharides and lignin which are resistant to hydrolysis by the digestive enzymes of man"[2], but although this definition represented an important conceptual advance in nutrition, it posed an impossible task for the analyst because the fraction of the diet which escapes digestion in the small bowel varies from individual to individual and includes many things other than cell wall and related polysaccharides. For example it has now become clear from experiments in man that quantitatively more starches than non-starch polysaccharides resist digestion in many foods[3]. NSP are the major component of the plant cell wall and the best single index of the "dietary fibre" concept[4,5].

4.2.2 Lignin is also a component of the plant cell wall traditionally included in "dietary fibre", but it is chemically different from the cell wall polysaccharides and in terms of the human diet is a minor component. Most analyses for lignin give gross overestimates of the amounts present.

4.2.3 The methods developed for the measurement of "dietary fibre" in food can broadly be divided into enzymatic-gravimetric and enzymatic-chemical methods. Enzymatic-gravimetric methods attempt to isolate a fraction of the diet which resists digestion in the human upper intestine[6–8], but actually measure an unspecified fraction of the diet which includes a variety of components. Furthermore gravimetric methods give no details of polysaccharide type or composition and currently do not allow subdivision into soluble and insoluble fractions.

4.2.4 Enzymatic chemical methods identify a chemically defined fraction of the diet ie non-starch polysaccharides[9–11]. Non-starch polysaccharides are a

Table 4.1 *Non-Starch Polysaccharides* (non alpha-glucan polysaccharides)

Class	Description	Solubility at pH 7.0	Monomers	Occurrence
CELLULOSE	Unbranched Beta 1–4 Glucan	Insoluble	Glucose	Very widely distributed especially leafy vegetables, peas, beans and rhubarb
NON-CELLULOSIC POLYSACCHARIDES	DIVERSE MIXTURE:			
	Pectins	Soluble	Galacturonic acid	Mainly fruit and vegetables
	Glucans	Soluble	Glucose	Oats, barley, rye
	Arabinogalactans, arabinoxylans	Partly soluble	Arabinose, xylose, galactose, glucose	Wheat, rye, barley
	Gums: gum arabic	Soluble	Galactose	Plant gums used as food additives
	sterculia	Soluble	Rhamnose, galactose, arabinose	
	Mucilages: ispaghula	Soluble	Arabinose, xylose	Seed mucilage of *Plantago ovata.*
	Storage: inulin guar	Soluble	Fructose	Jerusalem artichokes; to a lesser extent in other root vegetables
		Soluble	Galactose, mannose	As food additives mainly
	Fungal: chitin	Insoluble	Amino sugars	Mushrooms and other fungi, exoskeletons of crustacea eg shrimps and prawns

complex group of polymers which can be sub-divided in various ways (Table 4.1). Individual classes can be characterised with reference to the composition of the constituent sugars and uronic acids that make up these polymers. The Englyst technique has been the subject of four collaborative trials organised by the Ministry of Agriculture, Fisheries and Food (MAFF)[12-15] and can be modified to classify NSP into insoluble and soluble fractions. It has been recommended for food labelling purposes in the UK. The Panel therefore recommended that "dietary fibre" be defined for labelling purposes as NSP where this refers to non-alpha glucans as measured by the technique of Englyst and Cummings[11] or other comparable techniques. However, a number of NSP such as inulin, polydextrose and pyrodextrins are present in the diet, or are added to it in small amounts, but are not components of the plant cell wall and are not measured by any of the commonly used methods for determining dietary fibre. Foods containing these substances will need additional analyses to gain a complete estimate of their NSP content, though the number of such foods is limited.

4.3 Sources and intakes of NSP

4.3.1 Tables giving the detailed NSP composition of UK foods are available[16-20]. Detailed analysis of the composition of NSP in fruit, vegetables and cereals reveals major differences in the chemical identity of the various polysaccharides (Table 4.1). Cereals, especially whole grain foods, are a rich source of NSP. In wheat, maize and rice NSP is mainly insoluble, but in oats, barley and rye a significant proportion is soluble. Vegetables, containing more moisture than cereals, have a lower total NSP than whole grain cereals and different overall composition. Soluble and insoluble fractions are approximately equal. The proportion of cellulose is 30–40 per cent of NSP and is even greater in swede, broad beans and turnips. In fruit the ratio of soluble to insoluble varies widely with uronic acids the main contributor to soluble.

4.3.2 Few data exist on NSP intake in the UK or other world populations (see Table 4.2). Intakes of NSP in the UK are between 11 and 13 g/d with a range for other developed countries of between 10 and 18 g/d. In Britain 50 per cent of NSP is provided by vegetables and 40 per cent by cereals. 40–50 per cent of total NSP is soluble. Individual intakes appear to range from an average of 5 to 25 g/d (Table 4.2), but more information on the distribution of intakes of NSP between the various age and sex population groups is needed.

4.4 Appetite, satiety and energy intake

4.4.1 NSP-rich foods are generally less energy dense, more bulky, and may induce greater satiety than NSP-free foods[1]. It has been proposed that cell wall polysaccharides may be a barrier to consumption of energy and useful in the prevention and treatment of obesity. In single meal studies, with apples and oranges, it has been shown that removing NSP reduces satiety and increases post-prandial glucose and insulin levels. Studies of free choice high and low NSP diets have not provided consistent results. When isolated polysaccharides such as guar gum are added to controlled diets there is evidence of an effect on appetite but longer-term studies show that adaptation takes place. However, the amount of NSP in a diet is characteristic of a type of diet rather than a

Table 4.2 *Non starch polysaccharide intake (g/d)*

Country	Total	sd	Range	Soluble	Insoluble	Cellulose	Hexoses	Pentoses	Uronic acids	From cereals	From vegetables
Rural Finland[21]	18.4	7.8	—	—	—	4.2	5.3	7.4	1.9	—	—
Rural Denmark[21]	18.0	6.4	—	—	—	3.7	5.5	6.6	2.2	—	—
Helsinki[21]	14.5	5.4	—	—	—	3.4	3.7	5.5	2.0	—	—
Copenhagen[21]	13.2	4.8	—	—	—	3.2	3.6	4.5	1.9	—	—
UK—National Food Survey[22]	12.4	—	—	—	—	2.6	3.4	4.5	1.8	—	—
UK—Men[23]	11.2	3.5	5–19	5.2	6.1	3.1	2.2	4.0	1.7	4.4	5.6
UK—Women[23]	12.5	4.1	7–25	5.4	7.2	3.3	2.2	4.8	2.0		
Japan[24]	10.9	—	—	4.1	6.8	3.0	2.9	1.8	3.1	—	—

specific nutrient to affect appetite. Low NSP diets tend to be high in fat and sugar and it is difficult to ascribe to NSP *per se* an effect on food intake in humans.

4.4.2 NSP fermented in the large bowel are an energy source. In order to estimate the potential contribution of energy from dietary NSP the extent to which degradation occurs and the amount of short chain fatty acids produced from fermentation need to be known. Although there is some gain in energy from the fermentation of NSP, diets rich in NSP are associated with a lower apparent digestibility of fat and protein[1] and therefore of energy. At current intakes, this net gain from NSP is similar to the apparent loss from lower digestibility of fat and protein. Animal evidence suggests that the energy from short chain fatty acids may not lead to the deposition of body fat with the same efficacy as carbohydrate.

4.5 The large intestine

4.5.1 In population studies "dietary fibre" intakes have been related to the prevalence of diverticular disease, appendicitis, large bowel cancer, haemorrhoids and constipation[2]. However there are many confounding factors in the interpretation of these data, both in diet and in lifestyle. In the diet particularly, the nature and amount of starch has been virtually ignored, as has the fact that high NSP diets are usually low in fat and animal protein. Furthermore few reports are supported by measurements using modern methodology for dietary assessment or reliable analysis of the NSP content of foods eaten. It is clear that in some populations, such as the Japanese or urban South African blacks, low NSP intakes are not associated with high risk of large bowel diseases. Nevertheless no study has reported an association between high NSP and high risk of large bowel disease. It is not currently possible to identify NSP as a major dietary factor in the aetiology of these diseases. At best the aetiology may be ascribed to the consumption of a type of diet characterised by low starch, low NSP, high fat. Better epidemiological studies are needed.

4.5.2 In experimental studies in man cell wall material, measured by a variety of techniques, has been shown to have major effects on large bowel function. Dietary NSP escape digestion in the human stomach and small intestine[25]. Most forms of dietary NSP are fermented by the anaerobic flora of the large intestine to short chain fatty acids, carbon dioxide, hydrogen and methane, and stimulate bacterial growth. Most, if not all, aspects of large bowel function are affected by fermentation, for which dietary NSP is an important substrate[26].

4.5.3 The laxative effect of NSP has been well documented in many studies[27]. These include trials of purified sources of NSP such as ispaghula and cellulose, preparations containing concentrated NSP in brans, and diets rich in NSP-containing foods. In experimental studies of healthy people there is a simple linear relation between NSP intake and daily stool weight over a range of intakes from 4–32 g/d, other factors being constant. On NSP-free diets stool weights fall to 30–60 g/d and people may complain of constipation.

4.5.4 There is considerable variation in the response of bowel habit to NSP intakes, partly because not all sources of NSP increase stool weight to the same extent. In general insoluble forms of NSP, such as those found in cereal foods, are more effective than the more soluble types found in fruit and vegetables[28]. The response to NSP is also moderated by factors affecting large bowel function such as transit time, hormones and stress. Stool weight is inversely related to transit time up to a daily stool output of about 150 g/d. Above this there is little further decrease in transit time as stool weight increases[29]. These effects on bowel habit are probably not unique to NSP. It is not known to what extent these other dietary components such as certain starches can compensate for a total lack of NSP in the diet in terms of bowel habit.

4.5.5 The Panel considered the question of what constituted a healthy bowel habit, and whether there were any potential risks to health of a low stool output. There are no prospective data and only few temporal correlation studies relating bowel habit to morbidity or mortality. Despite this it has been suggested that the amount of stool passed, and in relation to it the frequency of defaecation and transit time, have a bearing on health, especially bowel disease. In the UK median stool weight is about 100 g/d. 95 per cent of the adult population passes between 30 and 260 g/d, 46 per cent less than 100 g/d, and 18 per cent less than 50 g/d[30]. On average women have lower stool weights than men. Constipation is a common symptom which impairs the quality of life of about 20 per cent of people aged over 65 years and around 10 per cent of the adult population[31-33]. It is commoner in women. Constipation is characterised by infrequent bowel habit (less than three times a week), transit time of five days or more and stool weight below 50 g/d (though in healthy volunteers complaints of constipation become common when stool weights fall below 100 g/d). In epidemiological studies stool weights below 150 g/d are associated with increased risks of bowel cancer[29,30,34], and diverticular disease[35]. Constipation and slow transit tend to coexist and are associated with increased levels of deoxycholic acid in bile, a risk factor for gallstones[36]. Experimentally deoxycholic acid levels can be reduced by shortening transit time.

4.6 **Carbohydrate metabolism and insulin** The effect of dietary NSP on carbohydrate metabolism is difficult to study because in altering the amount of NSP in the diet other components which may affect carbohydrate metabolism are often changed as well. Overall single meal experiments with gel-forming polysaccharides show lowering of blood glucose and insulin in both healthy and diabetic subjects[37]. However the amount of these polysaccharides that are needed are far outside the range usually found in UK diets. Long-term studies show less clearly beneficial effects of NSP, particularly in healthy people[38,39]. Epidemiological observations and trials of high NSP diets in diabetic subjects are confounded by many factors. Any role for decreased dietary NSP in the aetiology of non-insulin dependent diabetes mellitus remains to be established. Further studies on the mechanism of action of NSP on intermediary metabolism in diabetes are required. In the light of the evidence the Panel concluded that there was no sound basis for proposing reference values of NSP in the diet to moderate glucose and insulin metabolism.

4.7 **Plasma lipids and cardiovascular disease**

4.7.1 Although international studies show a high correlation between saturated fatty acid intake and CHD mortality, these studies are confounded by the inverse relationship between dietary fat and total carbohydrate, and the interaction between total carbohydrate and NSP. It has been suggested that in some populations low NSP intakes may contribute to the high rate of CHD. Four cohort studies have reported an inverse relationship between "dietary fibre" intake and CHD mortality. In two this relationship did not hold when "fibre" intake was expressed per 1,000 kcal[40–43].

4.7.2 In short term experimental studies isolated forms of NSP such as guar and pectin lower blood cholesterol[44,45]. Oats and beans, which are good sources of soluble NSP, also lower blood cholesterol, but this may be in part due to other constituents and associated dietary changes[46]. Oats and beans lower LDL cholesterol more than HDL cholesterol so that the HDL:LDL ratio is raised. Dietary NSP do not appear to affect serum levels of triglyceride or very low density lipoprotein. Wheat bran and most other insoluble forms of NSP so far tested do not affect serum cholesterol levels[47].

4.7.3 In cross sectional surveys there is a weak inverse association between blood pressure and cereal "fibre" intake independent of energy intake. This may be confounded by other aspects of health such as physical fitness and body weight. Randomised trials of cereal NSP supplements have failed to show any effect on blood pressure although none has been large enough to detect an effect as modest as that seen in observational studies.

4.7.4 *Conclusion* NSP is not the major dietary determinant of blood lipid patterns and may be acting as a marker of particular dietary habits. The Panel concluded that present evidence suggested that the benefits are from diets characterised by high NSP rather than only from NSP itself.

4.8 **Adverse effects of NSP** Even before "dietary fibre" was first proposed as a beneficial constituent of foods, potential adverse effects for wheat bran had been postulated. *In vitro* studies show that plant cell wall material acts as a cation exchanger and can bind divalent cations such as calcium, iron, copper and zinc[48]. Binding may be related to uronic acid residues of NSP[49], or to associated phytate[50]. *In vivo* studies in humans do not, on balance, show a significant reduction in mineral bioavailability except where phytate (or oxalate) is also high[51,52]. Furthermore, populations which habitually consume high NSP diets are not characterised by compromised mineral status. Interpretation of these studies is hampered by the lack of conformity in definition, study design and analytical techniques[53]. Any direct adverse effects of high NSP diets are therefore more likely to be seen in those members of the population whose diet is marginal with respect to mineral content, in particular the elderly, and in these cases care should be taken not to rely on phytate-rich sources. Indirect effects—ie the displacement of other nutrients from the diet—may be seen particularly in growing children. The Panel considered that neither the levels of NSP intake current in the UK, nor those proposed below, produce adverse effects on mineral status in adults. NSP should be derived from a variety of foods whose constituents contain it as a naturally integrated component, rather than as isolated supplements or as products enriched with NSP.

4.9 **Dietary Reference Values**

4.9.1 In the light of the above observations the Panel felt that there was a basis for DRVs for non-starch polysaccharide in the UK diet. Quantitatively the best evidence relates to bowel habit. Other factors may influence bowel habit, both dietary (such as resistant starches [see 8.4.3]) and non dietary, but NSP is usually the most effective. Stool weights of less than 100 g/d are associated with increased risk of bowel disease. These occur at NSP intakes below 12 g/d, which therefore should be the lower end of the reference range. NSP intakes of above 32 g/d have not been shown to increase stool weight further and are not found in populations so far studied. An increase in average dietary NSP intake from the current level of 13 to 18 g/day would be expected to increase average stool weight by 25 per cent. If the distribution of intakes remains unaltered, this would reduce the number of individuals with stool weights of 100 g/day or less. The Panel proposed that adult diets should contain an average for the population of 18 g/d (individual range 12–24 g/d) non-starch polysaccharide from a variety of foods whose constituents contain it as a naturally integrated component.

4.9.2 This recommendation is based on data from adults and is not applicable to children. There are no data on physiological effects of NSP in children. However it is likely that such effects are related to body size, and the Panel recommended that children should have proportionately lower NSP intakes. Children of less than two years should not take such foods at the expense of more energy-rich foods which they require for adequate growth.

4.9.3 The Panel made no specific recommendations for sub-groups of the adult population defined either by age or by sex. However people who have a tendency to constipation are particularly encouraged to increase their NSP intake especially from whole grain cereal sources.

4.9.4 *Guidance on high intakes* In view of the lack of evidence for benefit of intakes of NSP in excess of 32 g daily, the Panel saw no advantage in exceeding this level. Furthermore such intakes are not seen in self-selected diets and potentially undesirable effects cannot be excluded. Caution in the use of sources of NSP containing phytate (particularly unprocessed wheat bran) is advised, especially in elderly people.

4.10 **References**

[1] British Nutrition Foundation. *Complex Carbohydrates in Foods*. London: Chapman and Hall, 1990.

[2] Trowell H, Burkitt D, Heaton K, eds. *Dietary Fibre, Fibre-Depleted Foods and Disease*. London: Academic Press, 1985.

[3] Englyst H N, Cummings J H. Resistant starch, a 'new' food component: a classification of starch for nutritional purposes. In: Morton I, ed. *Cereals in a European Context*. Chichester: Ellis Horwood Ltd, 1987; 221–233.

[4] James W P T, Theander O. *The Analysis of Dietary Fiber in Food.* New York: Marcel Dekker, 1988.

[5] Englyst H N, Cummings J H. Non-starch polysaccharides (dietary fiber) and resistant starch. In: Furda I, Brine C, eds. *New Developments in Dietary Fiber. Physiological, Physiochemical and Analytical Aspects.* Advances in Experimental Medicine and Biology, 1990; **270:** 205–225.

[6] Asp A G, Johansson C G, Hallmer H, Siljestrom M. Rapid enzymatic assay of insoluble and soluble dietary fibre. *J Agric Food Chem* 1983; **31**: 476–482.

[7] Prosky L, Asp N G, Furda I, DeVries J W, Schweizer T F, Harland B F. Determination of total dietary fiber in foods and food products: collaborative study. *J Ass Off Anal Chem* 1985; **68**: 677–679.

[8] Prosky L, Asp N G, Schweizer T F, Devries J W, Furda I. Determination of insoluble, soluble and total dietary fiber in foods and food products: interlaboratory study. *J Ass Off Anal Chem* 1988; **71**: 1017–1023.

[9] Southgate D A T. Determination of carbohydrates in foods. II. Unavailable carbohydrates. *J Sci Food Agric* 1969; **20**: 331–335.

[10] Theander O, Aman P. Studies on dietary fibres. I Analysis and chemical characterization on water-soluble and water-insoluble dietary fibres. *Swed J Agric Res* 1979; **9**: 97–106.

[11] Englyst H N, Cummings J H. Improved method for measurement of dietary fiber as non-starch polysaccharides in plant foods. *J Ass Off Anal Chem* 1988; **71**: 808–814.

[12] Cummings J H, Englyst H N, Wood R. Determination of dietary fibre in cereals and cereal products—collaborative trials. Part I: Initial trial. *J Ass Off Anal Chem* 1985; **23**: 1–35.

[13] Englyst H N, Cummings J H, Wood R. Determination of dietary fibre in cereals and cereal products—collaborative trials. Part II: Studies of a modified Englyst procedure. *J Ass Publ Analysts* 1987a; **25**: 59–71.

[14] Englyst H N, Cummings J H, Wood R. Determination of dietary fibre in cereals and cereal products. Part III: Study of further simplified procedures. *J Ass Publ Analysts* 1987b; **25**: 73–110.

[15] Englyst H N, Hudson G J. Colorimetric method for routine measurement of dietary fibre as non-starch polysaccharides. A comparison with gas-liquid chromatography. *Food Chem* 1987; **24**: 63–76.

[16] Holland B, Unwin I D, Buss D H. *Cereals and Cereal Products.* Third Supplement to McCance and Widdowson's *The Composition of Foods.* Cambridge: The Royal Society of Chemistry, 1988.

[17] Holland B, Unwin I D, Buss D H. *Milk Products and Eggs.* Fourth Supplement to McCance and Widdowson's *The Composition of Foods.* Cambridge: The Royal Society of Chemistry, 1988.

[18] Englyst H N, Bingham S A, Runswick S A, Collinson E, Cummings J H. Dietary fibre (non-starch polysaccharides) in fruit, vegetables and nuts. *J Hum Nutr Dietet* 1988; **1**: 247–286.

[19] Englyst H N, Bingham S A, Runswick S A, Collinson E, Cummings J H. Dietary fibre (non-starch polysaccharides) in cereal products. *J Hum Nutr Dietet* 1989; **2**: 253–271.

[20] Holland B, Unwin I D, Buss D H. *Vegetables, Herbs and Spices.* Fifth Supplement to McCance and Widdowson's *The Composition of Foods.* Cambridge: The Royal Society of Chemistry, 1988.

[21] IARC. Report of the Second IARC Coordinated International Study on Diet and Large Bowel Cancer in Denmark and Finland. *Nutrition and Cancer* 1982; **4**: 3–79.

[22] Bingham S A, Williams D R R, Cummings J H. Dietary fibre consumption: new estimates and their relation to large bowel cancer mortality in Britain. *Br J Cancer* 1985; **52**: 399–402.

[23] Bingham S A, Pett S, Day K C. Non-starch polysaccharide intake of a representative sample of British adults. *J Hum Nutr Dietet* 1990; **3**: 333–337.

[24] Kuratsune M, Honda T, Englyst H N, Cummings J H. Dietary fiber in the Japanese diet as investigated in connection with colon cancer risk. *Jpn J Cancer Res* 1986; **77**: 736–738.

[25] Cummings J H, Englyst H N. Fermentation in the human large intestine and the available substrates. *Am J Clin Nutr* 1987; **45**: 1243–1255.

[26] MacFarlane G T, Cummings J H. The colonic flora, fermentation and large bowel digestive function. In: Phillips S *et al*, eds. *The large Intestine: Physiology, Pathophysiology and Diseases*. New York: Raven Press, 1991; (in press).

[27] Cummings J H. The effect of dietary fiber on fecal weight and composition. In: Spiller G, ed. *CRC Handbook of Dietary Fiber in Human Nutrition*. Boca Raton, Florida: C R C Press Inc. 1986; 211–280.

[28] Cummings J H, Southgate D A T, Branch W *et al*. The colonic response to dietary fibre from carrot, cabbage, apple, bran and guar gum. *Lancet* 1978; **1**: 5–8.

[29] Burkitt D P, Walker A R P, Painter N S. Effect of dietary fibre on stools and transit times, and its role in the causation of disease. *Lancet* 1972; **ii**: 1408–1412.

[30] Cummings J H, Bingham S A. Quantitative estimates of bowel habit, bowel disease risk and the role of diet. (Personal Communcation).

[31] Connell A M, Hilton C, Irvine G, Lennard-Jones J E, Misiewicz J J. Variation in bowel habit in two population samples. *Br Med J* 1965; **2**: 1095–1099.

[32] Thompson W G, Heaton K W. Functional bowel disorders in apparently healthy people. *Gastroenterology* 1980; **79**: 283–288.

[33] Royal College of General Practitioners. *Morbidity Statistics from General Practice—Third National Study*. **1981–1982.** London: HMSO, 1986. (Series MB5 No.1).

[34] Cummings J H, Branch W J, Bjerrum L, Paerregard A, Helms P, Burton R. Colon cancer and large bowel function in Denmark and Finland. *Nutrition and Cancer* 1982; **4**: 61–66.

[35] Findlay J M, Smith A N, Mitchell W D, Anderson A J B, Eastwood M A. Effects of unprocessed bran on colon function in normal subjects and in diverticular disease. *Lancet* 1974; **i**: 146–149.

[36] Marcus S N, Heaton K W. Intestinal transit, deoxycholic acid and the cholesterol saturation of bile—three inter-related factors. *Gut* 1986; **27**: 550–558.

[37] Jenkins D J A. Carbohydrates: dietary fiber. In: Shils M, Young V, eds. *Modern Nutrition in Health and Disease*. 7th Edn. Philadelphia: Lea and Febiger, 1988; 52–71.

[38] Goulder T J, Alberti K G, Jenkins D J A. Effect of added fiber on the glucose and metabolic response to a mixed meal in normal and diabetic subjects. *Diabetes Care* 1978; **1**: 351–355.

[39] Vinik A I, Jenkins D J A. Dietary fibre in management of diabetes. *Diabetes Care* 1988; **11**: 160–173.

[40] Morris J N, Marr J W, Clayton D G. Diet and Heart: a postscript. *Br Med J* 1977; **2**: 1307–1314.

[41] Yano K, Rhoads G K, Kagan A, Tillotson J. Dietary intake and the risk of coronary heart disease in Japanese men living in Hawaii. *Am J Clin Nutr* 1978; **31**: 1270–1279.

[42] Kromhout D, Bosschieter E B, Coulander C L. Dietary fibre and 10-year mortality from coronary heart-disease, cancer and all causes. The Zutphen Study. *Lancet* 1982; **ii**: 508–521.

[43] Kushi L H, Lew R A, Stare F J *et al*. Diet and 20-year mortality from coronary heart disease. The Ireland—Boston Diet—Heart Study. *New Engl J Med* 1985; **312**: 811–818.

[44] Jenkins D J A, Rainey-Macdonald C G, Jenkins A L, Benn G. Fibre in the treatment of hyperlipidemia. In: Spiller G, ed. *CRC Handbook of Dietary Fibre in Human Nutrition*. Boca Raton, Florida: CRC Press Inc, 1986; 327–344.

[45] Anderson J W, Deakins D A, Bridges S R. Soluble fibre; hypocholesterolemic effects and proposed mechanisms. In: Kritchevsky D *et al*, eds. *Dietary Fiber—Chemistry, Physiology and Health Effects* New York: Plenum Press, 1990; 339–347.

[46] Swain J F, Rouse I L, Curley C B, Sacks F M. Comparison of the effects of oat bran and low-fibre wheat on serum lipoprotein levels and blood pressure. *New Engl J Med* 1990; **322**: 147–152.

[47] Judd P A, Truswell A S. Dietary fibre and blood lipids in man. In: Leeds A, Avenell A, eds. *Dietary Fibre Perspectives: Reviews and Bibliography*. London: John Libbey, 1985; 23–39.

[48] Eastwood M A, Mitchell W D. Physical properties of fiber: a biological evaluation. In: Spiller G, Amen R. eds. *Fibre in Human Nutrition*. New York: Plenum Press, 1976; 109–129.

[49] James W P T, Branch W J, Southgate D A T. Calcium binding by dietary fibre. *Lancet* 1978; i: 638–639.

[50] Davies N T. The effects of dietary fibre on mineral availability. In: Heaton K, ed. *Dietary Fibre, Current Developments of Importance to Health*. London: Newman Publishing, 1978; 113–121.

[51] Kelsay J L. A review of research on effects of fiber intake on man. *Am J Clin Nutr* 1978; **31**: 142–159.

[52] Kelsay J L. Update on fibre and mineral availability. In: Vahouny G, Kritchevsky D, eds. *Dietary Fibre: Basic and Clinical Aspects*. New York: Plenum Press, 1986; 361–372.

[53] Gordon D T. Total dietary fiber and mineral absorbtion. In: Kritchevsky C *et al*, eds. *Dietary Fiber—Chemistry, Physiology and Health Effects*. New York: Plenum Press, 1990; 105–128.

5. Sugars

5.1 **Introduction** Sugars are soluble carbohydrates of fundamental importance in providing energy for the maintenance of life. Glucose, the most abundant sugar in nature, is a single sugar unit or monosaccharide, as are fructose and galactose. Sucrose, lactose, and maltose are disaccharides. Sucrose, the sugar most widely used as a food in the United Kingdom[1], is composed of glucose and fructose. Disaccharides are broken down in the intestine and absorbed as monosaccharides. The role of dietary sugars in human disease has recently been reviewed by COMA[1]. In their Report, sugars were classified on the basis of their availability for metabolism into *intrinsic* and *extrinsic* sugars (see 5.5). Intrinsic sugars are those naturally incorporated into the cellular structure of foods. Extrinsic sugars are those not so incorporated, whether natural and unprocessed, such as honey, or refined, such as table sugar. Extrinsic sugars in milk and milk products were deemed to be a special case, resulting in a sub-group of *non-milk extrinsic* sugars. The Panel endorsed the conclusions in that Report concluded that non-milk extrinsic sugars were a major cause of dental caries in the UK, and that their consumption by the population should be decreased.

5.2 **Metabolism of glucose** Glucose is distributed to the tissues as a fuel for many chemical processes. If there is insufficient dietary carbohydrate to meet this requirement, the liver releases glucose from stored glycogen or converts certain amino acids, lactate and glycerol into glucose. The brain and nervous system and red blood cells have an obligatory requirement for glucose as an energy source. If the diet is very low in carbohydrate, ketoacids formed in the liver from fatty acids may accumulate. Some dietary carbohydrate is therefore necessary to avoid ketoacidosis, but there is no specific dietary requirement for sugars.

5.3 **Current sugars consumption** Data on supplies of sugars in the UK come from the national food supply statistics of the Ministry of Agriculture, Fisheries and Food (MAFF). In 1987 sucrose, at 104 g/person/d, provided 14 per cent of food energy, honey and glucose at 16 g/person/d provided 2 per cent, and lactose, at 23 g/person/d, a further 3 per cent[2]. The National Food Survey provides data on domestic food purchases. Sucrose purchased as packet sugar was on average 26 g/person/d in 1989. Total sugars, at 95 g/person/d, contributed 18 per cent of food energy[3]. Surveys of individual food intakes give data on the variation of sugars intakes in individuals. Breast- or bottle-fed infants obtain 40 per cent of their energy from sugars (usually lactose). Pre-school children take 25–30 per cent of food energy as sugars. Older children and adults tend to take less sugars (17–25 per cent)[1]. In the recent representative dietary and nutritional survey of British adults, total sugars provided 18 per cent of energy[4]. Non-milk extrinsic sugars usually provide at least half of the intake of total sugars (45–73 per cent).

5.4 **Effects of sugars** In addition to chemical differences between sugars, physiological effects depend on the physical presentation of the sugars—whether free in solution, or an integral part of the cellular structure of a food (eg apple juice versus apples). When sugars are consumed as part of the cellular structure of foods, there has been no suggestion of any adverse effects. However, there have been suggestions that "refined", "fibre depleted" or "added" sugars may have adverse effects either indirectly, by reducing the "fibre" in the diet, or by their ability to be taken in quantities greater than in their "natural" form. These issues have recently been discussed by the COMA Panel on Dietary Sugars[1], whose report we endorse.

5.5 **Conclusions** The Panel agreed with the following conclusions of the COMA Panel on Dietary Sugars[1].

i. There is no evidence that sugars naturally incorporated in the cellular structure of foods (intrinsic sugars) or lactose in milk or milk products (milk sugars) have adverse effects on health.

ii. Apart from lactose in milk and milk products, extrinsic sugars in the UK, (principally sucrose), contribute to the development of dental caries. In societies where average total sugar supplies are less than 20 kg/person/year (approximately 60 g/person/d or 10 per cent of dietary energy) dental caries is rare. Those particularly at risk of dental caries are children, adolescents and the elderly. There is evidence from laboratory studies for the *potential* cariogenicity of fermentable carbohydrates other than sugars, but the epidemiological evidence implicates non-milk extrinsic sugars as the major dietary component contributing to dental caries. Factors other than dietary carbohydrate, in particular fluoridation, are also important in determining the incidence of dental caries (see Chapter 36).

iii. Non-milk extrinsic sugars may favour the consumption of food energy, and in predisposed individuals may have undesirable metabolic effects, but are not directly related to the development of cardiovascular disease, essential hypertension, diabetes mellitus or behavioural abnormalities.

iv. For the obese, consumption of non-milk extrinsic sugars should be restricted as part of a general reduction of dietary energy. For non-obese adults, consumption of non-milk extrinsic sugars up to about 30 per cent of food energy does not carry special metabolic risks.

v. Extreme intakes of sucrose, above about 200 g/day or about 30 per cent of food energy, may be associated in normal adults with elevations of cholesterol, blood glucose and insulin concentrations, all of which may be undesirable.

5.6 **Dietary Reference Values**

5.6.1 The Panel did not recommend that intake of intrinsic or milk sugars be limited. They can usefully contribute, with starch, to energy requirements not met by other restricted dietary components (see 6.6).

5.6.2 Infants who are breastfed receive about 40 per cent of energy from sugars (lactose) and the Panel recommended that infant formulas should contain similar amounts. As well as sugars, international guidelines allow the inclusion of maltodextrins and pre-cooked or gelatinised starch.

5.6.3 The Panel agreed that non-milk extrinsic sugars intake should be limited because of their role in dental caries. However, the Panel recognized that the data in support of any specific *quantified* targets for non-milk extrinsic sugars intake were scanty. In order to provide guidance for uses as specified in paragraph 1.4, the Panel agreed that sufficient evidence existed to make proposals for DRVs. The Panel accepted that the dental effects of non-milk extrinsic sugars were most likely to be related to the frequency, and so in practice absolute mass, of sugars consumption rather than the overall dietary composition, but considered that the value of DRVs would be greater if expressed not only as mass, but also as their contribution to dietary energy. This also allows DRVs for starches plus intrinsic sugars to be calculated. The Panel therefore proposed that the population's average intake of non-milk extrinsic sugars should not exceed about 60 g/d or 10 per cent of total dietary energy.

5.6.4 *Guidance on high intakes* When non-milk extrinsic sugars are consumed in excess of about 200 g/day or 30 per cent of dietary energy, undesirable elevations in plasma concentrations of glucose, insulin and lipids may occur[1]. Such intakes should be avoided, and those who have intakes of this order should replace the excess with starch or intrinsic sugars. For some people with low energy requirements and intakes, relatively high non-milk extrinsic sugars intake may compete with foods which provide other nutrients, and potentially compromise micronutrient intakes. Such individuals, particularly women or the elderly, should exercise special care in making dietary choices.

5.7 References

1 Department of Health. *Dietary Sugars and Human Disease*. London: HMSO, 1989. (Reports on health and social subjects; 37).

2 Central Statistical Office. *Annual Abstracts of Statistics*. London: HMSO, 1989.

3 Ministry of Agriculture, Fisheries and Food. *Household Food Consumption and Expenditure*: 1989. London: HMSO, 1990.

4 Gregory J, Foster K, Tyler H, Wiseman M. *The Dietary and Nutritional Survey of British Adults*. London, HMSO, 1990.

6. Starches

6.1 **Definition** Starches are alpha-glucan polysaccharides. They comprise two major types of polymer: amylose, which is linear with a molecular size ranging between 110 and 60 K daltons and is virtually completely alpha 1–4 linked, and amylopectin, which contains alpha 1–6 and alpha 1–4 linkages and is branched.

6.2 **Starches in the diet** Starches are present in the diet in a number of physical states which confer physiological properties whose nutritional significance is still a matter for current research. In uncooked foods starches are present in granules with a highly ordered crystalline structure characteristic of the plant source. Heat in the presence of water causes the granules to swell and rupture so that the linear amylose molecules leach out and form a sol which retrogrades on cooling. The crystalline aggregated and retrograded structures formed partially resist enzymatic hydrolysis ("resistant starch"). A range of chemically modified starches are used as food ingredients or additives but their nutritional significance is small.

6.3 **Intake and sources** There are few data on intakes of different starches by UK populations because dietary surveys have almost always reported total carbohydrate consumption with no distinction between sugars and starches. The information available suggests that the amounts consumed in Britain provide about half the total carbohydrate (Table 6.1). In the recent Dietary and Nutritional Survey of British Adults, starches provided 24 per cent of energy[1]. No direct information is available concerning the intake of starches in children.

6.4 **Physiology** When foods containing the same amount of starch from different sources are fed to healthy subjects, the subsequent rises in blood glucose and insulin vary depending on the type of starch and its processing. By means of measurements of peripheral plasma glucose concentrations following standardised test meals, Jenkins and others have developed the concept of a "glycaemic index" for foods[2]. Although the glycaemic index of a food is reproducible in groups of people, large variations are seen among individuals and it is difficult to apply the index to meals containing fat and protein, or when one meal closely follows another. Furthermore, whilst hyperinsulinaemia and insulin resistance are found in certain conditions (obesity, non-insulin dependent diabetes mellitus), evidence that they are primary pathogenetic rather than associated factors in diseases (eg hypertension, atherosclerosis) is conflicting. Moreover the changes seen are within normal physiological variance. The Panel considered that the ability to deal with short-term fluctuations of carbohydrate intake was a feature of normal function. The absence of this ability was a feature of disease, such as diabetes. For these reasons the Panel was unable to

Table 6.1 *Total starch consumption (g/d)*

Sample reference, age (n)	Average (range)	sd	Energy MJ	Starch Consumption as % total energy (range)
Cambridge[3]				
Men, 20–80 y (32)	118 (34–186)	39	10.0	19
Women, 20–80 y (31)	100 (41–175)	38	8.2	20
Both sexes, 20–80 y (63)	111 (34–186)	38	9.1	20 (7–26)
Men, 18–55 y (105)	137	42	11.8	19
Women, 18–55 y (112)	96	32	8.2	19
South Wales[4]				
Men, 45–50 y (512)	162	50	10.0	26
Northumberland[5]				
Boys, 11–14 y (184)	162*	—	9.4	28
Girls, 11–14 y	142*	—	8.5	27
Both sexes (405)	154*	—	8.9	28

*Calculated by difference between total carbohydrate and sugars.

ascribe at this stage any definite practical health effect to the physiological differences in glucose absorption in response to starches from different foods.

6.5 **Nutritional role** Starches are a major component of most diets throughout the world and may provide up to 80 per cent of total energy. Some very high starch diets may be associated with shortages of some vitamins and minerals in circumstances where other sources of food energy are scarce. However this is not a direct, negative effect of starch, but a result of the consumption of diets low in foods providing essential protein and vitamins. The Panel was unable to find any evidence of harm resulting from high starch intakes in normal individuals, so long as energy balance and essential nutrient intake were maintained. Starchy foods contain many other nutrients although the variety and amount vary from food to food. Carbohydrate is a necessary part of the diet, to avoid ketoacidosis (see para 5.2) and because there are substantial reasons why other sources of food energy, (fat, protein and alcohol) should not provide more than a certain proportion of total food energy (see Section 1). Although certain populations (eg Eskimo, Masai) survive on very low intakes of carbohydrate, the Panel agreed that carbohydrate should provide the major food energy requirement for UK populations. The Panel considered that starches together with intrinsic and milk sugars should provide the main source of carbohydrate food energy (Table 1.2). The Panel did not find sufficient evidence to propose what proportion of this should be derived from starches.

6.6 **Dietary Reference Values** The Panel therefore proposed that starches and intrinsic and milk sugars should provide the balance of dietary energy not provided by alcohol, protein, fat and non-milk extrinsic sugars, that is on average 37 per cent of total dietary energy for the population (Table 1.2). These values are based on data from adults. The Panel nevertheless recommended that the same principles be applied to children over 2 years old. The Panel endorsed the recommendation of the COMA Panel on Child Nutrition that breastfeeding provides the best infant nutrition[6]. Breastmilk does not contain starch.

6.7 References

[1] Gregory J, Foster K, Tyler H, Wiseman M. *The Dietary and Nutritional Survey of British Adults*. London: HMSO, 1990.

[2] Jenkins D J A. Carbohydrates: dietary fiber. In: Shils M, Young V, eds. *Modern Nutrition in Health and Disease*. 7th Edn. Philadelphia: Lea and Febiger, 1988; 52–71.

[3] Bingham S A, McNeil N I, Cummings J H. The diet of individuals. *Br J Nutr* 1981; **45**: 23–35, and unpublished.

[4] Fehily A M, Yarnell J W G, Butland B K. Diet and ischaemic heart disease. *Hum Nut: Appl Nut* 1987; **41A**: 319-326.

[5] Hackett A F, Rugg-Gunn A J, Appleton D R, Eastoe J E, Jenkins G N. A 2-year longitudinal nutritional survey of 405 Northumberland children initially aged 11.5 years. *Br J Nutr* 1984; **51**: 67–75.

[6] Department of Health and Social Security. *Present Day Practice in Infant Feeding: Third Report*. London: HMSO, 1988. (Report on health and social subjects; 32).

7. Protein

7.1 **Introduction** The Panel agreed that, with a few exceptions, protein requirements of all age groups would be based on the recommendations in the Report of the FAO/WHO/UNU expert consultation, in which the values were derived on the basis of estimates of the amounts of high-quality egg or milk protein required for nitrogen (N) equilibrium, as measured in nitrogen balance studies (Table 7.1). For infants and children, additions were made for growth, and in pregnancy and lactation additions were made to account for the growth of the fetus and to allow adequate breast milk production. The criteria used are the rate of weight gain or growth, the achievement of a suitably positive nitrogen balance, and the maintenance of a state of well-being[1].

7.2 **Maintenance requirement** Although the relatively few studies which were available to provide the maintenance values for the FAO/WHO/UNU Report[1] have been criticised, the Panel took the view that these remain the best estimates since there have subsequently been few new data. In children, both the short-term N-balance studies at several levels of protein intake and the few long-term studies at one level of protein intake, generally above the maintenance level, provided general confirmation of the adequacy of the safe level. In adults, there were both short-term N-balance studies over a range of intakes, and a small number of long-term N-balance studies at a single intake, all in young adults. This evidence suggested that there was relatively little change with age in the requirements for protein for maintenance, values falling from 120 mg N/kg/d at 1 year to 96 mg N/kg/d in adults. Values for intermediate age groups were determined by interpolation, and it was assumed that maintenance requirements in adults do not change with age[1].

7.3 **Growth requirements** Growth requirements in infants and children were calculated from estimated rates of nitrogen accretion calculated from rates of weight gain and from estimates of the N content of tissues[1]. A 50 per cent increment was added to account for day-to-day variability in growth, as it was assumed that growth rates in individuals are not constant but may vary from day to day; and the efficiency of dietary utilisation was assumed to be 70 per cent.

7.4 **Pregnancy** Requirements for pregnancy were calculated to allow for protein retention in the products of conception and in the maternal tissues associated with the birth of a 3.3 kg infant. A single value for the daily additional protein requirement throughout pregnancy was proposed. The maintainance needs of new maternal tissue were assumed to be accommodated within the calculated maternal needs.

Table 7.1 *Dietary Reference Values for Protein* [a]

Age	Weight	Estimated Average Requirement	Reference Nutrient Intake
	Kg	g/d[c]	g/d[c]
0–3 months	5.9	—[d]	12.5[d]
4–6 months	7.7	10.6	12.7
7–9 months	8.8	11.0	13.7
10–12 months	9.7	11.2	14.9
1–3 years	12.5	11.7	14.5
4–6 years	17.8	14.8	19.7
7–10 years	28.3	22.8	28.3
Males:			
11–14 years	43.0	33.8	42.1
15–18 years	64.5	46.1	55.2
19–50 years	74.0	44.4	55.5
50+ years	71.0	42.6	53.3
Females:			
11–14 years	43.8	33.1	41.2
15–18 years	55.5	37.1	45.4
19–50 years	60.0	36.0	45.0
50+ years	62.0	37.2	46.5
Pregnancy[b]			+6
Lactation[b]:			
0–6 months			+11
6+ months			+8

[a] Values from WHO[1]

[b] To be added to adult requirement through all stages of pregnancy and lactation.

[c] Milk or egg protein. These figures assume complete digestibility. For diets based on high intakes of vegetable proteins, a correction may need to be applied (see 7.7).

[d] No figures were given by WHO for infants aged 0–3 months[1], therefore no EAR has been derived. The RNI is calculated from the recommendations of COMA[2].

7.5 **Lactation** Requirements for lactation are based on estimates of the protein content of breast milk of healthy mothers (calculated as milk nitrogen × 6.25). The estimates reflect the fact that daily breast milk protein content is constant for the first 6 months and falls thereafter. FAO/WHO/UNU recommended an additional protein requirement for lactation which included a component to take into account the 70 per cent efficiency of dietary utilisation[1]. The Panel has not included such an addition since human breast milk contains considerable non-protein nitrogen (up to 25 per cent, of which the largest single component is urea[3]). The Panel decided that no extra dietary provision was necessary for the non-protein component since it should derive from the inefficiency of utilisation of the maternal maintenance protein requirement. The diet should only need to provide for milk protein *per se* (about 75 per cent of that estimated from total nitrogen), and hence this value, when corrected for an efficiency of dietary utilisation of 70 per cent, is close to the value of milk protein calculated from N × 6.25 and forms the basis of the Panel's additional requirement for lactation.

7.6 **Elderly** In the case of the elderly, the RNI is the same as for younger adults (0.75g protein/kg/d). However, because of the small amount of lean body mass per kg body weight in the elderly, this will result in a higher figure per unit lean body mass than in younger adults[1,4,15].

7.7 **Indispensible amino acid requirements and protein quality** The DRVs assume that the dietary protein pattern includes sufficient variety of different protein-containing foods, or sufficient high quality animal protein sources to provide for indispensible amino acid (IAA) requirements. Studies of the amino acid pattern of the British diet indicate that the average household consumes a diet which supplies adequate amounts of IAA[6]. The Panel took the view that it is unlikely that there were any groups in the UK who are consuming food which supplies sufficient protein and energy to satisfy overall requirements who would be deficient in IAA. For diets which contain considerable amounts of unrefined cereal grains and vegetables, a correction for digestibility of 85 per cent should be applied. For those based on refined cereals the correction should be 95 per cent[1].

7.8 **Areas of uncertainty**

7.8.1 In the case of childhood, adolescence, pregnancy and lactation the database used by FAO/WHO/UNU was limited in extent[1]. Considerable concern has been expressed about the methodologies involved in assessment of requirements, especially the adequacy of the nitrogen balance technique used in the determination of the values[1,7]. The derivation of the maintenance value for young children differed from that for adults in that for children the highest value from the reported range was chosen while the mean value was selected for adults. As a result it is possible to derive a lower value for children by calculating a value from the reported range closer to the mean value as has been suggested by some authors[8]. Furthermore it has been pointed out that at least one major short-term N-balance study was not included in the adult values listed by FAO/WHO/UNU[1], an omission which resulted in the calculation of a higher mean value than would otherwise have been derived[9,10].

7.8.2 However, maintenance needs for protein based on achievement of N equilibrium in nitrogen balance studies are considerably more (about 70 per cent) than minimum rates of nitrogen loss in individuals fed protein-free diets[1]. This is also the case for estimations of requirements for individual IAA in infants and children, and for total nitrogen and protein for all ages. The reason for this excess of apparent requirements over minimum needs is poorly understood and the extent to which adaptation to low intakes can occur is not resolved[1,11-13], although new metabolic models which attempt to account for dietary IAA needs are emerging[14-17]. In particular, adult values of FAO/WHO/UNU[1], which are based mainly on the studies by Rose, have been criticised as being too low on the grounds that excessive energy was used in the original N-balance studies, that inappropriate correction factors were used to assess miscellaneous losses and that in any case the N-balance technique is inadequate[15]. On the basis of theoretical arguments with some experimental support Young *et al* have proposed an alternative scoring pattern to be used for all ages, excluding infants, ie from pre-school to adulthood[15].

7.8.3 Millward and Rivers have described a metabolic model to account for human protein and IAA requirements, arguing that such requirements vary according to the food consumed and can only be defined unambiguously in terms of minimum values[18]. Furthermore, it has been suggested that these minimum values may be considerably less than the amounts needed for nitrogen equilibrium on normal diets since oxidative losses of IAA rise with increasing protein intake. These authors suggest that the age-dependent fall in the IAA requirement values[1] is largely an artefact of the different dietary designs used in the various original studies, and conclude that the FAO/WHO/UNU adult values for IAA requirements are likely to be closer to minimum values, ie lower values than those needed on normal diets. However they have argued that this is insufficient information from which to derive alternative values of practical use. In particular there is a lack of agreed criteria to replace nitrogen balance studies[18].

7.8.4 The Report of an FAO/WHO Expert Consultation on the assessment of protein quality adopted the method of protein scoring corrected for digestibility as the best method, and re-examined the values for IAA requirements in order to construct appropriate scoring patterns. After considering these arguments it decided that, strictly as an interim measure, it would adopt requirement values determined for pre-school children as a scoring pattern to be used for all ages with the exception of infants. However it issued the *caveat* that caution must be used in applying this scoring pattern to assess protein quality for the diets of older childen and adults, since the pattern might overestimate their needs and underestimate protein quality[17]. The Panel therefore took the view that the FAO/WHO/UNU values for protein quality for infants and children are the best estimates currently available[1], but that while the values for protein quality for adults may be too low, there is insufficient new reliable data to enable an alternative pattern to be derived. For adults consuming most mixed diets found in the UK, including vegetarians, there is little reason to be concerned about the amino acid composition. Nevertheless the Panel endorsed the view of the Report of the FAO/WHO Expert Consultation that further research should be conducted into amino acid requirements of children and adults[17].

7.9 Protein requirements of infants and young children

7.9.1 It is possible that the apparent excess of the protein requirement compared with minimum needs, as referred to above, might be important because of the regulatory influence of dietary amino acids on growth, development and body function[10,18]. This could be particularly important in the case of infants and young children, since it has been suggested that the requirement estimates for infants should be lowered[8]. This suggestion was based on the observation that in infants a factorial calculation of the safe protein intake is considerably higher than the average intake of breast-fed infants. If the NCHS standards are taken as representing desirable rates of growth, then infants of healthy, well-nourished mothers, consuming habitual amounts of breast milk, satisfy this target during the early months of life. This indicates that the average breast-milk protein intake is, in effect, a safe level.

7.9.2 However, the intake of protein and nitrogen from breast milk is lower, relative to the energy intake, than at later stages of life. Infancy is the period of most rapid growth, so the nitrogen in breast milk is utilised with unusual efficiency, indicating the poorly understood special properties and qualities of breast milk[19]. Whatever the explanation of this unique interaction of nutrients in breast milk, because of this enhanced efficiency of utilisation, it is unwise to use breast-milk protein intakes as the reference against which intakes from other infants foods can be compared[9]. The Panel also made this point in reference to the energy requirements of young children in comparison with the energy intakes from breast milk (see section 2.1).

7.10 **Guidance on high intakes**

7.10.1 It is important that the RNIs for protein are not overestimates, because among adults in the UK, protein intakes are on average higher than the 1979 RDAs—84g for men and 64g for women[20]—and there has been concern that excessive intakes of protein may be associated with health risks. There is some evidence that excessive dietary protein may contribute to demineralisation of bone[21], although the relationship is not a simple one[22] and increases in dietary phosphorus, which usually accompany increased dietary protein, may minimise any such effect[7]. Populations consuming vegetarian diets containing, on average, lower protein intakes than other groups, may exhibit lower blood pressure and there is firm evidence that excessive dietary protein contributes to deterioration of renal function in patients with renal disease, possibly by increasing intraglomerular pressure and glomerular filtration rate[23-25]. Dietary protein also increases glomerular filtration rate and this may be related to the age-related decline in renal function[23]. There is some evidence that animal protein exerts a greater such effect than vegetable protein[26].

7.10.2 Whilst there is at present relatively little firm evidence in this area and insufficient information to enable a safe upper limit to be defined, the Panel concluded that it was prudent for adults to avoid protein intakes of more than twice the RNI (ie 1.5g protein/kg/d).

7.10.3 For the population in general, this upper limit does not imply any change in dietary habits. However, for some groups involved in very intense physical activity at the workplace or during recreational activities, protein intakes can be in excess of this. This could be due to high food intakes to meet energy demands, or due to specific protein supplements consumed during athletic training. There is currently insufficient evidence for any benefit from high protein intakes in these groups. However, when considering the safety of such intakes it should be assumed that the potentially adverse influences discussed above will also apply. Care should also be taken in the consumption of specific amino acid supplements since it is desirable that dietary amino acids should be provided in a balanced mixture. Little is known about the possible toxic effects of supplements of individual amino acids or mixtures of them which are commercially available. In particular consumption of supplements containing tryptophan has recently been linked to the development of an eosinophilia-myalgia syndrome of unknown aetiology, though this seems likely to be related to a contaminant rather than to the tryptophan itself[27].

7.11 References

1 World Health Organization. *Energy and protein requirements. Report of a Joint FAO/WHO/UNU Meeting*. Geneva: World Health Organization, 1985. (WHO Technical Report Series; 724).

2 Department of Health and Social Security. *Artificial Feeds for the Young Infant*. London: HMSO, 1980. (Reports on health and social subjects; 18).

3 Harzer G, Franzke V, Bindels J G. Human milk nonprotein nitrogen components: changing patterns of free amino acids and urea in the course of early lactation. *Am J Clin Nutr* 1984; **40**: 303–309.

4 Munro H N. Protein nutriture and requirement in elderly people. *Biblthca Nutr Dieta* 1983; **33**: 61–74.

5 Munro H N, Suter P M, Russell R M. Nutritional requirements of the elderly. *Ann Rev Nutr* 1987; **7**; 23–49.

6 Buss D H, Ruck N F. The amino acid pattern of the British diet. *J Hum Nutr* 1977; **31**: 165–169.

7 Hegsted D M. Balance Studies. *J Nutr* 1976; **106**: 307–311.

8 Beaton G H, Chery A. Protein requirements of infants: reexamination of concepts and approaches. *Am J Clin Nutr* 1988; **48**: 1403–1412.

9 Millward D J. Protein requirements of infants. *Am J Clin Nutr* 1989; **50**: 406–407.

10 Millward D J, Price G M, Pacy P J H, Halliday D. Maintenance protein requirements: the need for conceptual re-evaluation. *Proc Nutr Soc* 1990; **49**: 473–487.

11 Nicol B M, Phillips P G. Endogenous nitrogen excretion and utilization of dietary protein, *Br J Nutr* 1976: **35**: 181–193.

12 Sukhatme P V, Margen S. Models for protein deficiency. *Am J Clin Nutr* 1978; **31**: 1237–1248.

13 Rand W M, Scrimshaw N S, Young V R. Retrospective analysis of data from five long-term, metabolic balance studies: implications for understanding dietary nitrogen and energy utilization. *Am J Clin Nutr* 1985; **42**: 1339–1350.

14 Millward D J, Rivers J P W. The nutritional role of indispensible amino acids and the metabolic basis of their requirements. *Eur J Clin Nutr* 1988; **42**: 367–393.

15 Young V R, Bier D M, Pellet P L. A theoretical basis for increasing current estimates of the amino acid requirements in adult man with experimental support. *Am J Clin Nutr* 1989; **50**: 80–92.

16 Millward D J. Amino acid requirements in adult man. *Am J Clin Nutr* 1990; **51**: 492–493.

17 Food and Agriculture Organization. *Report of the Joint FAO/WHO Expert Consultation on Protein Quality Evaluation, Bethesda, 1989*; Rome: Food and Agriculture Organization, 1990.

18 Millward D J, Rivers J P W. The need for indispensible amino acids: the concept of the anabolic drive. *Diabet Metab Rev* 1989; **5**: 191–212.

19 Jackson A A. Optimising amino acid and protein supply and utilisation in the newborn. *Proc Nutr Soc* 1989; **48**: 293–301.

[20] Gregory J, Foster K, Tyler H, Wiseman M. *The Dietary and Nutritional Survey of British Adults*. London: HMSO, 1990.

[21] Garn S M, Kangas J. Protein intake, bone mass and bone loss. In: Deluca H *et al.* eds. *Osteoporosis: Recent Advances in Pathogenesis and Treatment*. Baltimore: University Park Press, 1981; 257-263.

[22] Orwoll E S, Weigel R M, Oviatt S K, Meier D E, McClung M R. Serum protein concentrations and bone mineral content in aging normal men. *Am J Clin Nutr* 1987; **46**: 614–621.

[23] Brenner B M, Meyer T W, Hostetter T H. Dietary protein intake and the progressive nature of kidney disease: The role of hemodynamically mediated glomerular injury in the pathogenesis of progressive glomerular sclerosis in aging, renal ablation, and intrinsic renal disease. *New Engl J Med* 1982; **307**: 652–659.

[24] Wiseman M J, Bognetti E, Dodds R, Keen H, Viberti G C. Changes in renal function in response to protein restricted diet in Type 1 (insulin-dependent) diabetic patients. *Diabetologia* 1987; **30**: 154–159.

[25] Rudman D. Kidney senescence; a model for aging. *Nutr Rev* 1988; **46**: 209–214.

[26] Wiseman M J, Hunt R, Goodwin A, Gross J L, Keen H, Viberti G. Dietary composition and renal function in healthy subjects. *Nephron* 1987; **46**: 37–42.

[27] Belongia E A, Hedberg C W, Gleich G J *et al.* An investigation of the cause of the eosinophilia-myalgia syndrome associated with tryptophan use. *New Engl J Med* 1990; **323**: 357–365.

8. Vitamin A

8.1 **Functions and essentiality** Vitamin A is required for growth and for normal development and differentiation of tissues; prolonged deprivation results in death. Human vitamin A deficiency is common in some developing countries, particularly among young children. The most obvious deficiency signs are dryness of the conjunctiva and the cornea (xerophthalmia), which can lead to permanent eye damage. In the retina, the aldehyde form of vitamin A serves as the light-gathering part of the visual pigments. An early sign of deficiency is impaired adaptation to low-intensity light (night blindness)[1].

8.2 **Forms of vitamin A** Vitamin A can be obtained in two forms: as preformed vitamin A (retinol) and from some of the carotenoid pigments that can be cleaved in the body to give retinol. Preformed vitamin A (usually in the form of retinyl esters) occurs naturally only in animals, and the richest sources are liver, fish liver oils and dairy products. Between a quarter and a third of the dietary vitamin A in the United Kingdom is derived from carotenoids, mainly from plant foods and overwhelmingly as β-carotene; other carotenoids are probably of little quantitative importance in this country as dietary precursors of vitamin A. The Panel saw no reason to depart from the widely accepted convention that, taken over the range of foodstuffs in a normal mixed diet, 6 μg β-carotene can be regarded as nutritionally equivalent to 1 μg retinol, and that the vitamin A activity of the diet, whether preformed or from carotene, can be summed in retinol equivalents[2].

8.3 **Assessment of vitamin A status** Vitamin A absorbed in excess of immediate needs is stored in the liver in esterified form. The size of the liver reserves is therefore one objective measure of vitamin A status, but it cannot readily be determined in living subjects. Plasma retinol concentrations are insensitive indicators of vitamin A status, for a homeostatic mechanism maintains them reasonably constant over a large range of liver reserves. They fall unequivocally below 0.7 μmol/L (20 μg/100 ml) only in the later stages of deficiency, when other signs also appear.

8.4 **Procedures for establishing requirements**

8.4.1 Most assessments of the vitamin A requirements of adults have been based on repletion studies in vitamin A-depleted volunteers[3,4]. However, orthodox repletion studies tend to overestimate requirements slightly, because deficiency signs often take some time to improve[5], and there is understandable reluctance to keep volunteers on low intakes for long periods.

8.4.2 An alternative approach, based on body pool size, was adopted in the recent FAO/WHO recommendations[6] and this has also been chosen by the Panel. Adequate vitamin A status can be defined in terms of an adequate body pool, based on the amount of vitamin A in the liver, which contains the great majority of the vitamin A in the body. A liver concentration of 20 μg retinol (or the equivalent in esterified form) per gram wet weight was used as the basis of the FAO/WHO recommendations[6]. This meets the following criteria:

(i) no clinical or biochemical signs of deficiency have been noted in subjects with this liver concentration;

(ii) this concentration can maintain adequate plasma retinol concentrations;

(iii) this concentration should maintain an adult on a diet containing no vitamin A free from deficiency signs for a period of several months.

8.5 **Requirements**

8.5.1 *Adults* Studies with radioactive vitamin A in eight men gave a mean fractional catabolic rate, ie the percentage of total body stores lost per day, of 0.5 per cent[4,5]. From this the mean daily dietary intake needed to maintain a liver retinol concentration of 20 μg/g can be calculated, making the following assumptions[5]:

(i) the liver weight: body weight ratio is 0.03: 1 (the mean value in adults is 0.024);

(ii) the liver reserves represent 90 per cent of the total body vitamin A;

(iii) the efficiency of storage in the liver of an ingested dose of vitamin A is 50 per cent (reported values 40–90 per cent).

The mean dietary intake per kilogram body weight would then be 0.005 (fractional catabolic rate) x 20 μg retinol (concentration per g liver) x 1,000 (conversion to kilograms) x 0.03 (liver as proportion of body weight) x 1.11 (total body vitamin A: liver vitamin A) x 2 (50 per cent storage) = 6.7 μg retinol/kg body weight. This gives EARs of 496 μg/d for a 74 kg male and of 402 μg/d for a 60 kg female. As the coefficient of variation for the rate of depletion in the experimental subjects was 21 per cent, the LRNIs are 300 μg/d for men and 250 μg/d for women, and the RNIs are 700 μg/d for men and 600μg/d for women (Table 8.1). Although these calculations rest on assumptions that are somewhat arbitrary[5], the derived requirements are consistent with the effects on deficiency signs observed in depletion-repletion studies[3,4,7]. Most importantly, they provide some indication of what the range of individual requirements might be.

8.5.2 *Infants* RDAs for infants have usually been based on the vitamin A provided by breast milk. Breast fed infants do not show signs of vitamin A deficiency even on intakes little above 100 μg/d[8,9], although these would probably not be enough to maintain satisfactory reserves. The recent FAO/WHO Expert Group considered that a daily intake of 350 μg retinol equivalents would meet the needs of all healthy infants and allow the building and maintaining of sufficient liver stores[6], and the Panel has accepted this value as the RNI. If the coefficient of variation is assumed to be 20 per cent as in adults, the rounded value for the EAR becomes 250 μg/d and for the LRNI 150 μg/d (Table 8.1).

8.5.3 *Children* Children have a requirement for vitamin A for growth, in addition to the requirement (as in adults) to compensate for the loss of body stores. In the absence of data on which to set DRVs, the Panel have interpolated from the values for infants up to the adult values (Table 8.1). Intakes lower than those suggested here maintained satisfactory plasma retinol concentrations in preschool children in India[10].

8.5.4 *Pregnancy* In pregnancy extra vitamin A is required for the growth and maintenance of the fetus, for providing it with some reserves, and for maternal tissue growth. Much of the requirement for newborn infants seems to be for growth. The fetus, although smaller in size than the term infant, grows rapidly during the third trimester and presumably has needs rising towards those of the newborn. An increment of 100 μg/d throughout pregnancy (raising the maternal RNI to 700 μg/d) should enhance maternal storage and allow adequate vitamin A for the growing fetus in late pregnancy. Most pregnant women in the UK have a vitamin A intake in excess of this, and only a small number are likely to need supplementary vitamin A during pregnancy (see also 8.7).

8.5.5 *Lactation* The diet should contain an increment of 350 μg to cover that supplied in the milk (Table 8.1).

8.6 **Intakes** Surveys show that the mean intakes of groups of the UK population are in excess of the RNIs. The average daily intake by 35–49-year-old men, for example, is 1,834 μg retinol equivalent with a median of 1,118 μg, and for women of the same age it is 1,606 μg with a median of 926 μg. Mean serum retinol concentrations were 2.3 μmol and 1.8 μmol/L respectively[11]. Post mortem analyses of liver retinol show that almost all the population in Great Britain has substantial reserves[12].

8.7 **Guidance on high intakes**

8.7.1 Large amounts of retinol can cause liver and bone damage, hair loss, double vision, vomiting, headaches and other abnormalities. Single doses of 300 mg in adults or 100 mg in children are harmful, but toxicity usually arises from chronic ingestion of retinol or retinyl esters, not necessarily in very large amounts but sufficient over a period of time to build up stocks that exceed the liver's ability to destroy or store them. Regular intakes should not exceed 7,500 μg/d in adult women and 9,000 μg/d in adult men. Children are more sensitive, and the Panel agreed with the recommendations of others that regular daily intakes should not exceed 900 μg in infants; 1,800 μg between 1 and 3 years of age; 3,000 μg from 4 to 6 years old; 4,500 μg from 6 to 12 years old; or 6,000 μg for adolescents[13]. Therapeutic doses may exceed these limits, but only under medical supervision.

8.7.2 Retinol is teratogenic. A relationship has been suggested between the incidence of birth defects in infants and high vitamin A intakes (more than 3300 μg/day) during pregnancy. As a precautionary measure women in the UK who are, or might become, pregnant have therefore been advised not to take

Table 8.1 *Dietary Reference Values for Vitamin A** (μg retinol equivalent/d)

Age	Lower Reference Nutrient Intake	Estimated Average Requirement	Reference Nutrient Intake
0–3 months	150	250	350
4–6 months	150	250	350
7–9 months	150	250	350
10–12 months	150	250	350
1–3 years	200	300	400
4–6 years	200	300	400
7–10 years	250	350	500
Males			
11–14 years	250	400	600
15–18 years	300	500	700
19–50 years	300	500	700
50+ years	300	500	700
Females			
11–14 years	250	400	600
15–18 years	250	400	600
19–50 years	250	400	600
50+ years	250	400	600
Pregnancy			+100
Lactation:			
0–4 months			+350
4+ months			+350

* The LRNIs and EARs for children have been estimated from the RNIs on the assumption that the coefficient of variation of requirements is 20 per cent as for adults.

supplements containing vitamin A unless advised to do so by a doctor or antenatal clinic[14]. Furthermore, recent analyses of animal livers commonly consumed in the UK have shown them to contain on average 13,000 μg to 40,000 μg/100g depending on species, so women who are, or might become, pregnant are also advised as a matter of prudence not to eat liver or products made from it[14]. β-carotene, however, is not toxic although high intakes lead to a yellow appearance.

8.8 Carotenoids

8.8.1 Of the more than one hundred carotenoid pigments that have been identified in plants, only a few have structures that enable them to serve as precursors of vitamin A. It has been suggested, however, that they act as antioxidants in tissues, deactivating free radicals and excited oxygen[15], and specifically that a high dietary intake of carotenoids confers some protection against cancer[16]. There is an inverse relationship between the incidence of some cancers and the consumption of fruit and vegetables (many of which contain carotenoids), but there is no proof that carotenoids are the protective factor.

8.8.2 Prospective trials of the possible health effects of β-carotene other than as a precursor of vitamin A are in progress. The Panel considered the evidence insufficient to make any specific recommendations about the consumption of carotenoids beyond that needed to supply vitamin A.

8.9 **Research needs** There is scope for determining the needs of children as well as of adults using vitamin A labelled with deuterium. The possible relationship between the numerous carotenoids and other constituents of fruit and vegetables with the incidence of cancers needs further clarification.

8.10 References

[1] Wittpenn J, Sommer A. Clinical aspects of vitamin A deficiency. In: Bauernfeind J, ed. *Vitamin A Deficiency and its Control.* Orlando, Florida: Academic Press, 1986; 177–206.

[2] World Health Organization. *Requirements of Vitamin A, Thiamine, Riboflavine and Niacin.* Geneva: World Health Organization, 1967. (WHO Technical Report Series; 362).

[3] Hume E M, Krebs H A. *Vitamin A Requirement of Human Adults.* London: HMSO, 1949. (MRC Special Report Series; 264).

[4] Sauberlich H E, Hodges R E, Wallace D E *et al.* Vitamin A metabolism and requirements in the human studied with the use of labelled retinol. *Vitam Horm* 1974; **32:** 251–275.

[5] Olson J A. Recommended dietary intakes (RDI) of vitamin A in humans. *Am J Clin Nutr* 1987; **45:** 704–716.

[6] Food and Agriculture Organization. *Requirements of Vitamin A, Iron, Folate and Vitamin B_{12}.* Report of Joint FAO/WHO Expert Consultation. Rome: Food and Agriculture Organization, 1988. (FAO Food and Nutrition Series; 23).

[7] Hodges R E, Sauberlich H E, Canham J E *et al.* Hematopoietic studies in vitamin A deficiency. *Am J Clin Nutr* 1978; **31:** 876–885.

[8] Belavady B, Gopalan C. Chemical composition of human milk in poor Indian women. *Ind J Med Res* 1959; **47:** 234–245.

[9] Butte N F, Calloway D H. Evaluation of lactational performance of Navajo women. *Am J Clin Nutr* 1981; **34:** 2210–2215.

[10] Reddy V. Observations on vitamin A requirement. *Ind J Med Res* 1971; **59**(suppl): 34–37.

[11] Gregory J, Foster K, Tyler H, Wiseman M. *The Dietary and Nutritional Survey of British Adults.* London: HMSO, 1990.

[12] Huque T. A survey of human liver reserves of retinol in London. *Br J Nutr* 1982; **47:** 165–172.

[13] Bauernfeind J C. *The Safe Use of Vitamin A.* International Vitamin A Consultative Group. Washington DC: Nutrition Foundation, 1980.

[14] Chief Medical Officer. *Department of Health Press Release no 90/507.* Women cautioned: watch your vitamin A intake. London: Department of Health, 1990.

[15] Burton G W. Antioxidant action of carotenoids. *J Nutr* 1989; **119:** 109–111.

[16] Ziegler R G. Vegetables, fruits and carotenoids and the risk of cancer. *Am J Clin Nutr* 1991; **53**(suppl): 251–259.

9. Thiamin

9.1 **Functions and essentiality** Thiamin is required mainly during the metabolism of carbohydrate, fat and alcohol. Diets high in carbohydrate require more thiamin than diets high in fat[1,2], so symptoms of the deficiency disease beri-beri usually arise where there is dietary thiamin deficiency and where much of the dietary energy is derived from carbohydrate[3]. The Wernicke-Korsakov syndrome is characteristic of thiamin deficiency associated with alcoholism[4,5].

9.2 **Requirements** Estimations of thiamin requirements have been based on a variety of biochemical methods. However, the finding that urinary thiamin output falls below 15 μg/d in patients with beri-beri[6] provides the reference point against which other methods such as thiamin loading[7], glucose loading[8] and transketolase (TKL) activation[9,10] are all compared.

9.2.1 *Adult men* From early studies, Williams *et al* suggested that thiamin intakes of the order of 0.4 mg/d were close to the absolute minimum at low energy intakes[7], and epidemiological evidence indicated that beri-beri occurs when the intake of thiamin is 0.2 mg/1,000 kcal or less[6]. However, in other studies to establish the minimum requirement for thiamin, 0.4 mg/d (equivalent to 0.188 mg/1,000 kcal) was fed to sedentary elderly men for 2 years, and no incontrovertible alteration in clinical state was observed[8].

9.2.2 At higher energy intakes, the studies of Sauberlich *et al* confirmed the close relationship between thiamin requirements and energy intakes[10]. With liquid formula diets containing 2,800 kcal and 3,600 kcal fed to 3 and 4 young men respectively, thiamin was first depleted and then repleted in a stepwise fashion for periods of 11 to 14 d. At a thiamin intake of 0.16 mg/1,000 kcal, both urinary and TKL measurements were abnormal; increasing the intake to 0.20 mg/1,000 kcal and 0.23 mg/1,000 kcal moved first the urinary excretion and then the TKL activation values out of the deficient range. At thiamin intakes of 0.30 mg/1,000 kcal, both measurements were within the normal range. The assessment of thiamin status in these studies was made over a very short time span in comparison with earlier work[7,8], and this would probably lead to an overestimate of requirements since tissue thiamin may not have completely adapted to the successively changed intakes. These results were obtained with carbohydrate: fat ratios similar to those in most Western populations, and are thus particularly relevant to the British situation.

9.2.3 From these and other studies, the Panel accepted that thiamin requirements were related to energy metabolism and thus, in most people, to energy intake, and that the estimated average requirement to achieve both clinical and biochemical normality is 0.3 mg/1,000 kcal. With due allowance for variance, the RNI becomes 0.4 mg/1,000 kcal (Table 9.1). The Panel also agreed that the

Table 9.1 *Dietary Reference Values for Thiamin** (mg/1,000 kcal)

Age	Lower Reference Nutrient Intake	Estimated Average Requirement	Reference Nutrient Intake
0–3 months	0.2	0.23	0.3
4–6 months	0.2	0.23	0.3
7–9 months	0.2	0.23	0.3
10–12 months	0.2	0.23	0.3
1–3 years	0.23	0.3	0.4
4–6 years	0.23	0.3	0.4
7–10 years	0.23	0.3	0.4
Males			
11–14 years	0.23	0.3	0.4
15–18 years	0.23	0.3	0.4
19–50 years	0.23	0.3	0.4
50+ years	0.23	0.3	0.4
Females			
11–14 years	0.23	0.3	0.4
15–18 years	0.23	0.3	0.4
19–50 years	0.23	0.3	0.4
50+ years	0.23	0.3	0.4
Pregnancy	No increment		
Lactation:			
0–4 months	No increment		
4+ months	No increment		

* The LRNIs and EARs for children over 1 year have been assumed to be the same as for adults, to parallel the RNIs. RNIs in mg/day based on EARs for energy are given in Table 1.4.

absolute intake should not fall below 0.4 mg/d in people on very low energy diets.

9.2.4 *Adult women* Women are less frequently affected by beri-beri than men even when eating the same food[3,11] but there is no consistent indication from experimental work that the needs of women differ from those of men. Bamji suggested that thiamin requirements to normalise measurements of TKL and thiamin excretion were lower in young women (0.21–0.26 mg/1,000 kcal) than young men[9], but others reported that urinary thiamin excretion only approached normal values on 0.51 mg/1,000 kcal[12]. There is no influence of oral contraceptives on thiamin status[13,14].

9.2.5 *Infants* The mean thiamin concentration in human milk in Britain has been reported as 0.16 mg/L, which is equivalent to 0.23 mg/1,000 kcal[15]. An increase from 0.14 to 0.22 mg/L (ie from 0.2 to 0.32 mg/1,000 kcal) has also been reported between 1 and 6 weeks postpartum[16]. It is currently recommended that artificial feeds should contain not less than 0.2 mg thiamin/1,000 kcal[17]. The Panel agreed that the RNI should be 0.3 mg/1,000 kcal.

9.2.6 *Children* In upper middle class American children between 2 months and 5 years old, thiamin intakes steadily increased from 0.3 to

0.7 mg/1,000 kcal during the first year of life and there were no signs of deficiency[18]. Boyden and Erikson measured thiamin status in 7- to 9-year-old girls and found normal thiamin excretion when intakes were 0.28 to 0.39 mg/1,000 kcal[19]. Dick *et al* maintained eight boys aged between 14 and 17 years for 69 d on thiamin intakes ranging from 0.6 to 2.7 mg/d and calculated their minimum requirement as 1.41 ± 0.2 mg/d or 0.38 ± 0.06 mg/1,000 kcal[20]. The Panel found very little other evidence from which to determine thiamin requirements for children, particularly during the pre-school period, but what evidence there was suggested that the RNI should be the same for children as for adults (Table 9.1).

9.2.7 *Pregnancy and lactation* Oldham *et al* studied 15 American women who in all cases had uneventful pregnancies with normal deliveries. Dietary intakes were assessed using diaries and by dietary analysis. The absolute thiamin intake in four of the women was between 0.4 and 0.7 mg/d and, in all women, intake exceeded 0.5 mg/1,000 kcal. The authors concluded that there was no evidence of any increased need for thiamin during normal pregnancy[21]. There was also no influence of a generally poor nutritional status on pregnancy or obstetric performance in 150 Indian women in whom the mean thiamin intake was 0.74 mg/d, or 0.39 mg/1,000 kcal[22]. The loss of 0.14 mg thiamin/d in milk (from 850 ml/d containing 0.16 mg/L) would be met by the recommended increase in energy intake. The Panel therefore made no change to the RNI of 0.4 mg/1,000 kcal during pregnancy or lactation.

9.2.8 *The elderly* Horwitt *et al* maintained men aged from 66 to 74 years on a marginal intake of 0.188 mg/1,000 kcal (0.4 mg/d) for 2 years (paragraph 9.2.1) and found no evidence for an increase in thiamin requirements with age[8].

9.3 **Guidance on high intakes** Chronic intakes in excess of 50 mg/kg or more than 3g/d are toxic to adults with a wide variety of clinical signs including headache, irritability, insomnia, rapid pulse, weakness, contact dermatitis, pruritus and in one case death[4].

9.4 References

[1] Reinhold J G, Nicholson J T L, Elsom K O. The utilization of thiamin in the human subject: the effect of high intake of carbohydrate or of fat. *J Nutr* 1944; **28**: 51–62.

[2] Holt E, Snyderman S E. The influence of dietary fat on thiamin loss from the body. *J Nutr* 1955; **56**: 495–500.

[3] Platt B S. Clinical features of endemic beri-beri. *Fed Proc* 1958; **17** (suppl 2): 8–20.

[4] Iber F L, Blass J P, Brin M, Leevy C M. Thiamin in the elderly—relation to alcoholism and to neurological degenerative disease. *Am J Clin Nutr* 1982; **36**: 1067–1082.

[5] Wood B, Breen K J. Clinical thiamin deficiency in Australia: The size of the problem and approaches to prevention. *Med J Aust* 1980; **1**: 461–464.

[6] Williams R R. *Toward the Conquest of Beri-beri.* Cambridge, Massachusetts: Harvard University Press, 1961.

[7] Williams R D, Mason H L, Wilder R M. The minimum daily requirement of thiamine in man. *J Nutr* 1943; **25**: 71–97.

[8] Horwitt M K, Liebert E, Kreisler O, Wittman P. Investigations of human requirements for B-complex vitamins. *Bull Nat Res Council*. Washington DC: National Academy of Sciences, 1948.

[9] Bamji M S. Transketolase activity and urinary excretion of thiamin in the assessment of thiamin-nutrition status of Indians. *Am J Clin Nutr* 1970; **23:** 52–58.

[10] Sauberlich H E, Herman Y F, Stevens C O, Herman R H. Thiamin requirement of the adult human. *Am J Clin Nutr* 1979; **32:** 2237–2243.

[11] Tang C M, Wells J C, Rolfe M, Cham K. Outbreak of beri-beri in the Gambia. *Lancet* 1989; **ii:** 206–207.

[12] Oldham H G, Davis M V, Roberts L J. Thiamin excretions and blood levels of young women on diets containing varying levels of the B-vitamins, with some observations on niacin and pantothenic acid. *J Nutr* 1946; **32:** 163–180.

[13] Ahmed F, Bamji M S, Iyengar L. Effect of oral contraceptive agents on vitamin nutrition status. *Am J Clin Nutr* 1975; **28:** 606–615.

[14] Lewis C M, King J C. Effect of oral contraceptive agents on thiamin, riboflavin and pantothenic acid status in young women. *Am J Clin Nutr* 1980; **33:** 832–838.

[15] Department of Health and Social Security. *The Composition of Mature Human Milk*. London: HMSO, 1977. (Reports on health and social subjects; 12).

[16] Nail P A, Thomas M R, Eakin R. The effect of thiamin and riboflavin supplementation on the level of those vitamins in human breast milk and urine. *Am J Clin Nutr* 1980; **33:** 198–204.

[17] Department of Health and Social Security. *Artificial Feeds for the Young Infant*. London: HMSO, 1980. (Reports on health and social subjects; 18).

[18] Beal V A. Nutritional intake of children. III Thiamine, riboflavin and niacin. *J Nutr* 1955; **57:** 183–192.

[19] Boyden R E, Erikson S E. Metabolic patterns in pre-adolescent children. Thiamine utilisation in relation to nitrogen intake. *Am J Clin Nutr* 1966; **19:** 398–406.

[20] Dick E C, Chen S D, Bert M, Smith J M. Thiamine requirement of eight adolescent boys, as estimated from urinary thiamine excretion. *J Nutr* 1958; **66:** 173–188.

[21] Oldham H, Sheft B B, Porter T. Thiamine and riboflavin intakes and excretions during pregnancy. *J Nutr* 1950; **41:** 231–245.

[22] Bagchi K, Bose A K. Effect of low nutrient intake during pregnancy on obstetric performance and offspring. *Am J Clin Nutr* 1962; **11:** 586–592.

10. Riboflavin

10.1 **Functions and essentiality** Riboflavin plays an essential role in all the oxidative processes on which man and other organisms depend. A reduced activity of flavin-dependent enzymes therefore tends to manifest itself in reduced consumption of oxygen rather than in a single or specific block in intermediary metabolism. Riboflavin deficiency in man can result in lesions of the mucocutaneous surfaces of the mouth (angular stomatitis, cheilosis, atrophic lingual papillae, glossitis, magenta tongue), seborrhoeic skin lesions, surface lesions of the genitalia and vascularisation of the cornea.

10.2 Requirements

10.2.1 There are few epidemiological studies which can be used to determine minimum requirements, because the classical signs of clinical deficiency are not completely specific and respond only moderately to riboflavin supplements. They are also dependent on the status of other nutrients and precipitating factors[1]. Nevertheless, they indicate that group intakes of 0.5–0.8 mg/d are needed by adult men and women[2-6], and by adolescent youths[7]. This evidence is in agreement with the findings of Horwitt *et al* that subjects fed 0.55 mg/d for 4 months developed clinical symptoms of deficiency[8,9].

10.2.2 Biochemically, there are three main ways in which riboflavin status can be assessed: (i) by measurement of urinary riboflavin; (ii) by measurement of red cell riboflavin; and (iii) by determination of erythrocyte glutathione reductase activation coefficient (EGRAC). Urinary riboflavin was the first method to be used extensively[8,9], and the intersection of the excretion curves for a range of intakes of riboflavin enables the amount required to saturate tissues to be calculated[5]. Burch *et al* showed that 90 per cent of the riboflavin in blood is present in the red cells, and their results suggested that diets which achieve 85 per cent saturation of red cell riboflavin are associated with maximum growth[10]. The EGRAC test was first reported by Glatzle *et al*[11] and independently by Bamji[12] and by Beutler[13]. It is a measure of tissue saturation and long-term riboflavin status, and has the advantage of being both stable and extremely sensitive. EGRAC values below 1.3 represent more or less complete saturation of the tissues with riboflavin[14,15], and results obtained by this method were extensively used by the Panel to support many of the DRVs for riboflavin.

10.2.3 Since riboflavin and protein are intimately related in the formation and storage of flavoproteins in lean tissue, a negative nitrogen balance interferes with the assessment of riboflavin requirements. The accompanying tissue breakdown increases urinary excretion of riboflavin[16] and the saturation of red cell glutathione reductase[6,17]. Other components of the diet may also affect riboflavin status by promoting or inhibiting intestinal synthesis or by changing transit time. There is some evidence that riboflavin can be absorbed in the lower gastrointestinal tract[18], but intestinal synthesis does not appear to be an important source of riboflavin in Western diets[5].

10.2.4 *Adults* In the recent survey of British adults, the median intake of riboflavin by men was 2.03 mg/d, with 2.5 and 97.5 centiles of 0.92 and 4.32 mg. For women, it was 1.56 mg/d with 2.5 and 97.5 centiles of 0.59 and 4.04 mg[19]. EGRAC values of 1.3 or above were found in only about 1 and 2 per cent of the men and women respectively who were healthy and not slimming or taking supplements, and were mostly associated with riboflavin intakes below 1.3 mg/d in the men and 1.1 mg/d in the women[19]. The EAR for men is therefore more than the 0.5–0.8mg/d on which clinical symptoms of deficiency can arise (see para 10.2.1), but less than 2 mg/d, and between 0.8 mg/d and 1.6 mg/d for women. Riboflavin intakes greater than 0.44 mg/1,000 kcal are accompanied by a sharp rise in its excretion and possibly represent tissue saturation[20,21]. This led to earlier recommendations of 0.55 mg/1,000 kcal because individual variation was assessed as 25 per cent (2 sd of the BMR). This would translate into 1.35 mg and 0.95 mg/d for men and women respectively using the energy intakes recently found for British adults[19]. The Panel considered this approach, but, because the latter value was associated with high EGRAC values[19], it was decided to base the RNIs on those intakes above which there were only two EGRAC results (both men) greater than 1.3 in the Dietary and Nutritional Survey of British Adults, ie 1.3 mg/d for men and 1.1 mg/d for women. The LRNIs and EARs are as shown in Table 10.1.

10.2.5 *Infants* The riboflavin content of breast milk from a five-centre study in the UK was 0.31 mg/L[22]. However, a wide range of values has been reported both in the UK and America (0.2–0.79 mg/L), probably reflecting the strong influence of the mothers' intakes[23]. The unsupplemented intake of Gambian infants in the first 12 months of life provides only about 0.2 mg/d, producing EGRAC value between 1.23 to 1.45, but supplementing these intakes to 0.4 mg/d resulted in satisfactory biochemical status ie EGRAC values around 1.15[24]. The Panel therefore set this as the RNI for formula-fed infants.

10.2.6 *Children* The Panel set the RNIs for children by interpolation between the values for infants and those for adults (Table 10.1).

10.2.7 *Pregnancy and lactation* The extra need for riboflavin placed on the pregnant mother by the fetus has been estimated as 0.3 mg/d, and that needed to meet the riboflavin content of milk and the metabolic cost of its secretion is 0.5 mg/d[21]. The Panel agreed these as the increments to be added to the RNI for pregnancy and lactation. The Panel found insufficient evidence to interpret EGRAC data in pregnancy.

10.2.8 *The elderly* Thurnham found more abnormal EGRAC results in elderly men and women than in young adults, and intakes of 1.2–1.5 mg/d and 1.1–1.4 mg/d in elderly men and women respectively achieved EGRAC values below 1.3[26]. Resting metabolism and riboflavin intakes decrease with age, but

Table 10.1 *Dietary Reference Values for Riboflavin* (mg/d)

Age	Lower Reference Nutrient Intake	Estimated Average Requirement	Reference Nutrient Intake
0–3 months	0.2	0.3	0.4
4–6 months	0.2	0.3	0.4
7–9 months	0.2	0.3	0.4
10–12 months	0.2	0.3	0.4
1–3 years	0.3	0.5	0.6
4–6 years	0.4	0.6	0.8
7–10 years	0.5	0.8	1.0
Males			
11–14 years	0.8	1.0	1.2
15–18 years	0.8	1.0	1.3
19–50 years	0.8	1.0	1.3
50+ years	0.8	1.0	1.3
Females			
11–14 years	0.8	0.9	1.1
15–18 years	0.8	0.9	1.1
19–50 years	0.8	0.9	1.1
50+ years	0.8	0.9	1.1
Pregnancy			+0.3
Lactation:			
0–4 months			+0.5
4+ months			+0.5

the Panel saw no justification for reducing the RNIs for elderly people below those for younger adults.

10.3 **Guidance on high intakes** The low solubility of riboflavin prevents its absorption from the gastrointestinal tract in amounts sufficient to produce toxic effects. When 120 mg/d were used for 10 months to treat congenital methaemoglobinaemia, no adverse effects were reported[27].

10.4 **Research needs** Research is needed on the biochemical assessment of riboflavin status in pregnancy and in old age.

10.5 References

1 Thurnham D I, Migasena P, Vudhivai N, Supawan V. A longitudinal study on dietary and social influences on riboflavin status in pre-school children in Northeast Thailand. *SE Asian J Trop Med Publ Hlth* 1971; **2:** 552–563.

2 Adamson J D, Jolliffe M, Kruse H D, Lowry O H, Moore P E, Platt B S, Sebrell W H, Tice J W, Tisdall F F, Wilder R M. Medical survey of nutrition in Newfoundland. *Canad Med Assoc J* 1945; **52:** 227–250.

3 Burgess R C. Deficiency diseases in prisoners-of-war at Changi, Singapore. *Lancet* 1946; **251:** 411–418.

4 Nicol B M. Nutrition of Nigerian peasant farmers, with special reference to vitamin A and riboflavin deficiency. *Brit J Nutr* 1949; **3:** 25–43.

[5] Bro-Rasmussen F. The riboflavin requirements of animals and man and associated metabolic relations. Part I. Technique of estimating requirement and modifying circumstances. *Nutr Abs Rev* 1958; **28:** 1–23.

[6] Bates C J, Prentice A M, Paul A A *et al.* Riboflavin status in Gambian pregnant and lactating women and its implications for recommended dietary allowances. *Am J Clin Nutr* 1981; **34:** 928–935.

[7] Lo C S. Riboflavin status of adolescents in southern China: average intake of riboflavin and clinical findings. *Med J Austral* 1984; **141:** 635–637.

[8] Horwitt M K, Hills O W, Harvey C C *et al.* Effects of dietary depletion of riboflavin. *J Nutr* 1949; **39:** 357–373.

[9] Horwitt M K, Harvey C C, Hills O W, Liebert E. Correlations of urinary excretion with dietary intake and symptoms of ariboflavinosis. *J Nutr* 1950; **41:** 247–264.

[10] Burch H B, Bessey O A, Lowry O H. Fluorometric measurements of riboflavin and its natural derivatives in small quantities of blood serum and cells. *J Biol Chem* 1948; **175:** 457–470.

[11] Glatzle D, Weber F, Wiss O. Enzymatic test for the detection of a riboflavin deficiency. NADPH-dependent glutathione reductase of red blood cells and its activation by FAD in vitro. *Experientia* 1968; **24:** 1122.

[12] Bamji M S. Glutathione reductase activity in red blood cells and riboflavin nutritional status in humans. *Clin Chim Acta* 1969; **26:** 263–269.

[13] Beutler E. Effect of flavin compounds on glutathione reductase activity: *in vivo* and *in vitro* studies. *J Clin Invest* 1969; **48:** 1957–1966.

[14] Glatzle D, Korner W F, Christeller S, Wiss O. Method for the detection of a biochemical riboflavin deficiency. *Int J Vit Nutr Res* 1970; **40:** 166–183.

[15] Thurnham D I, Migasena P, Pavapootanon N. The ultramicro glutathione reductase assay for riboflavin status: its use in field studies in Thailand. *Mikrochim Acta* 1970; **5:** 988–993.

[16] Bro-Rasmussen F. The riboflavin requirements of animals and man and associated metabolic relations. Part II. Relation of requirement to the metabolism of protein and energy. *Nutr Abs Rev* 1958; **28:** 369–386.

[17] Bamji M S, Bhaskaram P, Jacob C M. Urinary riboflavin excretion and erythrocyte glutathione reductase activity in pre-school children suffering from upper respiratory infections and measles. *Ann Nutr Metab* 1987; **31:** 191–196.

[18] Jusko W J, Levy G. Absorption, protein binding and elimination of riboflavin. In: Rivlin R, ed. *Riboflavin.* New York: Plenum Press; 1975, 99–152.

[19] Gregory J, Foster K, Tyler H, Wiseman M. *The Dietary and Nutritional Survey of British Adults.* London: HMSO, 1990.

[20] Department of Health and Social Security. *Recommended Intakes of Nutrients for the United Kingdom.* London: HMSO, 1969. (Reports on public health and medical subjects; 120).

[21] Department of Health and Social Security. *Recommended Daily Amounts of Food Energy and Nutrients for Groups of People in the United Kingdom.* London: HMSO, 1979. (Reports on health and social subjects; 15).

[22] Department of Health and Social Security. *The Composition of Mature Human Milk.* London: HMSO, 1977. (Reports on health and social subjects; 12).

[23] Nail P A, Thomas M R, Eakin R. The effect of thiamin and riboflavin supplementation on the level of those vitamins in human breast milk and urine. *Am J Clin Nutr* 1980; **33:** 198–204.

[24] Bates C J, Prentice A M, Paul A A *et al.* Riboflavin status in infants born in rural Gambia, and the effect of a weaning food supplement. *Trans R Soc Trop Med Hyg* 1982; **76:** 253–258.

[25] Bates C J, Prentice A M, Watkinson M *et al.* Efficacy of a food supplement in correcting riboflavin deficiency in pregnant Gambian women. *Hum Nutr: Clin Nutr* 1984; **38C:** 363–374.

[26] Thurnham D I. The interpretation of biochemical measurements of vitamin status of the elderly. In: Kemm J, Ancill R, eds. *Vitamin Deficiency in the Elderly* London: Blackwell, 1985; 46–67.

[27] Hirano M, Matsuki T, Tanishima *et al.* Congenital methaemoglobinaemia due to NADH methaemoglobin reductase deficiency: successful treatment with oral riboflavin. *Br J Haematol* 1981; **47:** 353–359.

11. Niacin and Tryptophan

11.1 **Function and essentiality** The generic descriptor "niacin" includes nicotinic acid and nicotinamide, which functions as the reactive part of the nicotinamide nucleotide coenzymes, NAD and NADP. Nicotinamide can be synthesised from the amino acid tryptophan. The major metabolic role of NAD(P) is a coenzyme in oxidation and reduction reactions. Niacin is thus of central importance in intermediary metabolism, and the requirement is related to energy expenditure. Niacin deficiency results in pellagra, which is characterised by a severe sunburn-like skin lesion in areas of the body exposed to sunlight, and in areas such as the knees, ankles, wrists and elbows which are subjected to pressure. Diarrhoea is a characteristic, but not inevitable, symptom of pellagra. In advanced cases there may be dementia with intermittent periods of lucidity. Untreated pellagra is fatal.

11.2 **Tryptophan-niacin equivalence** The equivalence of dietary tryptophan and preformed niacin has been determined in volunteers maintained on controlled diets. There is a wide variation between individuals and from day to day in any one person. High dietary intake of tryptophan results in a greater apparent efficiency of conversion to niacin. Oestrogens reduce the rate of tryptophan metabolism, so that in areas where pellagra is or has been common, approximately twice as many women as men are affected although before puberty and after the menopause there is no sex difference. Kynureninase and kynurenine hydroxylase, two enzymes involved in tryptophan metabolism, are vitamin B_6 and riboflavin dependent; deficiency of either of these vitamins may result in secondary pellagra, despite an apparently adequate intake of tryptophan and niacin[1,2]. The Panel accepted the widely adopted convention that 60 mg tryptophan can be taken as equivalent to 1 mg dietary niacin[3]. This ratio includes an allowance for individual variation. The niacin equivalence of diets is then the amount of preformed niacin + (1/60 × tryptophan).

11.3 **Requirements** There is no wholly satisfactory laboratory assessment of niacin status. In experimental animals, measurement of whole blood NAD(P) can provide a sensitive index of niacin depletion[4], while the determination of the urinary excretion of N-methyl nicotinamide (NMN) and its onward metabolite methyl pyridone carboxamide (MPCX) offers the only other method available.

11.3.1 *Adults* The mean observed requirement for niacin to prevent or cure pellagra, or to normalise urinary excretion of NMN and MPCX, in experimental subjects maintained on niacin deficient diets and in energy balance, is 5.5 mg/1,000 kcal[3]. A coefficient of variation of 10 per cent gives an RNI of 6.6 mg/1,000 kcal and an LRNI of 4.4 mg/1,000 kcal (Table 11.1).

11.3.2 *Infants* The Panel accepted the DHSS Guidelines for Artificial Feeds for the Young Infant that infant milks should provide not less than 3.3–3.85 mg preformed niacin/1,000 kcal[5]. With the tryptophan present in cows' milk protein, infants would have similar intakes of niacin equivalent/1,000 kcal to those of adults, and the Panel saw no reason to set DRVs for infants or children at a different level than those for adults.

11.3.3 *Pregnancy* There are considerable changes in tryptophan metabolism in late pregnancy as a result of hormonal changes, such that 30 mg of tryptophan is equivalent to 1 mg dietary niacin[6]. The Panel agreed that any additional requirement for niacin would be met by changes in the metabolism of tryptophan, and that an increased dietary intake was unnecessary.

11.3.4 *Lactation* Mature human milk provides about 2.3 mg preformed niacin/d at a concentration of 2.7 mg/L. In the absence of information about the equivalence of dietary tryptophan and niacin in lactation, the Panel agreed that such an increase in dietary niacin plus tryptophan would be prudent to meet this extra need, above that appropriate for the increased energy intake (Table 11.1).

11.4 **Intakes** Under normal conditions for an adult in nitrogen balance, the amount of tryptophan present in dietary protein provides adequate niacin

Table 11.1 *Dietary Reference Values for Niacin** (mg niacin equivalent/1000 kcal)

Age	Lower Reference Nutrient Intake	Estimated Average Requirement	Reference Nutrient Intake
0–3 months	4.4	5.5	6.6
4–6 months	4.4	5.5	6.6
7–9 months	4.4	5.5	6.6
10–12 months	4.4	5.5	6.6
1–3 years	4.4	5.5	6.6
4–6 years	4.4	5.5	6.6
7–10 years	4.4	5.5	6.6
Males			
11–14 years	4.4	5.5	6.6
15–18 years	4.4	5.5	6.6
19–50 years	4.4	5.5	6.6
50+ years	4.4	5.5	6.6
Females			
11–14 years	4.4	5.5	6.6
15–18 years	4.4	5.5	6.6
19–50 years	4.4	5.5	6.6
50+ years	4.4	5.5	6.6
Pregnancy	No increment		
Lactation:			
0–4 months			+2.3 mg/d
4+ months			+2.3 mg/d

*RNIs in mg/d based on DRVs for energy are given in Table 1.4

without the need for any preformed vitamin at all. Median protein intakes in Britain are 84.0 g/d by men and 61.8 g/d by women[7] containing 12.6 mg tryptophan/g[8]. At an equivalence of 60 mg tryptophan: 1 mg niacin this alone is equivalent to 17.6 mg/d niacin for men and 13.0 mg/d for women.

11.5 **Guidance on high intakes** Very high doses of nicotinic acid (3–6 g/d) cause changes in liver ultra-structure and function, in carbohydrate tolerance and in uric acid metabolism, which may result in clinical signs of hepatotoxicity but which appear to be reversible on withdrawal of the vitamin. Doses of nicotinic acid but not of nicotinamide in excess of about 200 mg cause vasodilatation of cutaneous blood vessels, and hence flushing. Higher doses may also cause dilatation of other blood vessels, and a transient fall in blood pressure. The effect wears off after some days' repeated administration. There is no evidence that intakes of niacin above those required to prevent pellagra confer any benefit. Indeed, the main response to higher intakes of nicotinic acid, nicotinamide or tryptophan is an increase in the urinary excretion of their metabolites[9].

11.6 References

1 Bender D A. Biochemistry of tryptophan in health and disease. *Molec Aspects Med* 1983; **6**: 101–197.

2 Bender D A, Bender A E. Niacin and tryptophan metabolism: the biochemical basis of niacin requirements and recommendations. *Nutr Abs Rev* 1986; **56**: 695–719.

3 Horwitt M K, Harvey C C, Rothwell W S, Cutler J L, Haffron D. Tryptophan-niacin relationships in man. Studies with diets deficient in riboflavin and niacin together with observations on the excretion of nitrogen and niacin metabolites. *J Nutr* 1956; **60** (suppl 1): 1–43.

4 Magboul B I, Bender D A. Effects of a dietary excess of leucine on the synthesis of nicotinamide nucleotides in the rat. *Br J Nutr* 1983; **49**: 321–329.

5 Department of Health and Social Security. *Artificial Feeds for the Young Infant*. London: HMSO, 1980. (Reports on health and social subjects; 18).

6 Wertz, A W, Lojkin M I, Bouchard B S, Derby M B. Tryptophan-niacin relationships in pregnancy. *J Nutr* 1958; **64**: 339–353.

7 Gregory J, Foster K, Tyler H, Wiseman M. *The Dietary and Nutritional Survey of British Adults*. London: HMSO, 1990.

8 Buss D H, Ruck N. The amino acid pattern of the British diet. *J Hum Nutr* 1977; **31**: 165–169.

9 McCreanor G M, Bender D A. The metabolism of high intakes of tryptophan, nicotinamide and nicotinic acid in the rat. *Br J Nutr* 1986; **56**: 577–586.

12. Vitamin B_6

12.1 **Functions and essentiality** Vitamin B_6 is a mixture of pyridoxal, pyridoxine, pyridoxamine, and their 5'-phosphates, which are metabolically interconvertible. Pyridoxal phosphate (PLP) is a cofactor for a large number of enzymes catalysing reactions of amino acids. These are of central importance in the body's overall protein metabolism, and hence requirements are related to the total amount of amino acids to be metabolised. PLP is also the cofactor for glycogen phosphorylase. Gross clinical deficiency of vitamin B_6 is rare. In the early 1950s, however, an infant milk preparation which had undergone severe heating in manufacture lost much of its pyridoxine and the infants who were fed it developed a number of metabolic abnormalities and many convulsed. The symptoms responded to vitamin B_6 supplementation[1,2].

12.2 **Sources** The vitamin is widely distributed in foods, although much of the vitamin B_6 in some vegetables may be present as unavailable glycosides. Intestinal flora also synthesise relatively large amounts, at least some of which is absorbed.

12.3 **Requirements** Estimates of the total body pool of Vitamin B_6, based on very few studies, vary between 40–250 mg. Shane determined a half-life of 33 days for this pool, which implies an average requirement for replacement of between 0.6–3.78 mg/d[3]. More useful estimates of vitamin B_6 requirements have come from studies of changes in tryptophan and methionine metabolism, and blood vitamin B_6, during depletion and repletion of adults maintained on controlled diets. Deficiency develops faster on relatively high protein intakes (80–160 g/d) than on lower intakes (30–50 g/d). During repletion of deficient subjects, tryptophan and methionine metabolism and blood vitamin B_6 are normalised faster at low than at high levels of protein intake[4–7].

12.3.1 *Adults* By interpolation from the above studies, which used a relatively wide range of vitamin B_6 intakes with two different intakes of protein, the Panel agreed with most other committees that the RNI for vitamin B_6 is 15 μg/g dietary protein. With the variance of 20 per cent, the LRNI and the EAR become 11 μg and 13 μg per gram of protein respectively (Table 12.1). Because requirements will depend upon actual protein intake, the Panel considered it inadvisable to set absolute DRVs for this nutrient. If, however, the energy intake of the group was at the EARs in this Report and protein provided 14.7 per cent of this energy as in the recent dietary survey of British adults[8], then the absolute RNIs would be as in Table 1.4.

12.3.2 *Infants* Of the infants fed overheated formula (see para 12.1), 0.3 per cent convulsed when their pyridoxine intake was 60 μg/d. Provision of

Table 12.1 *Dietary Reference Values for Vitamin B_6* (μg/g protein*)

Age	Lower Reference Nutrient Intake	Estimated Average Requirement	Reference Nutrient Intake
0–3 months	3.5	6	8
4–6 months	3.5	6	8
7–9 months	6	8	10
10–12 months	8	10	13
1–3 years	11	13	15
4–6 years	11	13	15
7–10 years	11	13	15
Males			
11–14 years	11	13	15
15–18 years	11	13	15
19–50 years	11	13	15
50+ years	11	13	15
Females			
11–14 years	11	13	15
15–18 years	11	13	15
19–50 years	11	13	15
50+ years	11	13	15
Pregnancy	No increment		
Lactation:			
0–4 months	No increment		
4+ months	No increment		

*RNIs as mg/d based on actual protein intakes are given in Table 1.4 (see 12.3.1)

260 μg/d prevented or cured these symptoms, and 300 μg/d normalised tryptophan metabolism[1,2]. However, those amounts overestimate infants' requirements because the pyridoxal-lysine which was formed in this formula has anti-vitamin activity[9]. Based on the composition of pooled mature human milk, the DHSS Guidelines on Artificial Feeds for the Young Infant recommend a concentration of vitamin B_6 not less than 5 μg/100 ml and a protein concentration between 1.5–2.0 g/100 ml, which gives a vitamin B_6 intake of 2.5–3.5 μg/g protein[10]. The Panel equated this to the LRNI up to the age of 6 months, and set an RNI of 8 μg/g protein which is the amount calculated for human milk from the data of Paul and Southgate[11]. These values are lower than for adults, in part because some of the protein is used for tissue growth rather than metabolised for energy.

12.3.3 *Pregnancy* Plasma pyridoxal phosphate falls markedly in pregnancy, but there is no evidence that it is necessary or desirable to raise the plasma PLP of pregnant women to that considered normal for non-pregnant women.

12.3.4 *Oral contraceptive users* There is no evidence that use of oral contraceptive steroids increases the requirement for vitamin B_6, although pharmacological doses of the vitamin may overcome some of the side-effects of contraceptive steroids[12,13].

12.3.5 *The elderly* There is a fall in plasma PLP of some 3.6 nmol/L per decade of life. It is not clear whether this represents a decline in vitamin B_6 status with age, or simply a change in the blood concentration of the vitamin; erythrocyte aspartate aminotransferase activity does not show a similar change with age[14,15]. Middle-aged women fed a constant diet providing 2.3–2.4 mg/d vitamin B_6 show lower plasma PLP and higher urinary 4-pyridoxic acid than young women fed the same diet[16]. It seems likely that there are age related changes in the absorption and metabolism of the vitamin, but although the elderly may have a higher absolute requirement than younger people, there is insufficient evidence from which to quantify an increased RNI, especially as some studies have failed to show any beneficial effect of supplements as high as 20 mg/d.

12.4 **Guidance on high intakes** Schaumburg *et al* reported the development of sensory neuropathy in 7 patients taking 2–7 g/d pyridoxine. Although there was residual damage in some patients, withdrawal of these extremely high doses resulted in a considerable recovery of sensory nerve function[17]. Dalton and Dalton reported peripheral sensory neuropathy in 60 per cent of 172 women taking between 50–500 mg vitamin B_6/d for 6 to 60 months, but even among women taking only 50 mg/d, 40 per cent reported symptoms of peripheral sensory neuropathy[18]. Within 6 months after withdrawal of these vitamin B_6 supplements, all patients reported recovery. Although one study has demonstrated no teratogenic effect of vitamin B_6 in experimental animals[19], the safety of high intakes in human pregnancy has not been established.

12.5 References

[1] Bessey O A, Adam D J D, Hansen A E. Intake of vitamin B_6 and infantile convulsions: a first approximation of requirements of pyridoxine in infants. *Paediatr*. 1957; **20:** 33–44.

[2] Coursin D B. Vitamin B_6 metabolism in infants and children. *Vitamins and Hormones* 1964; **22:** 755–786.

[3] Shane B. Vitamin B-6 and blood. In: *Human Vitamin B_6 requirements*, Committee on Dietary Allowances, Food and Nutrition Board, National Research Council Washington DC: National Academy of Sciences, 1978; 111–128.

[4] Miller L T, Linkswiler H. Effect of protein intake on the development of abnormal tryptophan metabolism by men during vitamin B_6 depletion. *J Nutr* 1967; **93**: 53–59.

[5] Kelsay J, Miller L T, Linkswiler H. Effect of protein intake on the excretion of quinolinic acid and niacin metabolites by men during vitamin B_6 depletion. *J Nutr* 1968; **94**: 27–31.

[6] Kelsay J, Baysal A, Linkswiler H. Effects of vitamin B_6 depletion on the pyridoxal, pyridoxamine and pyridoxine content of the blood and urine of man. *J Nutr* 1968; **94**: 490–494.

[7] Canham J E, Baker E M, Harding R S, Sauberlich H E, Plough I C. Dietary protein; its relationship to vitamin B_6 requirements and function. *Ann NY Acad Sci* 1969; **166**: 16–29.

[8] Gregory J, Foster K, Tyler H, Wiseman M. *The Dietary and Nutritional Survey of British Adults*. London: HMSO, 1990.

[9] Gregory J F. Effects of ϵ-pyridoxyl-lysine bound to dietary protein on the vitamin B_6 status of rats. *J Nutr* 1980; **110**: 995–1005.

[10] Department of Health and Social Security. *Artificial Feeds for the Young Infant*. London: HMSO, 1980. (Reports on health and social subjects; 18).

[11]Paul A A, Southgate D A T. *McCance and Widdowson's The Composition of Foods*, 4th edn. London: HMSO, 1987.

[12] Rose D P, Braidman I P. Excretion of tryptophan metabolites as affected by pregnancy, contraceptive steroids and steroid hormones. *Am J Clin Nutr* 1971; **24**: 673-683.

[13] Bender D A. Oestrogens and vitamin B_6: actions and interactions. *Wld Rev Nutr Diet* 1987; **51**: 140–188.

[14] Hamfelt A. Age variation of vitamin B_6 metabolism in man. *Clin Chim Acta* 1964; **10**: 48–54.

[15] Rose C S, Gyorgy P, Butler M *et al*. Age differences in the vitamin B_6 status of 617 men. *Am J Clin Nutr* 1976; **29**: 847–853.

[16] Lee C M, Leklem J E. Differences in vitamin B_6 status indicator responses between young and middle-aged women fed constant diets with two levels of vitamin B_6. *Am J Clin Nut* 1985; **42**: 226–234.

[17] Schaumburg H, Kaplan J, Windebank A *et al*. Sensory neuropathy from pyridoxine abuse: a new megavitamin syndrome. *New Engl J Med* 1983; **309**: 445–448.

[18] Dalton K, Dalton M J T. Characteristics of pyridoxine overdose neuropathy syndrome. *Acta Neurol Scand* 1987; **76**: 8–11.

[19] Khera K S. Teratogenicity study in rats given high doses of pyridoxine (vitamin B_6) during organogenesis. *Experientia* 1975; **31**: 469–470.

13. Vitamin B_{12}

13.1 Functions and essentiality

13.1.1 Compounds with vitamin B_{12} activity consist of a corrinoid ring surrounding an atom of cobalt, the sole function known for cobalt in humans. Vitamin B_{12} is involved in the recycling of folate coenzymes through involvement in methionine synthesis and the degradation of valine via methylmalonyl CoA. Interactions with the folate group of co-enzymes are responsible for the haematological abnormality of megaloblastic anaemia, in which vitamin B_{12} deficiency results in the same syndrome as folate deficiency. In addition, vitamin B_{12} is needed for nerve myelination, and prolonged deficiency leads to irreversible neurological damage.

13.1.2 Food sources of vitamin B_{12} include almost all animal products, and certain algae (eg seaweeds) and bacteria, which can synthesize it. Green plants, however, contain none at all, unless they become contaminated by bacteria or algae. The natural forms of vitamin B_{12} are the methyl, adenosyl, hydroxo or aquo-cobalamins, and the usual commercially available form, cyanocobalamin, is readily converted to these *in vivo*. For normal vitamin B_{12} absorption in the terminal ileum, the vitamin must bind to salivary haptocorrin and then to "intrinsic factor", a protein cofactor which is secreted by the parietal cells of the stomach. The most common reason for B_{12} deficiency in humans is not dietary, but a failure of intrinsic factor secretion, leading to pernicious anaemia[1,2]. Diet-related vitamin B_{12} deficiency has, however, been observed in some very strict vegetarians and vegans, who obtain essentially no vitamin B_{12} from food or from microbial sources.

13.2 **Requirements** About 80 per cent of the body store is in the liver, and turnover is extremely slow (0.05–0.2 per cent of the body pool per day). Conservation by the kidney and during enterohepatic circulation is very efficient. As a result, no experimental human depletion studies have been undertaken to produce vitamin B_{12} deficiency, or to measure the daily requirement directly since these would take too long and be considered too hazardous. The usual criterion for vitamin B_{12} inadequacy is a serum level below 130 pg/ml or about 100 pmol/L[3].

13.2.1 *Adults* The average requirement to prevent or cure the megaloblastic anaemia of vitamin B_{12} deficiency in adults appears to be less than 1 μg/d, and this is the intake now recommended by FAO[4]. The evidence for this estimate was derived from 3 main types of study: a) the absence of anaemia or macrocytosis from Australian Seventh Day Adventist vegetarians, whose vitamin B_{12} intakes were estimated as 0.26 ± 0.23 (sd) μg/d, and from Swedish vegans with vitamin B_{12} intakes estimated as 0.3–0.4 μg/d[5,6]; b) a slow but "adequate" haematological response by South Indian subjects with diet-related B_{12}-deficiency anaemia when given 0.3–0.65 μg/d[7]; and c) a haematological response to parenteral doses of vitamin B_{12} between 0.1 and 0.2 μg/d by pernicious anaemia patients[8,9]. The LRNI was therefore set at 1 μg/d (Table 13.1), but the Panel considered that the RNI of 1.5 μg/d for adults would not only reduce the risk of megaloblastic anaemia in all normal subjects but also provide sufficient stores to withstand a period of zero intake. Although the incidence of pernicious anaemia is increased among elderly people, there is no evidence that normal healthy elderly subjects have increased vitamin B_{12} requirements.

13.2.2 *Pregnancy and lactation* There is little or no information about requirements during pregnancy, and the 1.5 μg/d intake was considered to be sufficient to cover the needs of pregnant women, on the assumption that their body stores would not be depleted at the outset of pregnancy. For lactation, an increment of 0.5 μg/d should ensure an adequate supply for breast milk, which is estimated to contain 0.2–1.0 μg vitamin B_{12}/L unless it comes from deficient or from supplemented subjects[10].

13.2.3 *Infants* Since a daily supplement of 0.1 μg cures megaloblastic anaemia in infants receiving less than 60 ng/d from breast milk[11], the Panel set the LRNI at 0.1 μg/d. The RNI is, however, set at 0.3 μg/d which is the intake required to normalise methyl malonic acid excretion[12]. Amounts for children have been interpolated between these and the values for adults.

Table 13.1 *Dietary Reference Values for Vitamin B_{12}* (μg/d)

Age	Lower Reference Nutrient Intake	Estimated Average Requirement	Reference Nutrient Intake
0–3 months	0.1	0.25	0.3
4–6 months	0.1	0.25	0.3
7–9 months	0.25	0.35	0.4
10–12 months	0.25	0.35	0.4
1–3 years	0.3	0.4	0.5
4–6 years	0.5	0.7	0.8
7–10 years	0.6	0.8	1.0
Males			
11–14 years	0.8	1.0	1.2
15–18 years	1.0	1.25	1.5
19–50 years	1.0	1.25	1.5
50+ years	1.0	1.25	1.5
Females			
11–14 years	0.8	1.0	1.2
15–18 years	1.0	1.25	1.5
19–50 years	1.0	1.25	1.5
50+ years	1.0	1.25	1.5
Pregnancy	No increment		
Lactation:			
0–4 months			+0.5
4+ months			+0.5

13.3 **Guidance on high intakes** Vitamin B_{12} has extremely low toxicity; it is toxic only at g/kg intakes in experimental animals, and no toxic effects have been encountered in man. Injections of as much as 3 mg/d have been used in attempts to treat fatigue and various neurological disorders, and 1 mg/d has been used to treat vitamin B_{12}-responsive inborn errors of metabolism.

13.4 **Research needs** There is scope for the development of improved functional tests of marginal deficiency, and further exploration of the relationship between the haematological and the neurological aspects of deficiency. Requirements during pregnancy and lactation and those of infants and children need to be clarified.

13.5 References

[1] Chanarin I. *The Megaloblastic anaemias*, 2nd ed. Oxford: Blackwell Scientific, 1979.

[2] Grasbeck R, Salonen E-M. Vitamin B_{12}. *Prog Fd Nutr Sci* 1976; **2**: 193–231.

[3] Herbert V, Colman N, Palat D *et al.* Is there a 'gold standard' for human serum vitamin B_{12} assay? *J Clin Med* 1984; **104**: 829–841.

[4] Food and Agriculture Organization. *Requirements of Vitamin A, Iron, Folate and Vitamin B_{12}.* Report of a joint FAO/WHO Consultation. Rome: Food and Agriculture Organization, 1988. (FAO Food and Nutrition Series; 23).

[4] Food and Agriculture Organization. *Requirements of Vitamin A, Iron, Folate and Vitamin B_{12}.* Rome: Food and Agriculture Organization, 1988. (FAO Food and Nutrition Series; 23).

[5] Armstrong B K, Davies R E, Nicol D J, Van Merwyk A J, Larwood C J. Hematological vitamin B_{12} and folate studies on Seventh Day Adventist vegetarians. *Am J Clin Nutr* 1974; **27**: 712–718.

[6] Abdulla M, Anderson I, Asp N-G. *et al.* Nutrient intake and health status of vegans. Chemical analysis of diets using the duplicate portion sampling technique. *Am J Clin Nutr* 1981; **34**: 2464–2477.

[7] Baker S J, Mathan V I. Evidence regarding the minimal daily requirement of dietary vitamin B_{12}. *Am J Clin Nutr* 1981; **34**: 2423–2433.

[8] Sullivan L W, Herbert V. Studies on the minimum daily requirement for vitamin B_{12}. Hematopoietic responses to 0.1 micrograms of cyanocobalamin or coenzyme B_{12} and comparison of their relative potency. *New Engl J Med* 1965; **272**: 340–346.

[9] Cooper B A, Lowenstein L. Vitamin B_{12}-folate interrelationships in megaloblastic anaemia. *Brit J Haematol* 1966; **12**: 283–296.

[10] Bates C J, Prentice A. Vitamins, minerals and essential trace elements. In: Bennett P *et al*, eds. *Drugs and Human Lactation*. Amsterdam: Elsevier, 1988; 433–493.

[11] Jadhav M, Webb J K G, Vaishnava A, Baker S J. Vitamin B_{12} deficiency in Indian infants. A clinical syndrome. *Lancet* 1962; **2**: 903–907.

[12] Specker B L, Black A, Allen L, Morrow F. Vitamin B_{12}: low milk concentrations are related to low serum concentrations in vegetarian women and to methyl-malonic aciduria in their infants. *Am J Clin Nutr* 1990; **52**: 1072–1076.

14. Folate

14.1 **Functions and essentiality** Folic acid (pteroyl glutamic acid) is the parent molecule for a large number of derivatives collectively known as folates. They are involved in a number of single carbon transfer reactions, especially in the synthesis of purines, pyrimidines, glycine and methionine. The characteristic sign of folate deficiency is megaloblastosis, with abnormal, multilobed neutrophil nuclei and giant platelets in peripheral blood[1]. Other rapidly regenerating tissues such as the intestinal mucosa may also suffer, while in babies and young children, growth may be affected.

14.2 **Forms and bioavailability**

14.2.1 Although most experimental studies of human requirements have used free pteroyl glutamic acid, this chemical species is not present in food or human tissues unless added as a dietary supplement. It is physiologically inactive until it has been reduced to dihydrofolic acid, when it can enter the body's folate pool. The main naturally occurring forms are tetrahydrofolate (THF), 5-methyl tetrahydrofolate (5MeTHF), and 10-formyltetrahydrofolate, each with side chains of up to 11 glutamic acid residues. Polyglutamate forms based mainly on 5MeTHF predominate in fresh food, but on storage these slowly break down to monoglutamates and oxidise to less available folates. Before polyglutamates can be absorbed, they must be hydrolysed by the τ-glutamyl hydrolase ("conjugase") present in the small intestine. The main circulating form is the monoglutamate 5-methyl tetrahydrofolate, but polyglutamates are the forms that are active inside cells, including those of liver, where folates are present in relatively large amounts.

14.2.2 Rich food sources of folate include liver, yeast extract and green leafy vegetables and a diet that is rich in other B vitamins and in vitamin C is usually rich in folate too. However, many estimates of human folate intakes are unreliable. This is partly because the amounts in food measured with *Lactobacillus casei* may be incorrect unless the assay conditions are exactly appropriate. Some assays have separately reported "free" and "total" folate (the fractions reacting in the *L. casei* assay before and after deconjugation), but the concept of "free" folate has now been abandoned since its measurement is unreliable and humans can deconjugate and utilise polyglutamates to a considerable extent. Microbiological assessment of "total" folate is gradually being superseded by HPLC measurements of all the different forms, of which 5-MeTHF may be the best utilised.

14.3 **Requirements** Biochemical evidence of folate status can be obtained from a variety of indices. The lower limit of normal serum folate concentration is usually accepted as 3 ng/ml[2]. Tissue levels are better indicated by the concentration of folate in red cells, which is buffered against short-term changes. Red cell levels below 100 ng/ml are considered to be severely deficient, while values between 100 and 150 ng/ml (μg/L) indicate marginal status[3]. Liver levels greater than 3 μg/g indicate adequate reserves[4].

14.3.1 *Adults* When folate deficiency was induced experimentally in a human subject by eliminating practically all known sources of folate from an otherwise well-balanced diet to leave an intake of only 5 μg/d, the symptoms were reversed by 50 μg pteroylglutamic acid/d[5,6]. Pteroyl-glutamic acid at intakes of 50–100 μg/d also cured naturally-occurring folate-deficiency megaloblastic anaemia, and maintained small but stable folate stores in cancer patients whose treatment necessitated precise control of their folate supply[7]. The Panel set the LRNI at 100 μg/d.

14.3.2 Careful estimates of folate intakes and the distribution of folate status indices in Canada have shown that with a mean folate intake from food of 150–200 μg/d, the folate content of autopsied liver samples was consistently greater than 3 μg/g[4,8]. No more than 8–10 per cent of this population's red cell folate levels were below 150 μg/ml, and overt signs of clinical or haematological folate deficiency were (as in the UK) very uncommon[9]. Median folate intakes in Britain were 300 μg/d by men (range 145–562 μg/d) and 209 μg/d by women (range 95–385 μg/d)[10]. The Panel saw no reason for men and women to have different reference values, because the arguably smaller requirement by women, based on their smaller lean body mass, was offset by a potentially greater need during reproduction, especially during the periconceptunal period (see 14.3.4). The same RNI, of 200 μg/d, was therefore set for adults of both sexes (Table 14.1).

14.3.3 *Infants and children* Folate-deficiency anaemia has not been reported in breast-fed infants, and even folate-deficient mothers secrete sufficient to cover the needs of their infants. Breast milk provides 40 μg/d, but a formula containing 60–70 μg/L (50–60 μg/d) produced lower red cell folate levels than did breast milk, but no differences in haemoglobin concentrations, weight gain or growth rate[11]. The Panel therefore decided to set an RNI of 50 μg/d for formula-fed infants. For older children, the Panel interpolated values between this and the RNI for adults (Table 14.1) The values were well above 3.6 μg folate/kg body weight—an amount which has been shown to maintain plasma folate levels at a low but acceptable level and to ensure freedom from overt folate deficiency in children[12].

14.3.4 *Pregnancy* There is evidence for an increase in folate requirements in late pregnancy, as indicated by the widespread occurrence of bone marrow megaloblastosis, even in otherwise well-nourished Western societies, before maternal folate supplementation during pregnancy became widespread during the 1960s[13]. The mean amount of extra folic acid needed to maintain plasma and red cell folate levels at or above those of non-pregnant women was 100 μg/d[14,15], and the Panel raised the DRV by this amount throughout pregnancy. The Medical Research Council is currently investigating the possibility that folate supplements during the periconceptunal period may reduce the incidence of neural tube defects in infants.

Table 14.1 *Dietary Reference Values for Folate* (μg/d)

Age	Lower Reference Nutrient Intake	Estimated Average Requirement	Reference Nutrient Intake
0–3 months	30	40	50
4–6 months	30	40	50
7–9 months	30	40	50
10–12 months	30	40	50
1–3 years	35	50	70
4–6 years	50	75	100
7–10 years	75	110	150
Males			
11–14 years	100	150	200
15–18 years	100	150	200
19–50 years	100	150	200
50+ years	100	150	200
Females			
11–14 years	100	150	200
15–18 years	100	150	200
19–50 years	100	150	200
50+ years	100	150	200
Pregnancy			+100
Lactation:			
0–4 months			+60
4+ months			+60

14.3.5 *Lactation* The amount of folate secreted in breast milk averages about 40 μg/d at peak breast-milk production, and this needs to be replaced from the diet during lactation[16]. The Panel decided to increase the DRV by 60 μg/d to allow for incomplete absorption and utilisation of folates from the diet.

14.3.6 *The elderly* Although folate deficiency occurs more frequently in the elderly than in young adults[17], there is little evidence that healthy elderly people have an increased requirement. Many elderly people have low intakes of folate-containing foods, however, and they may have a variety of medical conditions which increase their requirements[13].

14.4 **Guidance on high intakes** Claims have been made that very high folate intakes may result in mood changes[18] but have received little or no subsequent support. High intakes may reduce zinc absorption[19], and folate supplements given to patients with developing vitamin B_{12} deficiency may obscure a correct diagnosis and delay the appropriate treatment. Nevertheless, both the dangers of toxicity and the possible benefits from folate megadosage seem slight.

14.5 **Research needs** There is a need for improvements in the techniques for the measurement of food folates and the estimation of their availability, and for new studies of the relationship between food folate intakes and indices of folate status, especially for "high risk" groups such as pregnant women. Because folates apart from folic acid itself are readily destroyed by nitrite under acid conditions, the dependence of dietary folate requirements on the nitrite content of the food and water supply needs further exploration.

14.6 References

[1] Rodriguez M S. A conspectus of research on folacin requirements of man. *J Nutr* 1978; **108**: 1983–2103.

[2] Ratnas Thien K, Blair J A, Leeming R J, Cooke W T, Melikian V. Serum folates in man. *J Clin Path* 1977; **30**: 438–448.

[3] Sauberlich H E, Skala J H, Dowdy R P. *Laboratory Tests for the Assessment of Nutritional Status*. Cleveland: CRC Press, 1974; 49–60.

[4] Hoppner K, Lampi B. Folate levels in human liver from autopsies in Canada. *Am J Clin Nutr* 1980; **33**: 862–864.

[5] Herbert V. Experimental nutritional folate deficiency in man. *Trans Assoc Am Phys* 1962; **75**: 307–320.

[6] Herbert V. Folic acid requirement in adults (including pregnant and lactating females). In: *Folic acid, Biochemistry and Physiology in Relation to the Human Nutrition Requirement*. Washington DC: National Academy of Sciences, 1977; 247–255.

[7] Gailani S D. Studies of folate deficiency in patients with neoplastic diseases. *Cancer Res* 1970; **30**: 327–333.

[8] Hoppner K, Lampi B, Smith D C. Data on folacin activity in foods: availability, applications and limitations. In: *Folic acid, Biochemistry and Physiology in Relation to the Human Nutrition Requirement*. Washington DC: National Academy of Sciences, 1977; 69–81.

[9] Cooper B A. Reassessment of folic acid requirements. In: White P, Selvey N, eds. *Nutrition in Transition: Proceedings of the Western Hemisphere Congress* no 5. Monroe, W I: American Medical Association, 1978; 281–288.

[10] Gregory J, Foster K, Tyler H, Wiseman M. *The Dietary and Nutritional Survey of British Adults*. London: HMSO, 1990.

[11] Foged N, Lillquist K, Rolschau J, Blaabjerg O. Effect of folic acid supplementation on small-for-gestational age infants born at term. *Eur J Paediat* 1989; **149**: 65–67.

[12] Asfour R, Wahbeh N, Waslien C I, Guindi S, Darby W J. Folacin requirement of children. III. Normal infants. *Am J Clin Nutr* 1977; **30**: 1098–1105.

[13] Chanarin I. *The Megaloblastic Anaemias* (2nd ed). Oxford: Blackwell Scientific, 1979.

[14] Hanson H, Rybo G. Folic acid dosage in prophylactic treatment during pregnancy. *Acta Obst Gyn Scand* 1967; **46** (suppl. 17): 107–112.

[15] Chanarin I, Rothman D, Ward A, Perry J. Folate status and requirement during pregnancy. *Br Med J* 1968; **2**: 390–394.

[16] Ek J. Plasma, red cell and breast milk folacin concentration in lactating women. *Am J Clin Nutr* 1983; **38**: 929–935.

[17] Sneath P, Chanarin I, Hodkinson H M, McPherson C K, Reynolds E H. Folate status in a geriatric population and its relation to dementia. *Age, Ageing*. 1973; **2**: 177–182.

[18] Hunter R, Barnes J, Oakley H F, Matthews D M. Toxicity of folic acid given in pharmacological doses to healthy volunteers. *Lancet* 1970; **1**: 61–62.

[19] Simmer K, Iles C A, James C, Thompson R P H. Are iron-folate supplements harmful? *Am J Clin Nutr* 1987; **45**: 122–125.

15. Pantothenic Acid

15.1 **Function and essentiality** Pantothenic acid is a part of the coenzyme A molecule which plays an essential role in the catabolism of all the macronutrients to yield energy. Pantothenic acid is very widely distributed in animal and plant tissues. Experimental dietary deficiency of pantothenic acid in humans leads to fatigue, headache, dizziness, muscle weakness and gastrointestinal disturbances[1]. There is, however, no convincing evidence of pantothenic acid deficiency in humans other than when fed an experimental diet.

15.2 **Intakes** Estimates from National Food Survey records gave mean daily intakes of pantothenic acid of 5.1 mg in 1979[2] and 6.07 mg in 1986[3]. The median intake from food sources by British adult males was 6.1 mg/d and 4.4 mg/d for adult females. British mothers have been reported to have mean intakes of pantothenic acid between 3.4 and 5.3 mg/d during pregnancy and lactation, though these values could have underestimated intakes by up to 0.6 mg/d[4].

15.3 **Requirements** No biochemical method has yet been accepted for determining pantothenate status in humans. Measurements have been made of blood levels and urinary excretion of pantothenic acid but it is difficult to interpret them in terms of dietary needs[5]. The Panel therefore derived no DRVs, but as there are no signs of pantothenic acid deficiency in the UK, intakes between 3 and 7 mg/d must be adequate, even during pregnancy and lactation.

15.4 **Infants** The DHSS recommend that infant formulas should contain at least 2.0 mg pantothenic acid/L, which would provide 1.7 mg/d[6]. The concentration is equivalent to about 3 mg pantothenic acid/1,000 kcal and is similar to the 2.9 mg/1,000 kcal of the average diet in this country. The Panel endorsed this recommendation.

15.5 **Guidance on high intakes** Ralli and Dumm reported no toxic signs after giving young men 10 g calcium pantothenate daily for six weeks[7], although such doses may cause diarrhoea and gastrointestinal disturbances[8].

15.6 **References**

[1] Hodges R E, Øhlson M A, Bean W B. Pantothenic acid deficiency in man. *J Clin Invest* 1958; **37**: 1642–1657.

[2] Bull N L, Buss D H. Biotin, pantothenic acid and vitamin E in the British household food supply. *Hum Nutr: App Nutr* 1982; **36A**: 190–196.

[3] Lewis J, Buss D H. Trace nutrients. 5. Minerals and vitamins in the British household food supply. *Br J Nutr* 1988; **60**: 413–424.

[4] Black A E, Wiles S J, Paul A A. The nutrient intakes of pregnant and lactating mothers of good socioeconomic status in Cambridge, United Kingdom: some implications for recommended daily allowances of minor nutrients. *Br J Nutr* 1986; **56:** 59–72.

[5] Fox H M. Pantothenic acid. In: Machlin L, ed. *Handbook of Vitamins: Nutritional Biochemical and Clinical Aspects.* New York: Marcel Dekker, 1984; 437–457.

[6] Department of Health and Social Security. *Artificial Feeds for the Young Infant.* London: HMSO, 1980. (Reports on health and social subjects; 18).

[7] Ralli E P, Dumm M E. Relation of pantothenic acid to adrenal cortical function. *Vitam Horm* 1953, **11:** 133–158.

[8] Miller D R, Hayes K C. Vitamin excess and toxicity. In: Hathcock J, ed. *Nutritional Toxicology.* Vol 1. New York: Academic Press, 1982; 81–133.

16. Biotin

16.1 **Function and essentiality** Biotin was originally discovered as part of a complex which promoted the growth of yeast. It was also found to be the protective or curative factor in "egg white injury" which can be caused in man and experimental animals by feeding large amounts of raw egg white: the glycoprotein avidin in egg white binds biotin with a remarkably high affinity. Metabolically, biotin is of central importance in lipogenesis, gluconeogenesis and the catabolism of branched chain amino acids. Apart from patients maintained on total parenteral nutrition for long periods, deficiency is not known in man except in people who consumed large amounts of uncooked eggs and thus of avidin. They developed a fine scaly dermatitis and hair loss (alopecia). Histology of the skin showed an absence of sebaceous glands and atrophy of the hair follicles. In experimental studies of biotin depletion, diets providing up to 30 per cent of energy intake from raw egg white have been used. The subjects developed glossitis, anorexia, nausea, hallucinations, depression and somnolence, as well as a fine scaly desquamating dermatitis. Urinary excretion of biotin fell to about 10 per cent of that in subjects eating a normal diet. Injection of biotin reversed all the clinical signs[1].

16.2 **Sources** The vitamin is widely distributed in many foods, and is also synthesised by intestinal flora. Studies *in vivo* show that there is significant absorption of biotin from the proximal and mid-transverse colon, suggesting that biotin from intestinal bacteria can be absorbed[2]. The extent to which it is available is, however, not known, for the faecal excretion of biotin is 3–6 times greater than the intake.

16.3 **Requirements** The signs of biotin deficiency that have been observed in patients receiving total parenteral nutrition for prolonged periods after major resection of the gut have resolved following the provision of 60–200 μg biotin, but there have been no studies of the actual amounts of biotin needed[3]. The average intake by British men is 39 μg/d (range 15–70 μg) and by women is 26 μg/d (range 10–58 μg)[4]. These amounts prevent deficiency, and the average requirement must lie below these values. Although the Panel could set no DRVs on such limited evidence, they agreed that biotin intakes between 10 and 200 μg/d were both safe and adequate.

16.4 References

1 Sydenstricker V P, Singal S A, Briggs A P, DeVaughn N M, Isbell H. Observations on the 'Egg White Injury' in man and its cure with a biotin concentrate. *J Am Med Assoc* 1942; **118:** 1199–1120.

2 Bowman B B, Rosenberg I H. Biotin absorption by distal rat small intestine. *J Nutr* 1987; **117:** 2121–2126.

[3] Mock D M, Baswell D L, Baker H, Holman R T, Sweetman L. Biotin deficiency complicating parenteral alimentation: diagnosis, metabolic repercussions and treatment. *J Pediatr* 1985; **106:** 762–769.

[4] Gregory J, Foster K, Tyler H, Wiseman M. *The Dietary and Nutritional Survey of British Adults.* London: HMSO, 1990.

17. Vitamin C

17.1 **Functions and essentiality**

17.1.1 Essential and undisputed roles of vitamin C (ascorbic acid) in man are to prevent scurvy and to aid wound healing. It also assists in the absorption of non-haem iron, and because of its potential for reaction with destructive free radical containing oxygen, it is an important antioxidant. However, ascorbic acid may exhibit pro-oxidant properties in the presence of certain metal ions and oxygen, and these pro-and anti-oxidant activities are reflected in its role as a cofactor, modulator or protective agent in a series of essential mixed function oxidase enzyme reactions.

17.1.2 Vitamin C is one of the most labile nutrients in the diet, easily destroyed by oxygen, metal ions, increased pH, heat or light. The richest sources are citrus and soft fruits and the growing points of vegetables, whereas unsprouted cereals and their products contain virtually none.

17.1.3 The most definitive evidence for essentiality has come from experimental depletion and repletion studies in adult human volunteers. In the MRC Sheffield study[1] and in Iowa[2] the most characteristic clinical signs of diet-induced vitamin C deficiency were failure of hair follicle eruption, the occurrence of petechial haemorrhages spreading to sheet haemorrhage on the limbs, and bleeding gums. Impairment of connective tissue formation within wound repair tissue was frequently seen, and a wide range of other signs and symptoms was reported, but less often.

17.1.4 Many studies have raised the question of whether vitamin C has beneficial effects on normal human subjects at intakes and tissue levels considerably greater than those needed to prevent or cure scurvy. These studies have included examination of indices as diverse as histamine removal[3]; cholesterol turnover[4]; physical working capacity[5,6]; immune function[7]; male fertility[8]; gingival collagen[9]; nitrosamine and carcinogenesis prevention[10] and selenium or iron utilisation[11,12]. Despite scientific concern about such questions, it is impossible to base estimates of requirements directly upon the evidence of these studies, partly because the evidence is conflicting in many areas, partly because those studies which have noted a positive benefit of vitamin C supplements have not defined the minimum dietary requirement needed to achieve it, and partly because specific design features have made the interpretation difficult in many cases. Because of these and other difficulties, the Panel decided to base their estimates of vitamin C requirements mainly upon the prevention of scurvy, on vitamin C turnover studies, and on biochemical indices of vitamin C status in man.

17.2 **Requirements**

17.2.1 In normal adults, about 2.7 per cent of the exchangeable body pool of ascorbic acid is degraded each day[13,14]. This is independent of body pool size, so that at zero intake there is a first-order rate of loss from the tissues. When the body pool falls to 300 mg or less there is evidence of impaired function[2]. Leukocyte or buffy coat vitamin C levels generally change in parallel with those of most other organs and tissues, and a lower limit of 15 $\mu g/10^8$ cells is frequently accepted as an indicator of deficiency. Plasma vitamin C levels are more sensitive to recent intake, with values less than 11 $\mu mol/L$ (0.2 mg/100 ml) indicating biochemical depletion[15].

17.2.2 The amount of vitamin C required by human adults (mainly males) to prevent and cure scorbutic signs and symptoms has been carefully investigated. Nearly all individuals who received no more than 1 mg/d for 3–6 months from a specially vitamin C-depleted but otherwise adequate diet developed mild clinical signs of scurvy, whereas those who received 10 mg/d did not. 10 mg/d was also sufficient to cure clinical signs of scurvy in an already-depleted group[1]. Although three subjects who received 10 mg/d for 23 weeks and then only 3.2–4.5 mg/d for 28 weeks showed no clinical signs, a recent study has indicated that an intake of 5 mg/d may be insufficient for gum protection[16].

17.2.3 These studies indicated that the requirement to prevent and cure scurvy in men is less than 10 mg/d. The minimum requirement of women has not been determined, but as women maintain higher blood levels of vitamin C for a given intake than men, their requirements, except perhaps during reproduction, are likely to be less. However, although 10 mg/d is sufficient to protect against scurvy, it is not sufficient to maintain measurable amounts of ascorbate in the plasma, and it leads to a low buffy coat ascorbate level. The Panel therefore judged the safety margin to be insufficient with this intake, and turned to the consideration of biochemical indices.

17.2.4 *Adults* Figure 17.1 shows the sigmoidal relationship between vitamin C intake and plasma ascorbate levels[17,19]. Both men and women exhibit very low plasma levels at intakes between 0 and 30 mg/d, which rise steeply between 30 and 70 mg/d, and approach an upper plateau between 70 and 100 mg/d. Measurable amounts of ascorbic acid begin to circulate in the plasma of most people at an intake of 40 mg/d, and this is available for transfer between the tissues and to sites of depletion or damage. The Panel therefore selected this as the RNI for both men and women. Women probably need less when not in a reproductive cycle, but more during reproduction, including the periconceptual period. An adult will maintain an exchangeable body pool of about 900 mg at this intake, which can provide at least 1 month's safety interval, even on a zero intake, before the pool falls to 300 mg[20]. An LRNI of 10 mg/d for adults is compatible with studies of scurvy prevention in the UK[1], and elsewhere, on the basis that protection against clinical deficiency signs is provided but no margin of safety against further loss. By interpolation, the EAR was calculated as 25 mg/d (Table 17.1).

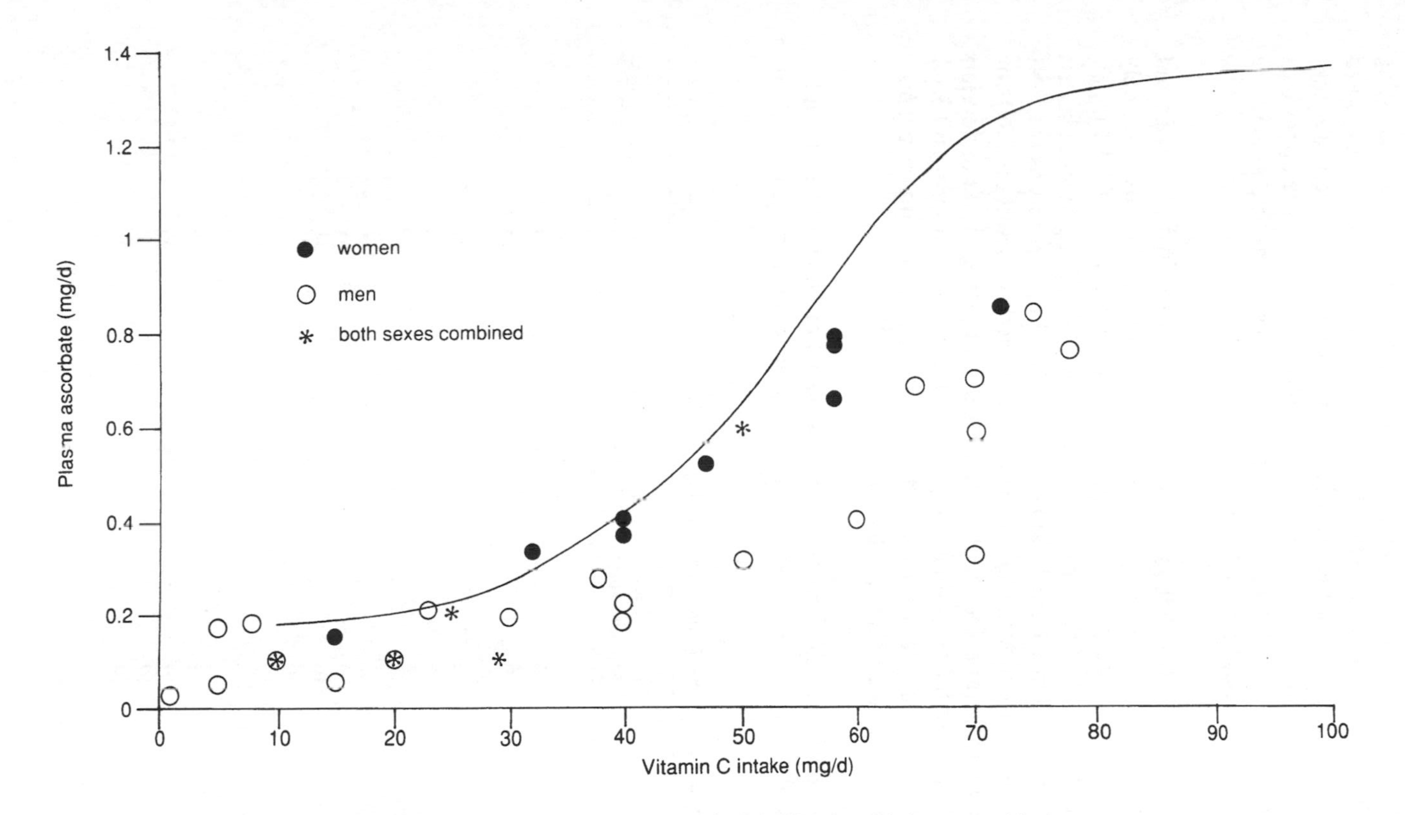

Figure 17.1 Relationship between plasma ascorbic acid concentration and vitamin C intake, in adult human subjects

The continuous line represents a study of elderly women by Newton *et al*[23]. The individual points are mean values compiled from other published studies on this relationship in adult subjects (the data from these represented only part of the range being considered).

● :women O:men
X:both sexes combined.

17.2.5 *Pregnancy and lactation* During pregnancy there is a moderate extra drain on tissue stores, especially towards the final stages of pregnancy, since the fetus concentrates the vitamin at the expense of maternal stores and circulating vitamin levels. The Panel has increased the RNI by 10 mg/d during the third trimester for this purpose. During lactation, an intake of 70 mg/d ensures that maternal stores are maintained and that breast milk levels are in the upper half of the physiological range for human milk. This represents an increase in the DRVs of 30 mg/d throughout lactation.

17.2.6 *Children* Clinical scurvy has not been observed in fully breast-fed infants, even in communities where mothers' vitamin C intakes are extremely low. Although ascorbate in breast milk may vary from 30 to 80 mg/L depending on the intake of the mother[21], the provision of 25 mg/d from breast milk appears to be adequate for infants, and the Panel has set this as the RNI for infants. RNIs for children were interpolated between this and the RNI for adults (Table 17.1). Infants fed on dried milks providing 5 mg/d do not develop scurvy, and this, together with their body pool size estimates, support an LRNI of 6 mg/d for infants. Values for children have been scaled down proportionately from those for adults (Table 17.1).

17.2.7 *The elderly* In the UK, elderly people may have low blood vitamin C levels, low body stores, and occasionally even overt clinical deficiency signs.

Table 17.1 *Dietary Reference Values for Vitamin C* (mg/d)

Age	Lower Reference Nutrient Intake	Estimated Average Requirement	Reference Nutrient Intake
0–3 months	6	15	25
4–6 months	6	15	25
7–9 months	6	15	25
10–12 months	6	15	25
1–3 years	8	20	30
4–6 years	8	20	30
7–10 years	8	20	30
Males			
11–14 years	9	22	35
15–18 years	10	25	40
19–50 years	10	25	40
50+ years	10	25	40
Females			
11–14 years	9	22	35
15–18 years	10	25	40
19–50 years	10	25	40
50+ years	10	25	40
Pregnancy			+10*
Lactation:			
0–4 months			+30
4+ months			+30

*Last trimester only.

However, most deficient individuals have persistently low intakes, and there is no compelling evidence for an increased requirement in old age[23,24].

17.2.8 *Smokers* Several recent studies have indicated that smokers have an increased turnover of vitamin C. To maintain their body pool and circulating levels near those of non-smokers, their intake would need to be greater by up to 80 mg/d[25,26].

17.3 Guidance on high intakes Claims that intakes of vitamin C above those necessary to cure scurvy can protect from, or cure, various diseases, tissue damage or improve general health, are still being assessed. Possible risks associated with high intakes include diarrhoea at intakes of grams/d; increased production of oxalate, and hence of kidney stones in a small group of individuals with an unusually high propensity for oxalate synthesis[27]; and 'systemic conditioning', whereby the sudden cessation of high intakes may precipitate scurvy, through enhanced turnover.

17.4 Research needs Future research effort should include a) further classification of the biological functions of vitamin C; b) further studies on vitamin C turnover; c) studies of the requirements of different groups within the population, and d) identification of possible benefits or detrimental effects of high intakes.

17.5 References

[1] Bartley W, Krebs H A, O'Brien J R P. *Vitamin C Requirement of Human Adults.* London: HMSO, 1953. (MRC Special Report Series; 280).

[2] Hodges R E, Baker E M, Hood J, Sauberlich H E, March SC. Experimental scurvy in man. *Am J Clin Nutr* 1969; **22:** 535-548.

[3] Clemetson C A B. Histamine and ascorbic acid in human blood. *J Nutr* 1980; **110:** 662-668.

[4] Ginter E, Cerna O, Budlovsky J *et al.* Effect of ascorbic acid on plasma cholesterol in humans in a long-term experiment. *Int J Vit Nutr Res* 1977; **47:** 123-124.

[5] Suboticanec-Buzina K, Buzina R, Brubacher G, Sapunar J, Christeller S. Vitamin C status and physical working capacity in adolescents. *Int J Vit Nutr Res* 1984; **54:** 55-60.

[6] van der Beek E J, van Dokkum W, Schrijver J, Wesstra A, Kistemaker C, Hermus R J. Controlled vitamin C restriction and physical performance in volunteers. *J Am Coll Nutr* 1990; **9:** 332-339.

[7] Anderson R, Oosthuizen R, Maritz R, Theron A, van Reusberg A J. The effects of increasing weekly doses of ascorbate on certain cellular and humoral immune functions in normal volunteers. *Am J Clin Nutr* 1980; **33:** 71-76.

[8] Dawson E B, Harris W A, Powell L C. Relationship between ascorbic acid and male fertility. *World Rev Nutr Diet* 1990; **62:** 1-26.

[9] Buzina R, Aurer-Kozelj J, Srdak-Jorgic E, Buhler E, Gey K F. Increase of gingival hydroxproline and proline by improvement of ascorbic acid status in man. *Int J Vit Nutr Res* 1986; **56:** 367-372.

[10] Tannenbaum S R, Wishnok J S. Inhibition of nitrosamine formation by ascorbic acid. *Ann N Y Acad Sci* 1987; **498:** 354-363.

[11] Martin R F, Young V R, Blumberg J, Janghorbani M. Ascorbic acid-selenite interactions in humans studied with an oral dose of $^{74}SeO_3^{2-}$. *Am J Clin Nutr* 1989; **49:** 862–869.

[12] Hunt J R, Mullen L M, Lykken G I, Gallagher S K, Nielson F H. Ascorbic acid: effect on ongoing iron absorption and status in iron-depleted young women. *Am J Clin Nutr* 1990; **51:** 649–655.

[13] Baker E M, Hodges R E, Hood J, Sauberlich H E, March S C, Canham J E. Metabolism of ^{14}C- and ^{3}H- labelled L-ascorbic acid in human scurvy. *Am J Clin Nutr* 1971; **24:** 444–454.

[14] Kallner A, Hartmann D, Hornig D. Steady state-turnover and body pool of ascorbic acid in man. *Am J Clin Nutr* 1979; **32:** 530–539.

[15] Sauberlich H E. Vitamin C status: methods and findings. *Ann N Y Acad Sci* 1975; **258:** 438–500.

[16] Jacob R A, Omaye S T, Skala J H, Leggott P J, Rothman D L, Murray P A. Experimental vitamin C depletion and supplementation in young men. Nutrient interactions and dental health effects. *Ann N Y Acad Sci* 1987; **498:** 333–346.

[17] Basu T K, Schorah C J. *Vitamin C in Health and Disease.* Westport, Connecticut: AVI Publishing Co Inc, 1982; 61–92.

[18] Newton H M V, Morgan D B, Schorah C J, Hullin R P. Relation between intake and plasma concentration of vitamin C in elderly women. *Br Med J* 1983; **287:** 1429.

[19] Bates C J, Rutishauser I H E, Black A E, Paul A A, Mandal A R, Patnaik B K. Long-term vitamin status and dietary intake of healthy elderly subjects. *Br J Nutr* 1979; **42:** 43–56.

[20] Olson J A, Hodges R E. Recommended dietary intakes (RDI) of vitamin C in humans. *Am J Clin Nutr* 1987; **45:** 693–703.

[21] Bates C J, Prentice A. Vitamins, minerals and essential trace elements. In: Bennett P *et al*, eds. *Drugs and Human Lactation.* Amsterdam: Elsevier, 1988; 433–493.

[22] Bates C J, Prentice A M, Prentice A, Lamb W H, Whitehead R G. The effect of vitamin C supplementation on lactating women in Keneba, a West African rural community. *Int J Vit Nutr Res* 1983; **53:** 68–76.

[23] Newton H M V, Schorah C J, Habibzadeh N, Morgan D B, Hullin R P. The cause and correction of low blood vitamin C concentrations in the elderly. *Am J Clin Nutr* 1985; **42:** 656–659.

[24] Neale R J, Lim H, Turner J, Freeman C, Kemm J R. The excretion of large vitamin C loads in young and elderly subjects: an ascorbic acid tolerance test. *Age Ageing* 1988; **17:** 35–41.

[25] Kallner A, Hartmann D, Hornig D. On the requirements of ascorbic acid in man: steady-state turnover and body pool in smokers. *Am J Clin Nutr* 1981; **34:** 1347–1355.

[26] Smith J L, Hodges R E. Serum levels of vitamin C in relation to dietary and supplemental intake of vitamin C in smokers and non-smokers. *Ann N Y Acad Sci* 1987; **498:** 144–152.

[27] Balcke P, Schmidt P, Zazgarnik J, Kopsa H, Haubenstock A. Ascorbic acid aggravates secondary hyper-oxalemia in patients on chronic hemodialysis. *Ann Intern Med* 1984; **100:** 344–345.

18. Vitamin D

18.1 Function and essentiality

18.1.1 The two main forms of vitamin D are ergocalciferol (vitamin D_2) and cholecalciferol (vitamin D_3). The only role of vitamin D is as a precursor of 25-hydroxyvitamin D (25-OHD) and 1,25-dihydroxyvitamin D (1,25-$(OH)_2$D). 25-OHD occurs almost exclusively in plasma, while 1,25-$(OH)_2$D is formed in the kidney (and placenta of pregnant animals) and is the active form of the vitamin which is involved in calcium homeostasis. Plasma calcium is maintained within narrow limits, in part by varying the proportions of dietary calcium absorbed and excreted, thereby ensuring a plentiful supply of this element for bone mineralisation (see Chapter 22). In addition, 1,25-$(OH)_2$D may have a direct effect on bone.

18.1.2 Prolonged deficiency of vitamin D in children results in rickets, the main signs of which are skeletal deformity with bone pain or tenderness, and muscle weakness. In florid rickets there may be hypocalcaemia and tooth eruption may be delayed. Rachitic children show reduced bone growth, are anaemic, and are prone to respiratory infections. Plasma 25-OHD concentrations in rickets range from not detectable to about 8 ng/ml[1].

18.1.3 In adults, hypovitaminosis D presents as osteomalacia, with muscle weakness and bone tenderness or pain in the spine, shoulder, ribs or pelvis. Plasma 25-OHD concentrations in osteomalacia are less than 4 ng/ml and plasma levels of calcium and phosphate may be reduced.

18.2 Vitamin D formation

18.2.1 Ergocalciferol is derived by ultraviolet (UV) irradiation of the ergosterol that is widely distributed in plants, fungi and lower life-forms but it does not occur naturally in higher vertebrates. Cholecalciferol is derived from the action of UV irradiation on 7-dehydrocholesterol in the skin in animals including man. Hypovitaminosis arises both from inadequate exposure to UV radiation and from increased metabolism of vitamin D due to factors such as low calcium intake or calcium absorption[2]. It can normally be corrected by adequate exposure to sunlight or by vitamin D in non-pharmacological doses.

18.2.2 There are few dietary sources of vitamin D. Fatty fish such as herring, mackerel, pilchards, sardines and tuna are rich sources but are not major contributors to the diet. The only other useful sources are eggs and fortified foods including margarine (which is required by law to contain vitamin D), some yogurts and breakfast cereals. The amount of vitamin D in meat is uncertain, as modern analytical methods have not been applied to obtaining this information, but it is believed to be very low. The average dietary intake of vitamin D by adults in Britain is about 3 μg/d, ranging from 0.5 to 8 μg/d[3]. For most people in the UK the main source is from the action of sunlight on the skin.

18.2.3 Solar UV radiation varies with latitude, time of year and time of day. Complete cloud cover reduces the energy of the radiation by 50 per cent and about 40 per cent of available UV radiation can be detected in shade. There is no UV radiation of the appropriate wavelength (290 nm–310 nm) in Britain from the end of October to the end of March. For the remaining months of the year 60 per cent of the effective UV radiation occurs between 11.00 am and 3.00 pm, but is lower in the north than the south. Thus for normal individuals exposed only to natural UV radiation there is a seasonal variation in plasma 25-OHD concentrations[4], with summer levels correlated with the amount of UV radiation available, the extent of the exposure to sunlight, and the amount of skin exposed, and winter levels dependent upon the amount of vitamin D_3 formed during the previous summer[5]. Vitamin D status in the UK therefore depends very much on the time spent out of doors during the day, which itself depends on mobility, institutionalization, inclement weather and cultural influences on skin exposure.

18.3 **Requirements**

18.3.1 *Adults (18–65 years of age)* Plasma 25-OHD normally ranges from 15 ng/ml to 35 ng/ml in summer and from 8 ng/ml to 18 ng/ml in winter[4]. No dietary intake is therefore necessary for individuals living a normal life-style, for whom the Panel set no DRVs (Table 18.1). For those confined indoors the Panel agreed an RNI for vitamin D of 10 μg/d.

18.3.2 *Infants and children* Term infants who are receiving infant formula and who are weaned at the normal time to a normal British diet do not develop nutritional rickets because they receive about 8.5 μg/d from the infant formula and in general this maintains plasma 25-OHD concentration at an acceptable 20 ng/ml[6]. Breast-fed babies show a seasonal variation in plasma 25-OHD, and for babies born in the autumn the concentration can decline to very low levels because winter milk contains little vitamin D[7,8]. The Panel therefore endorsed the view of the Third COMA Report on Present Day Practice in Infant Feeding that lactating mothers should receive supplementary vitamin D to ensure continuing adequate levels of the vitamin in their breast milk[9]. Vitamin D intakes usually decline on weaning because most weaning foods (excluding manufactured products which are fortified) are low in vitamin D as is whole cow milk. Therefore plasma 25-OHD may be lower in the second 6 months of life than in the first 6 months[10]. Those between 6 months and 3 years may be particularly vulnerable to vitamin D depletion because of the rate at which calcium is being laid down in bone at this time, and the limited availability of UV radiation for many children. After this age, children (apart from some of Asian origin) have a satisfactory vitamin D status with plasma 25-OHD ranging from 13 ng/ml in mid winter to over 20 ng/ml in late summer[11], and need no dietary vitamin D (Table 18.1). The Panel endorsed the view of COMA that it remains prudent for infants and young children up to at least 2 years of age to receive supplementary vitamin D (currently providing 7 μg/d)[9].

Table 18.1 *Dietary Reference Values for Vitamin D* (μg/d)

Age	Reference Nutrient Intake†
0–3 months	8.5
4–6 months	8.5
7–9 months	7
10–12 months	7
1–3 years	7
4–6 years	0*
7–10 years	0*
Males	
11–14 years	0*
15–18 years	0*
19–50 years	0*
50+ years	10**
Females	
11–14 years	0*
15–18 years	0*
19–50 years	0*
50+ years	10**
Pregnancy	10
Lactation:	
0–4 months	10
4+ months	10

†May require supplementation of the diet.
*Certain at-risk individuals or groups may require dietary vitamin D (para 18.3.6).
**For the population aged 65 or more only.

18.3.4 *Pregnancy* Plasma 25-OHD in pregnancy shows a seasonal variation with different ranges reported by different studies. There is a significant correlation between maternal and cord blood 25-OHD, with the values in cord blood being lower than in the maternal circulation. In Scotland but not in the south of England infants of women not taking vitamin D supplements have a higher incidence of hypocalcaemia, hyperparathyroidism and a defect of dental enamel which has been related to vitamin D-deficiency[12]. Neonatal hypovitaminosis D in pregnant women can be avoided by dietary supplementation with vitamin D. The Panel endorsed the view of COMA that pregnant women should receive supplementary vitamin D to achieve an intake of 10 μg/d.

18.3.5 *Lactation* A decline in plasma 25-OHD values and an increase in 1,25-$(OH)_2$D concentrations has been observed. These are changes which may indicate reduced vitamin D status. The Panel therefore recommended supplementation to achieve an intake of 10 μg/d to maintain vitamin D status at adequate levels during lactation (see 18.3.2).

18.3.6 *Asian community* Low vitamin D status is relatively more common among Asians especially children, adolescents and women. A combination of factors including the type of vegetarian diet, low calcium intake and limited solar radiation appear to underlie the greater risk[13,14]. The Panel agreed with the recommendations of the COMA Working Party on the Fortification of Food with Vitamin D that Asian women and children in the UK should take supplementary vitamin D[15].

18.3.7 *The elderly* Mean plasma 25-OHD concentrations in those over 75 years old may average less than 5 ng/ml[16] and never rise above 10 ng/ml at any time of the year. Levels are lower in women than in men. However, the main reason for the lower plasma 25-OHD levels in the elderly in Britain is because they expose insufficient skin to sunlight for an inadequate time in the summer. Thirty minutes exposure of the face and legs at 37° latitude increased plasma 25-OHD levels by about 7.4 μg/ml[17]. This observation suggests that for Northern Britain (latitude 55°) about 1–2 hours exposure daily is necessary to achieve a similar response. To maintain winter 25-OHD levels at or above 8 ng/ml would require summer values to reach 16 ng/ml, which is 2 to 3 times higher than the elderly, particularly those over 75 years, reach in practice.

18.3.8. Histologically proven osteomalacia occurs in 2–5 per cent of the elderly presenting to hospitals[18,19]. Low plasma 25-OHD is found in up to 40 per cent of the elderly living in homes and hospitals[20], and the Panel concluded that dietary or supplementary vitamin D is an effective means of maintaining the vitamin D status of the elderly. The Panel recommended that the population aged over 65 years should consume 10 μg of vitamin D daily to achieve plasma 25-OHD values at the lower end of the normal range found in younger adults.

18.4 **Guidance on high intakes** Infants are most at risk of developing hypervitaminosis D[15]. There are some reports of hypercalcaemia from 50 μg/d, and mild hypercalcaemia was also found from 15 mg vitamin D orally every 3 to 5 months[21].

18.5 **Research needs** The reason for poor vitamin D status in some Asians needs further exploration. The effect on vitamin D status of UV radiation at different latitudes and under different cloud conditions needs more accurate quantification.

18.6 References

1 Arnaud S B, Stickler G B, Haworth J C. Serum 25-hydroxyvitamin D in infantile rickets. *Pediatrics* 1976; **57:** 221–225.

2 Clements M R, Johnson S, Fraser D R. A new mechanism for induced vitamin D deficiency in calcium deprivation. *Nature* 1987; **335:** 62–65.

3 Gregory J, Foster K, Tyler H, Wiseman M. *The Dietary and Nutritional Survey of British Adults.* London: HMSO, 1990.

4 McLaughlin M, Fairney A, Lester E, Raggatt P R, Brown D J, Wills M R. Seasonal variations in serum 25-hydroxycholecalciferol in healthy people. *Lancet* 1974; **i:** 536–537.

[5] Lawson D E M, Davie M. Aspects of the metabolism and function of vitamin D. *Vitamin Horm* 1979; **37:** 1-67.

[6] Brooke O G. Supplementary vitamin D in infancy and childhood. *Arch Dis Childh* 1983; **58:** 573-574.

[7] Greer F R, Ho M, Dodson D, Tsang R C. Lack of 25-hydroxyvitamin D and 1,25-dihydroxyvitamin D in human milk. *J Pediat* 1981; **99:** 233-235.

[8] Markestad T, Kolmannskog S, Arntzen E, Toftegaard L, Haneberg B A, Aksnes L. Serum concentrations of vitamin D metabolites in exclusively breast-fed infants at 70 degrees north. *Acta Ped Scand* 1984; **73:** 29-32.

[9] Department of Health and Social Security. *Present Day Practice in Infant Feeding: Third Report.* London: HMSO, 1988. (Reports on health and social subjects; 32).

[10] Belton N R. Rickets—not only the 'English disease'. *Acta Ped Scand* 1986; **323** (suppl): 68-75.

[11] Poskitt E M E, Cole T J, Lawson D E M. Diet, sunlight and 25-hydroxyvitamin D in healthy children and adults. *Brit Med J* 1979; **1:** 221-223.

[12] Cockburn F, Belton N R, Purvis R J *et al.* Maternal vitamin D intake and mineral metabolism in mothers and their new born infants. *Br Med J* 1980; **281:** 11-14.

[13] Henderson J B, Dunnigan M G, McIntosh W B, Abdul-Motaal A A, Gettinby G, Glekin B M. The importance of limited exposure to ultraviolet radiation and dietary factors in the aetiology of Asian rickets: a risk-factor model. *Quart J Med* 1987; **63:** 413-425.

[14] Clements M R. The problem of rickets in UK Asians. *J Hum Nutr Dietet* 1982; **2:** 105-116.

[15] Department of Health and Social Security. *Rickets and Osteomalacia.* London: HMSO, 1980. (Reports on health and social subjects; 19).

[16] Lawson D E M, Paul A A, Black A E, Cole T J, Mandal A R, Davie M. Relative contribution of diet and sunlight to vitamin D state of the elderly. *Br Med J* 1979; **2:** 303-308.

[17] Read I R, Gallagher D J A, Bosworth J. Prophylaxis against vitamin D deficiency in the elderly by regular sunlight exposure. *Age Ageing* 1986; **15:** 35-40.

[18] Campbell G A, Kemm J R, Hosking D J, Boyd R V. How common is osteomalacia in the elderly? *Lancet* 1984; **ii:** 386-388.

[19] Hodkinson H M, Stanton B R, Round P, Morgan C. Sunlight, vitamin D and osteomalacia in the elderly. *Lancet* 1973; **i:** 910-912.

[20] Davies M, Mawer E B, Hann J T, Taylor J L. Seasonal changes in the biochemical indices of vitamin D deficiency in the elderly: A comparison of people in residential homes, long stay wards and attending a day hospital. *Age Ageing* 1976; **15:** 77-83.

[21] Markestad T, Hesse V, Siebenhuner M *et al.* Intermittent high dose vitamin D prophylaxis during infancy: effect on vitamin D metabolites, calcium and phosphorus. *Am J Clin Nutr* 1987; **46:** 652-658.

[22] Burns J, Patterson C R. Single dose vitamin D treatment for osteomalacia in the elderly. *Br Med J* 1985; **290:** 281-282.

19. Vitamin E

19.1 **Function and essentiality** The biological activity of vitamin E results principally and possibly entirely from its antioxidant properties, and *in vivo* it appears to be the major lipid-soluble antioxidant in membranes. The first vitamin E deficiency state to be clearly demonstrated was in premature infants as a specific syndrome comprising haemolytic anaemia, thromobocytosis and oedema. Infant formulas now contain adequate vitamin E concentrations[1]. Those children and adults unable to absorb or utilise vitamin E adequately may develop a characteristic and progressive neurological syndrome involving the central and peripheral nervous system, retina and skeletal muscles. Appropriate treatment with vitamin E, if given sufficiently early, can prevent the neurological features or, if they are already present, halt or sometimes reverse their progression[2]. All other children and adults virtually never show any signs of clinical deficiency.

19.2 **Vitamin E-active compounds** Vitamin E activity is manifested by two series of compounds, the more important being the tocopherols while the tocotrienols are less potent. The most active compound of all is the natural isomer (RRR) of α-tocopherol, which accounts for about 90 per cent of the vitamin E present in human tissues. Vitamin E activity is conventionally summed in terms of the equivalent value (in milligrams) of RRR-α-tocopherol[3].

19.3 **Indicators of vitamin E status**

19.3.1 Vitamin E status can be measured as the plasma tocopherol concentration, but increased concentrations of serum lipids appear to cause tocopherol to partition out of cellular membranes into the circulation thereby increasing blood levels. For this reason plasma tocopherol concentrations are generally expressed in relation to circulating lipids. If a single lipid is to be used it is probably most conveniently expressed as the serum tocopherol: cholesterol ratio[4].

19.3.2 Below a plasma tocopherol concentration of about 0.5 mg/dl (11.6 μmol/L), or a tocopherol:cholesterol ratio of about 2.25 μmol/mmol, erythrocytes tend to haemolyse after exposure to oxidizing agents such as dilute hydrogen peroxide. This is sometimes taken as an indication of biochemical deficiency, but is not indicative of a clinical deficiency of vitamin E. A substantial decrease below this concentration is, for example, necessary to reduce red cell survival time[5], and neurological signs of deficiency are not seen until the plasma tocopherol concentration has been undetectable or extremely low for a number of years. Nevertheless the Panel considered a serum tocopherol:cholesterol ratio of 2.25 μmol/mmol to be the lowest satisfactory value, and took the dietary requirement of vitamin E as being that necessary to keep the ratio above this level.

19.4 Requirements The requirement for vitamin E is determined to a large extent by the polyunsaturated fatty acid (PUFA) content of tissues, which in turn reflects the PUFA content of the diet. A number of studies has shown that increasing the PUFA content of a diet low in vitamin E reduces plasma tocopherol concentrations[6,7]. The dependence of an individual's vitamin E requirement on dietary PUFA intake makes it difficult to set group DRVs because the range of PUFA intakes in this country is wide. Furthermore, the relationship between PUFA intake and vitamin E requirement is not a simple linear one. In a recent survey, the 2.5 and 97.5 centile intakes of n-6 PUFA by men were 5.1 and 29 g/d[8], and the amount of vitamin E sufficient for those with the higher PUFA intakes would be quite large. To give such a value as the RNI would be undesirable as it might suggest that groups with a much lower, but adequate, PUFA intake should increase their consumption of vitamin E when they had no need to do so.

19.4.1 The Panel decided that since vitamin E requirements depend on PUFA intake, which varies widely, it was impossible to set DRVs of practical value and there was little merit or utility in giving more than ranges of acceptable intakes. Some indication of what these might be can be obtained from the results of the recent survey in this country. Of 1,629 adult subjects only 11 (0.7 per cent) had serum tocopherol:cholesterol ratios below 2.25 μmol/mmol. The 2.5 and 97.5 centiles of intakes from the 7-day weighed dietary records were 3.5 and 19.5 (median 9.3) mg α-tocopherol equivalents/d for men, and 2.5 and 15.2 (median 6.7) mg/d for women[8]. Black *et al* reported that intakes of 3.8 to 6.2 mg/d appeared to be satisfactory for pregnant and lactating women[9]. The Panel concluded that these ranges were safe, and that daily intakes of 4 mg and 3 mg α-tocopherol equivalents can be adequate for men and women respectively. Potential hazards cannot, however, be totally ruled out if the lower intakes are maintained over prolonged periods.

19.4.2 Some Committees have chosen to calculate requirements for vitamin E from the PUFA content of the diet. Although there is no general agreement on what factor should be used, 0.4 mg α-tocopherol equivalents/g dietary PUFA in a normal American diet appears to be satisfactory[10,11], and the ratio has been recommended in this country for infant formulas[12]. Using this, it is possible to calculate what might be the mean requirements of adults consuming the amounts of PUFA recommended by the Panel in Table 1.2 (6 per cent of dietary energy intake). For 18–50 year old males with an intake of 2,550 kcal/d, the average vitamin E requirement would be about 7 mg/d, and for 18–50 year old women with an intake of 1,940 kcal it would be about 5 mg/d. In practice, average intakes are in excess of this[8]. Furthermore, because foods rich in PUFA also tend to contain large amounts of vitamin E, high intakes of PUFA are usually accompanied by corresponding amounts of the vitamin. Thus the mean dietary ratio of α-tocopherol equivalent (mg):PUFA (g) in Britain was over 0.6[8], which is above any estimate of what would be adequate. However, if supplements of PUFA are taken, they should contain adequate amounts of vitamin E.

19.4.3 *Infants* Normal breast fed infants show a steady increase in serum tocopherol concentrations, usually reaching the range seen in older children within 2 to 3 weeks. Human milk has a vitamin E content which varies during early lactation, having a maximum concentration of 1 mg α-tocopherol equivalent/100 ml in colostrum which decreases to a mean concentration of 0.32 mg/100 ml at 12 days and then remains constant[13]. A breast fed infant consuming 850 ml milk/d would therefore have an average daily intake of 2.7 mg. The Panel endorsed the DHSS recommendations that the vitamin E content of milk formulas should not be less than 0.3 mg α-tocopherol equivalents/100 ml reconstituted feed and not less than 0.4 mg α-tocopherol equivalents/g PUFA[12].

19.5 **Increased intake of antioxidants** There is some evidence that increased tissue levels of antioxidants, and in particular vitamin E, may protect against conditions such as ischaemic heart disease and cancer[14-17]. The Panel was not persuaded that the evidence was yet sufficiently strong to provide a basis for making proposals, but recommended that this area be kept under review.

19.6 **Guidance on high intakes** Few adverse effects have been reported from doses of vitamin E up to 3200 mg/d, and none were observed consistently[18].

19.7 References

1 Muller D P R. Free radical problems of the newborn. *Proc Nutr Soc* 1987; **46**: 69–75.

2 Muller D P R. Vitamin E—its role in neurological function. *Postgrad Med J* 1986; **62**: 107–112.

3 Diplock A T. Vitamin E. In: Diplock A, ed. *Fat-Soluble Vitamins, Their Biochemistry and Applications*. London: Heinemann, 1985; 154–224.

4 Thurnham D I, Davies J A, Crump B J, Situnayake R D, Davis M. The use of different lipids to express serum tocopherol: lipid ratios for the measurement of vitamin E status. *Ann Clin Biochem* 1986; **23**: 514–520.

5 Horwitt M K. Interpretation of human requirements for vitamin E. In: Machlin L, ed. *Vitamin E, A Comprehensive Treatise*. New York: Marcel Dekker, 1980; 621–636.

6 Horwitt M K. Status of human requirements for vitamin E. *Am J Clin Nutr* 1974; **27**: 1182–1193.

7 Bunnell R H, de Ritter E, Rubin S H. Effect of feeding polyunsaturated fatty acids with a low vitamin E diet on blood levels of tocopherol in men performing hard physical labor. *Am J Clin Nutr* 1975; **28**: 706–711.

8 Gregory J, Foster K, Tyler H, Wiseman M. *The Dietary and Nutritional Survey of British Adults*. London: HMSO, 1990.

9 Black A E, Wiles S J, Paul A A. The nutrient intakes of pregnant and lactating mothers of good socio-economic status in Cambridge, UK: some implications for recommended daily allowances of minor nutrients. *Br J Nutr* 1986; **56**: 59–72.

10 Beiri J G, Evarts R P. Tocopherols and fatty acids in American diets: The recommended allowance for vitamin E. *J Am Diet Assoc* 1973; **62**: 147–151.

11 Witting L A, Lee L. Dietary levels of vitamin E and polyunsaturated fatty acids and plasma vitamin E. *Am J Clin Nutr* 1975; **28**: 571–576.

12 Department of Health and Social Security. *Artificial Feeds for the Young Infant*. London: HMSO, 1980. (Reports on health and social subjects; 18).

[13] Jansson L, Åkesson B, Holmberg L. Vitamin E and fatty acid composition of human milk. *Am J Clin Nutr* 1981; **34**: 8–13.

[14] Stähelin H B, Gey K F, Eichholzer M, Ludin E, Brubacher G. Cancer mortality and vitamin E status. *Ann NY Acad Sci* 1989; **570**: 391–399.

[15] Esterbauer H, Dieber-Rotheneder M, Striegl G, Waeg G. The role of vitamin E in preventing the oxidation of low density lipoprotein. *Am J Clin Nutr* 1991; **53** (suppl): 314–321.

[16] Gey K F, Puska P, Jordan P, Moser U K. Inverse correlation between plasma vitamin E and mortality from ischemic heart disease in cross-cultural epidemiology. *Am J Clin Nutr* 1991; **53** (suppl): 326–334.

[17] Riemersma R A, Wood D A, Macintyre C C A, Elton R A, Gey K F, Oliver M F. Risk of angina pectoris and plasma concentrations of vitamins A, C, E and carotene. *Lancet* 1991; **1**: 1–5.

[18] Bendich A, Machlin L J. Safety of oral intake of vitamin E. *Am J Clin Nutr* 1988; **48**: 612–619.

20. Vitamin K

20.1 **Functions and essentiality**

20.1.1 Vitamin K activity is shown both by the plant (phylloquinone) and by the related menaquinones which are synthesised by intestinal bacteria. Once thought to play a role only in the hepatic synthesis of the four procoagulant factors II (prothrombin), VII, IX and X, vitamin K is now known to be needed for the gamma-carboxylation of at least two coagulation inhibitors as well as serveral proteins of unknown function located in a variety of calcified and non-calcified tissues[1]. In its severest form, vitamin K deficiency results in a bleeding syndrome due to the lowering of circulating levels of the procoagulant factors and their replacement by undercarboxylated species.

20.1.2 Overt vitamin K deficiency is almost never seen after the first few months of life except as a consequence of underlying disease affecting absorption or utilisation of the vitamin. In contrast, infants are born with hepatic reserves of phylloquinone which are on average about one fifth the adult levels and with no menaquinones[2]. The adult complement and pattern of hepatic menaquinones seem to be reached slowly over several weeks[2,3]. Vitamin K deficiency may occur spontaneously as haemorrhagic disease of the newborn or as an idiopathic late-onset form which typically occur in totally breast-fed infants during the third to eighth week of life. Most of the infants presenting after one month with acute intracranial haemorrhage die, and those who survive have severe neurological sequelae[4].

20.2 **Requirements** There have been few if any satisfactory studies of the vitamin K requirements of humans because of the difficulties in inducing deficiency through dietary deprivation alone. At the present time the only widely accepted criterion for vitamin K sufficiency is the maintenance of normal plasma concentrations of the vitamin K-dependent coagulation factors. This is usually assessed by relatively insensitive functional coagulation assays such as the prothrombin time. Most estimates of the amount of phylloquinone needed to correct induced clotting changes suggest that requirements are between 0.5 and 1.0 µg/kg/day[1].

20.3 **Intakes** There is limited quantitative information on vitamin K in foods and diets because early bioassays in the chick were unreliable[1]. The predominant dietary form is phylloquinone, with green leafy vegetables being by far the richest sources although other vegetables, fruits, dairy produce, vegetable oils, cereals and meats can also provide significant amounts. HPLC assays of phylloquinone have mostly been limited to vegetables[5,6], but Suttie *et al* have estimated from the analysis of duplicate food portions that the normal intake of phylloquinone in 10 male college students was about 80 µg/d[7]. Menaquinones produced by the intestinal bacteria may also be important, for recent measurements by HPLC have shown that while vitamin K circulates mainly as phylloquinone, hepatic reserves are mainly menaquinones[2,8].

20.4 Requirements

20.4.1 *Infants* The vitamin K in human milk consists almost entirely of phylloquinone, and may vary between 1 and 10 μg/L[9,10]. In contrast to most nutrients, however, DRVs for vitamin K for infants are not based on normal intakes from breast milk because of the epidemiological association of haemorrhagic disease of the newborn with total breast feeding[11]. The Panel felt that it would be prudent to base any DRV on the highest value for breast milk, which for infants consuming 850 ml would be 8.5 μg phylloquinone/d, and to round this up to account for the uncertain but low concentrations of menaquinones. The safe intake of 10 μg/d is higher in relation to body weight (~2 μg/kg) than for adults (see below), but is justified by the absence of hepatic menaquinones in early life and presumed reliance on dietary vitamin K alone.

20.4.2 The Panel agreed with the growing consensus that to protect the few babies who develop haemorrhagic disease, all babies need to be given prophylactic vitamin K at birth.

20.4.3 *Adults* Too few studies have been carried out to determine the range of variance of adult vitamin K requirements, but 1 μg/kg/d is both safe and adequate since it maintains vitamin K dependent clotting factors at normal concentrations and in their fully carboxylated form.

20.5 Guidance on high intakes Natural K vitamins seem remarkably free from toxic side effects when taken orally even in milligram quantities. On the other hand, synthetic preparations of menadione are best avoided for nutritional purposes. Besides lacking intrinsic biological activity, the high reactivity of its unsubstituted 3-position has been linked to haemolysis and liver damage in the newborn.

20.6 References

[1] Suttie J W. Vitamin K. In: Diplock A, ed. *The Fat-Soluble Vitamins, their Biochemistry and Applications*. London: Heinemann, 1985; 225–311.

[2] Shearer M J, McCarthy P T, Crampton O E, Mattock M B. The assessment of human vitamin K status from tissue measurements. In: Suttie J, ed. *Current Advances in Vitamin K Research*. New York: Elsevier, 1988; 437–452.

[3] Kayata S, Kindberg C, Greer F R, Suttie J W. Vitamin K_1 and K_2 in infant human liver. *J Pediatr Gastroenterol Nutr* 1989; **8**: 304–307.

[4] Lane P T A, Hathaway W E. Vitamin K in infancy. *J Pediat* 1985; **106**: 351–359.

[5] Shearer M J, Allan V, Haroon Y, Barkhan P. Nutritional aspects of vitamin K in the human. In: Suttie J, ed. *Vitamin K Metabolism and Vitamin K-Dependent Proteins*. Baltimore: University Park Press, 1980; 317–327.

[6] Langenberg J P, Tjaden U R, de Vogel E M, Langerak D I. Determination of phylloquinone (vitamin K_1) in raw and processed vegetables using reversed phase HPLC with electrofluorometric detection. *Acta Alimentaria* 1986; **5**: 187–198.

[7] Suttie J W, Mummah-Schendel L L, Shah D V, Lyle B J, Greger J L. Vitamin K deficiency from dietary restriction in humans. *Am J Clin Nutr* 1988; **47**: 475–480.

[8] Usui Y, Tanimura H, Nishimura N, Kobayashi N, Okanoue T, Ozawa K. Vitamin K concentrations in the plasma and liver of surgical patients. *Am J Clin Nutr* 1990; **51**: 846–852.

[9] von Kries R, Shearer M, McCarthy P T, Haug M, Harzer G, Gobel U. Vitamin K_1 content of maternal milk: influence of the stage of lactation, lipid composition and vitamin K_1 supplements given to the mother. *Pediatr Res* 1987; **22**: 513–517.

[10] Canfield L M, Hopkinson J M. State of the art vitamin K in human milk. *J Ped Gastroenterol Nutr* 1989; **8**: 430–441.

[11] von Kries R, Shearer M J, Gobel U. Vitamin K in infancy. *Eur J Pediatr* 1988; **147**: 106–112.

21. Other Organic Substances sometimes reported to be Essential Dietary Components

21.1 Foods contain thousands of other organic constituents. They are made by, or accumulate in, the plant or animal from which the food was derived, and many have some functional role in that plant or animal or are by-products of its metabolism. Among the trace constituents are enzymes, hormones, alkaloids, colours and many simpler compounds including free sugars, amino acids, fatty acids, alcohols, and cholesterol and other sterols. Some of these, such as caffeine, solanine and digitalis, have biological effects in humans, and some, including taurine, are essential for some animal species.

21.2 Humans can synthesise taurine, choline, carnitine, inositol and cholesterol, and human breast milk contains these and a number of other minor constituents. There is, however, no convincing evidence that it is necessary to include any of these in the normal human diet except possibly for taurine and carnitine in diets for low birth weight or preterm infants[1,2]. The Panel therefore gave no further consideration to these or to other unnecessary substances including ornithine, orotic acid, lecithin, 'vitamin B_{15}' (pangamic acid), 'vitamin B_{17}' (laetrile), bioflavonoids (eg rutin, hesperidin), ubiquinones (coenzyme Q)s nucleotides and para-amino benzoic acid.

21.3 References

1 Galeano N F, Darling P, Lepage G *et al.* Taurine supplementation of a premature formula improves fat absorption in preterm infants. *Pediat Res* 1987; **22**: 67–71.

2 Olson A L, Nelson S E, Rebouche C J. Low carnitine intake and altered lipid metabolism in infants. *Am J Clin Nutr* 1989; **49**: 624–628.

22. Calcium

22.1 **Function and essentiality** Of the approximately 1.2 kg (300 mmol) calcium (Ca) in the human body, about 99 per cent is in the bones and teeth where its primary role is structural. One per cent is in tissues and fluids, where it is essential for cellular structure and inter-and intracellular metabolic function and signal transmission.

22.2 **Metabolism**

22.2.1 Calcium absorption occurs predominantly in the jejunum but also, to a lesser extent, in the ileum and colon.[1-3] Uptake occurs by active transport and simple passive diffusion. At low Ca intakes active transport predominates but as intakes increase, more is absorbed by non-specific pathways. A metabolite of vitamin D, calcitriol (1,25-dihydroxycholecacliferol), enhances the active phase of absorption by stimulating the biosynthesis of a specific intestinal calcium binding protein which is involved in cellular transport. Some individuals can adapt to a prolonged low intake by increasing the efficiency of absorption[4]. A higher proportion of dietary Ca is absorbed by young growing persons than by adults. Pregnancy likewise results in increased efficiency of absorption[5].

22.2.2 Calcium is lost mainly through renal excretion. Losses also occur via faeces, sweat, skin, hair and nails. Calcium also enters the gut via the bile, which is relatively rich in Ca, in the pancreatic secretions and as part of the desquamated cells from the mucosal lining and may be reabsorbed from the ileum and colon. Because of this endogenous secretion, net absorption is less than gross dietary absorption by roughly 100 mg (2.5 mmol)/d[1].

22.3 **Plasma calcium** Total plasma Ca is 90–105 mg/L (2.25–2.60 mmol/L)[3] of which 50 per cent is ionised. The plasma ionised Ca compartment is maintained by a combination of humoral factors which regulate intestinal absorption, renal loss and deposition or mobilisation of Ca from bone. There are no data to indicate that any dietary variable affects plasma Ca concentration significantly in healthy people.

22.4 **Urinary excretion** Available data suggest that 97 per cent of the filtered Ca load is reabsorbed by the renal tubules[3]. Most authors have assumed that the remaining 3 per cent, which is excreted in the urine represents *obligatory* loss but there is doubt whether it is truly obligatory. A major determinant of urinary Ca excretion is dietary Ca intake. Urinary Ca excretion is higher when protein and sodium intakes are high than when intakes of these nutrients are low[6-10]. However, the effects of protein on Ca excretion may be partly offset by higher phosphorus intake[11,12]. Urinary Ca excretion decreases in old age with glomerular filtration rate, and as intestinal absorption declines due to reduction in the efficiency of parathyroid hormone (PTH) and vitamin D metabolism.

However, it increases in women at the menopause, reflecting increased mobilisation of bone Ca[3].

22.5 **Bone metabolism** The average adult human has something over 1 kg of Ca in the bones. It is difficult to separate the influence on bone metabolism of dietary Ca from that of other nutrients, since adequate intakes of protein, energy and many other nutrients are also necessary for bone growth.

22.6 **Peak bone mass** Peak bone mass (PBM) is achieved on average at age 35–40 years for cortical bone; somewhat earlier for trabecular bone[13]. Some 90–95 per cent of PBM is contributed during growth and it becomes only 5–10 per cent greater during consolidation. The main influences on PBM are sex (25–30 per cent greater in males than in females) and genetics (10 per cent greater in Afro-Carribean than in Caucasians). Within these groups there is wide individual variation which has been ascribed to genetic, hormonal and nutritional influences[13]. The few studies bearing on the question of how nutrition might affect PBM are, however, inadequate to draw firm conclusions[14–16].

22.7 **Age-related bone loss** The loss of bone usually begins within a few years of achieving PBM. The average loss of cortical bone is about 0.3 per cent of PBM per year in males and in females up to the menopause, with acceleration for about 5 years in females after the menopause[13]. Most studies have failed to show a relationship between usual Ca intakes and the rate of postmenopausal bone loss. In supplementation studies with healthy subjects, some have claimed a clear and significant reduction of bone loss with additional dietary Ca alone[17–19] or with combined Ca and oestrogen supplements[20]. Some studies have demonstrated a weak effect of Ca when bone loss was measured at one site but not another[21], in cortical but not trabecular bone[22], or by one method of measurement of bone mass but not another[23]. Other studies have shown no change whatsoever in bone loss with Ca supplementation[24,25]. No studies in patients with osteoporosis have demonstrated a significant improvement with dietary Ca alone[26–29]. There is some evidence that seasonal increases in PTH may contribute to cumulative bone loss[30]. Whether higher Ca or vitamin D intakes, or both, during the winter would affect this is not known.

22.8 **Significance of the Ca/P ratio** At customary Ca intakes the level of phosphorus (P) intake (other than that present specifically as phytate which strongly complexes Ca and inhibits its absorption) has no significant influence on calcium absorption or retention. Excessive P intakes of 1.0–1.5 g/d (30–50 mmol/d) with low Ca: P molar ratios (1:3) alter Ca metabolism causing hypocalcaemia and secondary hyperparathyroidism (ie over-secretion of PTH).

22.9 **Perspectives on calcium requirements** In spite of the clear biological essentiality of Ca, the very diversity of its functions makes it difficult to define the appropriate end-point to use for assessing the adequacy either of the dietary supply or of its delivery to the relevant tissues. The Panel recognised a number of possible parameters which could be used.

22.9.1 Plasma Ca, in particular the ionised component, is the most conserved of all the physiological features of Ca metabolism and it may be possible to monitor changes in the variety of hormonal factors which come into play when perturbation of plasma Ca is threatened. The Panel would have regarded such data as the preferred basis for the DRVs, but found no useful studies in the literature.

22.9.2 The maintenance of positive balance is necessary to preserve the skeleton and this can be measured. However the data so far available have come only from relatively short term studies mostly carried out among hospital patients with limited ability to exercise, poor exposure to sunlight and which have not allowed for any adaptation that might occur to a lower or higher Ca intake[4].

22.9.3 In the factorial approach, theoretical calculations can be made of the needs for Ca for growth and maintenance. However, the calculation of the 'obligatory losses' may depend on balance studies with their inherent flaws and, as urinary Ca excretion is highly dependent on dietary intake, it is not clear whether these losses would be the same under experimental conditions where dietary Ca intakes were different or minimally adequate.

22.9.4 As development of osteoporosis is seen by some as an outcome of Ca deficiency, its occurence might be a possible end point because dietary Ca may be critical in the development of peak bone mass. Some current data are consistent with this hypothesis, though fall far short of proof. Osteoporosis can also be ameliorated by reducing bone loss in later life particularly in post menopausal women, but in both situations dietary Ca is only one, and probably not the chief, modulating factor, exercise, body build and other dietary factors being other candidates. For these reasons the Panel did not consider peak bone mass or changes in bone density to be appropriate parameters for the basis of DRVs for Ca. The Panel agreed that, in the absence of robust evidence on Ca requirements in the elderly, it was not possible to say whether intakes by the elderly higher than those by younger people might be advantageous or disadvantageous.

22.9.5 Data from studies of actual dietary Ca intakes of populations which show no apparent Ca deficiencies can be used to estimate Ca requirements. The Panel noted that average Ca intakes for adults in Great Britain are 940 and 730 mg/d (23.5 and 18.3 mmol/d) for men and women respectively[31]. These figures are approximately the same as those obtained by calculating requirements by either the balance or factorial methods. The Panel considered these intakes to represent apparent requirements under the particular dietary and other circumstances pertaining to the period and circumstances in which they were measured.

22.9.6 In order to derive DRVs for Ca the Panel agreed that no single approach was satisfactory, and have opted for the factorial approach. In doing so they concede that the EARs do not represent true basal dietary requirements, but rather they describe the apparent Ca requirements of healthy people in the UK under the prevailing dietary circumstances.

22.10 **Bioavailability** The bioavailability of Ca is extremely important in the setting of DRVs as the calculations given in table 22.1 indicate. The few values regarded as reliable are summarised in table 22.2. Several populations of the world consume Ca at levels lower than the current RDA for the UK[32] yet show no evidence of adverse effects. It is possible that such intakes may be acceptable in any society[33], but the Panel could not be sure of this. Systemic and intestinal adaptation in response to changes in Ca intake has not been adequately characterised in terms of bioavailability and other dietary and non-dietary factors (See Annex 8).

Table 22.1 *Dietary intakes necessary to achieve calcium absorption of 160 mg (4 mmol)/d assuming different net absorption efficiencies*

Assumed absorption %	Dietary intake mg/d (mmol/d)
20	800 (20.0)
25	640 (16.0)
30	550 (13.8)
35	460 (11.5)
40	400 (10.0)
45	360 (9.0)
50	320 (8.0)
55	290 (7.3)
60	270 (6.8)
65	250 (6.3)
70	230 (5.8)

Table 22.2 *Average figures for calcium absorption from mixed diets*

True absorption %		radioactively labelled food	calcium intake mg/d (mmol/d)	subjects	reference
mean	sd				
30	6	milk	1,024 (25.6)	8 women	42
36	9	milk	744 (18.6)	premenopause	
23	6	milk	821 (20.5)	13 women	25
24	7	milk	801 (20.0)	post-	
24	6	milk	679 (17.0)	menopause	
18	6	milk	1,471 (36.8)		
27	6	watercress	1,207 (30.2)	10 adult	43
46	9	skim milk	1.207 (30.2)	males	
36	10	Ca-enriched milk	1.207 (30.2)		

22.11 **Dietary Reference Values** In each group for which there is a Ca requirement for growth or reproduction, the EARs are based on published figures for the retention of Ca. Urinary excretion has not been regarded as obligatory. The RNIs are based on the EARs by adding a notional 2 standard deviations (see para 1.3.6). The LRNIs are set for calcium at the other end of the distribution; that is 2 notional standard deviations below the EARs (Table 22.3).

22.11.1 *Infants* Although in early infancy Ca balance data can be negative, the rate of Ca retention is about 160 mg (4 mmol)/d[34]. Absorption efficiency from breast milk is about 66 per cent so intakes in the first year of about 240 mg (6 mmol)/d would be adequate. Calcium absorption from infant formula is only about 40 per cent[10,35,36], on which basis the EAR would be achieved on an intake of 400 mg (10 mmol)/d with the RNI 2 sd above this at 525 mg (13.1 mmol)/d. This may be higher than that available from some infant formulas (see para 1.3.16).

22.11.2 *Children* Between one and 10 years average daily Ca retention needed for skeletal growth has been estimated to rise from 70 to 150 mg/d (1.8 to 3.8 mmol/d)[34]. Assuming net absorption of 35 per cent (slightly lower than that used for infants), this level of Ca retention can be maintained on a Ca intake of about 275 mg (6.9 mmol)/d at age 2 and 425 mg (10.6 mmol)/d at age 10 years. Allowing for 2 sd above these EARs, the RNIs are therefore 30 per cent higher at 350 and 550 mg/d (8.8 and 13.8 mmol/d) respectively, and the RNIs for other ages have been interpolated (Table 22.3).

22.11.3 *Adolescents* Assuming a mean retention in adolescence of 250 mg (6.3 mmol)/d for girls and 300 mg (7.5 mmol)/d for boys, and a net absorption of 40 per cent, the EARs are 625 and 750 mg/d (15.6 and 18.8 mmol/d) respectively. Corresponding RNIs are 2 sd above these means at 800 and 1,000 mg/d (20 and 25 mmol/d) (Table 22.3).

22.11.4 *Adults* Despite the Panel's decision not to accept urinary losses necessarily as obligatory, there is probably some requirement for Ca in adulthood when growth has ceased. The EAR derived here is based on average urinary losses in adults of 150 mg (3.8 mmol)/d plus an estimated 10 mg (0.25 mmol)/d for losses via skin, sweat, hair and nails. The Panel assumed a mean absorption of 30 per cent from mixed diets providing a normal range of Ca intakes (Table 22.2). Therefore the EAR is 525 mg (13.1 mmol)/d and the RNI is plus 2 sd, that is 700 mg (17.5 mmol)/d and the LRNI is 400 mg (10 mmol)/d (Table 22.3). The EAR thus derived is similar to that derived from balance studies[10].

22.11.5 *Pregnancy* There is no evidence for a spontaneous increase in food consumption by pregnant women, and the satisfactory outcomes lend support to the view that mobilisation of maternal Ca depots rather than a dietary increment is an appropriate source of the additional Ca needed for fetal growth[37]. There is evidence that bone density diminishes in the first 3 months of both pregnancy and lactation to provide an internal Ca reservoir which is

Table 22.3 *Dietary Reference Values for Calcium mg/d (mmol/d*)*

Age	Lower Reference Nutrient Intake	Estimated Average Requirement	Reference Nutrient Intake
0–12 months	240 (6.0)	400 (10.0)	525 (13.1)
1–3 years	200 (5.0)	275 (6.9)	350 (8.8)
4–6 years	275 (6.9)	350 (8.8)	450 (11.3)
7–10 years	325 (8.1)	425 (10.6)	550 (13.8)
11–14 years, male	480 (12.0)	750 (18.8)	1,000 (25.0)
11–14 years, female	450 (11.3)	625 (15.6)	800 (20.0)
15–18 years, male	480 (12.0)	750 (18.8)	1,000 (25.0)
15–18 years, female	450 (11.3)	625 (15.6)	800 (20.0)
19–50 years	400 (10.0)	525 (13.1)	700 (17.5)
50+ years	400 (10.0)	525 (13.1)	700 (17.5)
Pregnancy: no increment	–	–	–
Lactation	–	–	+ 550 (+14.3)

*1 mmol = 40 mg

replenished by 6 months[37]. In any case, the efficiency of Ca absorption rises during pregnancy over and above that for normal women, but among adolescents pregnancy is a special case where two risk factors for Ca deficiency coincide[38]. Higher maternal Ca intakes would be advisable in these circumstances[38].

22.11.6 *Lactation* Most lactating women increase their food intakes, and hence their Ca intakes, spontaneously thus providing the additional Ca required for milk production. If it is assumed that this should be derived entirely from the diet, then an additional 300 mg/d (850 ml milk/d × 0.35 mg Ca/ml = 298 mg/d) must be absorbed by the mother. There is some evidence which suggests that the increased bioavailability of Ca during pregnancy is maintained during lactation, although as yet, there is little data available to quantify this precisely[44]. The Panel therefore assumed an absorption efficiency of 40 per cent. The EAR is 160 ÷ 0.4 = 400 mg (10.0 mmol)/d and the extra requirement for lactation is 300 ÷ 0.4 = 750 mg (18.8 mmol)/d. The RNI for lactation is therefore 400 × 1.3 (+ 2 sd) + 750: that is 1270 mg—rounded to 1250 mg (31.8 mmol)/d—giving an increment of 550 mg (14.3 mmol)/d (Table 22.3). Adolescent mothers might be expected to require higher intakes[38].

22.11.7 *Postmenopause* The Panel could find no evidence that significant benefits would be derived from increasing dietary Ca sources alone. However the increasing prevalence of osteoporosis, with associated fractures, has been ascribed by some to dietary Ca deficiency[39]. Osteoporosis results, however, from loss of all components of bone (atrophy) not just of Ca. The postmenopausal increase in bone loss, which is the main cause of osteoporosis, results from oestrogen deficiency. Oestrogen replacement can prevent, and possibly restore, bone loss. Calcium supplementation alone has not been shown to be effective in preventing significant bone loss. The achievement of Ca balance in the peri-and postmenopausal periods in the absence of oestrogen replacement may therefore be an inappropriate goal. However there is some evidence that if Ca intakes are high the oestrogen dose can be reduced without loss of efficacy[20].

22.11.8 *Elderly* The Panel could find no evidence to justify a recommendation for increased Ca intakes in the elderly. The Panel has recommended an increased allowance for vitamin D since declining kidney function in ageing people results in poorer metabolism of vitamin D and reduced Ca absorption (see Section 18). In the absence of further information the Panel felt unable to recommend any increase in Ca intakes by those aged 60 or more years, and stressed that data which could help to quantify Ca requirements in the elderly were particularly scanty.

22.12 **Intakes**

22.12.1 In the UK, supplies of Ca were 1,062 mg (26.6 mmol)/person/d in 1987, with 665 mg (16.6 mmol) (62 per cent) from milk and milk products and 58 mg (1.5 mmol) (5 per cent) from vegetables. However, because most flour in the UK is required by law to be fortified with calcium carbonate, a further 235 mg (5.9 mmol) (22 per cent) is derived from cereals (Ministry of Agriculture, Fisheries and Food, unpublished). In addition, hard water can provide typically 200 mg (5 mmol)/d and occasionally as much as 500 mg (12.5 mmol)/d while in very soft water areas it provides essentially none.

22.12.2 The NFS show some regional variation in Ca intakes from 820 mg (20.5 mmol) in Wales to 910 mg (22.8 mmol)/person/d in the West Midlands but there is greater variation with family composition. In 1987, the intake in households with two adults ranged from 950 mg (23.8 mmol)/person/d where there were no children to 770 mg (19.3 mmol)/person/d where there were 3 or more children[40].

22.12.3 Secondary schoolboys consumed an average of 833 mg (20.8 mmol)/d when aged 10–11 and 925 mg (23.1 mmol)/d when 14–15 years, while at the same ages girls, whose intakes of milk and cereal products were lower, consumed 702 and 692 mg/d (17.6 mmol and 17.3 mmol/d)[41]. The Dietary and Nutritional Survey of British Adults showed average Ca intakes of 940 and 730 mg/d (23.5 and 18.3 mmol/d) in men and women respectively[31].

22.13 **Guidance on high intakes** Body Ca metabolism is under such close homeostatic control that an excessive accumulation in blood or tissues from overconsumption is virtually unknown. Where accumulation in blood or the tissues does occur it results from a failure of the control mechanisms, either generally or locally, and has little relevance to dietary recommendations[3]. The Panel were unconvinced that high intakes of around 2g (50 mmol)/d sometimes recommended were of value in the prevention or treatment of osteoporosis. In oestrogen deficiency, increased Ca loss is most effectively treated by oestrogen replacement not by Ca supplementation. However, in view of the lack of Ca toxicity and the equivocal nature of the data relating to benefit, the Panel agreed that in people who are considered to be at high risk of osteoporosis, a diet richer in Ca than the DRVs proposed for the general population might be prudent.

22.14 **Research needs** The Panel considered that much further research was necessary to give data on which to base future recommendations, and identified as deserving priority the need to characterise more thoroughly the mechanisms for controlling and regulating Ca homeostasis and the need to understand the pathophysiology of osteoporosis. The Panel recommended that further research be carried out into ways of identifying those individuals at special risk of developing osteoporosis.

22.15 References

[1] Nordin B E C. *Calcium, Phosphate and Magnesium Metabolism*. London: Churchill Livingstone, 1976.

[2] Nordin B E C. *Calcium in Human Biology*. London: Springer Verlag, 1988.

[3] British Nutrition Foundation *Report of Task Force on Calcium*. British Nutrition Foundation: London, 1989.

[4] Malm O J. Calcium requirements and adaptation in adult men. *Scand J Clin Lab Invest* 1958; **10** (suppl 36): 1-290.

[5] Hegsted D M. Symposium on human calcium requirements. *J Am Med Assoc* 1963; **185**: 588-593.

[6] Linkswiler H M, Zemel M B, Hegsted M, Schouette S. Protein induced hypercalciuria. *Fed Proc* 1981; **40**: 2429-2433.

[7] Goulding A, Lim P E. Effects of varying dietary salt intake on the fasting urinary excretion of sodium, calcium and hydroxyproline in young women. *NZ Med J* 1983; **96**: 853–854.

[8] Parfitt A M. Dietary risk factors for age-related bone loss and fractures. *Lancet* 1983; **ii**: 1181–1185.

[9] Sabto J, Powell M J, Breidahl M J, Gurr F W. Influence of urinary sodium on calcium excretion in normal individuals, or redefinition of hyperealciuria. *Med J Aust* 1984; **140**: 354–356.

[10] Nordin B E C. Calcium. *J Food Nutr* 1986; **42**: 67–82.

[11] Heaney R P, Recker R R. Effect of nitrogen, phosphorus and caffeine on calcium balance on women. *J Lab Clin Med* 1982; **99**: 46–55.

[12] Spencer H, Kramer L. The calcium requirement and factors causing calcium loss. *Fed Proc* 1986; **45**: 2758-2762.

[13] Parfitt A M. Bone remodeling: Relationship to the amount and structure of bone and the pathogenesis and prevention of fractures. In: Riggs B, Melton L, eds. *Osteoporosis: Etiology, Diagnosis and Management*. New York: Raven Press, 1988; 45–93.

[14] Garn S M. *The earlier gain and the later loss of cortical bone in nutritional perspective.* Springfield: C C Thomas, 1970.

[15] Matkovic V, Kostial K, Simonovic I, Buzina R, Broarec A, Nordin B E C. Bone status and fracture rates in two regions of Yugoslavia. *Am J Clin Nutr* 1979; **32**: 540–549.

[16] Sandler R B, Slemenda C W, LaPorte R E *et al.* Post menopausal bone density and milk consumption in childhood and adolescence. *Am J Clin Nutr* 1985; **42**: 270–274.

[17] Albanese A A, Edelson A H, Lorenz E J, Woodhall M L, Wein E H. Problems of bone health in the elderly. *New York State Journal of Medicine* 1975; **75**: 326–336.

[18] Nordin B E C, Polley K J. Metabolic consequences of the menopause. A cross-sectional, longitudinal and itervention study on 557 normal postmenopausal women. *Calcif Tissue Intl* 1987; **41** (suppl 1): S1–S59.

[19] Polley K J, Nordin B E C, Baghurst P A, Walker C J, Chatterton B E. Effect of calcium supplementation on forearm bone mineral content in postmenopausal women: a prospective sequential controlled trial. *J Nutr* 1987; **117**: 1929–1935.

[20] Ettinger B, Genant H K, Cann C E. Postmenopausal bone loss is prevented by treatment with low dosage estrogen with calcium. *Ann Intern Med* 1987; **106**: 40–45.

[21] Horsman A, Gallagher J C, Simpson M, Nordin B E C. Prospective trial of oestrogen and calcium in postmenopausal women. *Br Med J* 1977; **2**: 789–792.

[22] Riis B, Thomsen K, Christiansen C. Does calcium supplementation prevent postmenopausal bone loss? *N Engl J Med* 1987; **316**: 173–177.

[23] Recker R R, Saville P D, Heaney R P. Effects of estrogens and calcium carbonate on bone loss in postmenopausal women. *Ann Intern Med* 1977; **87**: 649–655.

[24] Nilas L, Christiansen C, Rodbro P. Calcium supplementation and postmenopausal bone loss. *Br Med J* 1984; **289**: 1103–1107.

[25] Recker R R, Heaney R P. The effect of milk supplements on calcium metabolism, bone metabolism and calcium balance. *Am J Clin Nutr* 1985; **41**: 254–263.

[26] Smith D A, Anderson J J B, Aitken J M, Shimmins J. The effects of calcium supplements of the diet on bone mass measurements in women. In: Kuhlencordt F, Kruse H, eds. *Calcium Metabolism and Metabolic Bone Disease.* Berlin: Springer Verlag, 1975; 278–282.

[27] Lamke B, Sjoberg H E, Sylven M. Bone mineral content in women with Colles fracture. Effect of calcium supplementation. *Acta Orthopaedica Scandinavica* 1978; **49**: 143–146.

[28] Nordin B E C, Horsman A, Crilly R G, Marshall D H, Simpson M. Treatment of spinal osteoporosis in postmenopausal women. *Br Med J* 1980; **280**: 451–455.

[29] Shapiro J R, Moore W T, Jorgensen H, Reid J, Epps C H, Whedon D. Osteoporosis: evaluation of diagnosis and therapy. *Arch Intern Med* 1975; **135**: 563–567.

[30] Krall E A, Sahyoun N, Tannenbaum S *et al.* Effect of vitamin D intake on seasonal variations in parathyroid hormone secretion in postmenopausal women. *New Engl J Med* 1989; **321**: 1777–1783.

[31] Gregory J, Foster K, Tyler H, Wiseman M. *The Dietary and Nutritional Survey of British Adults*. London: HMSO, 1990.

[32] Department of Health and Social Security. *Recommended Daily Intakes of Food Energy and Nutrients for Groups of People in the United Kingdom*. London: HMSO, 1979. (Reports on health and social subjects; 15).

[33] Hegsted D M, Moscoso I, Collazos C. A study of the minimum calcium requirements of adult men. *J Nutr* 1952; **46**: 181–201.

[34] Leitch I, Aitken F C. Estimation of calcium requirement: a re-examination. *Nut Abst Rev* 1959; **29**: 393–411.

[35] American Academy of Pediatrics Committee on Nutrition. Calcium requirements in infancy and childhood. *Paediatrics* 1978; **62**: 826–834.

[36] Widdowson E M. Nutritional requirement and its assessment with special reference to energy, protein and calcium. *Biblthca Nutr Dieta* 1979; **28**: 148–154.

[37] Purdie D W. Bone mineral metabolism and reproduction. *Contemporary Reviews in Obstetrics and Gynaecology* 1989; **1**: 214–221.

[38] Chan G M, McMurray M, Westover K, Engelbert-Fenton K, Thomas M R. Effects of increased dietary calcium intake upon calcium and bone mineral status in lactating adolescent and adult women. *Am J Clin Nutr* 1987; **46**: 319–323.

[39] Nordin B E C, Heaney R P. Calcium supplementation of the diet: justified by present evidence. *Br Med* J 1990; **300**: 1056–1060

[40] Ministry of Agriculture, Fisheries and Food. *Household Food Consumption and Expenditure, 1987*. London: HMSO, 1989.

[41] Department of Health. *The Diets of British Schoolchildren*. London: HMSO, 1989. (Reports on health and social subjects; 36).

[42] Heaney R P, Recker R R, Saville P D. Menopausal changes in calcium balance performance. *J Lab Clin Med* 1978; **92**: 953–963.

[43] Fairweather-Tait S J, Johnson A J, Eagles J, Ganatra K, Kennedy H, Gurr M I. Studies on calcium absorption from milk using a double label stable isotope method. *Br J Nutr* 1989; **62**: 379–388.

[44] Heaney R P, Skillman T G. Calcium metabolism in normal human pregnancy. *J Clin Endocrin Met*, 1971; **33**: 661–70.

23. Magnesium

23.1 **Function and essentiality** The physiological importance of magnesium (Mg) lies in its role in skeletal development and in the maintenance of electrical potential in nerve and muscle membranes. Biochemically Mg acts as a co-factor for enzymes requiring ATP, in the replication of DNA and the synthesis of RNA[1]. Magnesium is intimately involved with calcium in metabolism. Calcium homeostasis is controlled in part by a Mg-requiring mechanism which releases parathyroid hormone. Several Mg activated enzymes are inhibited by calcium while in others Mg can be replaced by manganese[2]. Hypomagnesaemia induced by starvation, malabsorption syndromes, acute pancreatitis, alcoholism, prolonged diarrhoea or vomiting is almost always accompanied by hypocalcaemia[3]. The body contains about 25 g (1 mol) of Mg, and roughly 60 per cent is in the skeleton[4, 5].

23.2 **Metabolism** Magnesium deficiency is characterised by progressive muscle weakness, failure to thrive, neuromuscular dysfunction, tachycardia, ventricular fibrillation, coma and death[3, 6]. Because of these cardiac effects, a low level of dietary intake has been postulated as a risk factor in CHD. However evidence for this is circumstantial, for while ventricular arrhythmia has been shown to be associated with low levels of Mg in heart tissue, in most cases the deficiency appears to have been induced by other factors (alcohol abuse and diuretics) not nutritional inadequacy, and associated with hypocalcaemia[7]. Epidemiological evidence linking low Mg levels in soft water supplies with a higher incidence of CHD is also conflicting[8].

23.3 **Absorption** Magnesium is absorbed both by a facilitated process and by passive diffusion[9]. Excretion is primarily through the kidneys and increases with dietary intake up to about 2 g (82 mmol)/d. Intakes in excess of this have been shown to pass through the intestine unabsorbed[1]. When intake decreases, however, the kidney is very efficient at conserving Mg and the skeleton acts as a store. Because of these homeostatic mechanisms it is very difficult to demonstrate either deficiency symptoms or toxic effects in normal healthy people[1].

23.4 **Requirements**

23.4.1 *Adults* Physiological data suggest that Mg balance is achieved in adults on about 50 mg (2.1 mmol)/d[10]. The efficiency of absorption increases from 25 per cent on high Mg diets to about 75 per cent on Mg restricted diets.[11]. Early balance studies suggested that adult requirements may be as high as 700 mg (28.8 mmol)/d[12], but interpretation of these is difficult because of the long time needed to reach equilibrium[13]. One study suggested that normal adults could maintain positive balance on 3.0 mg (0.12 mmol)/d over a 6 to 9 day experimental period but that an intake of 3.4 mg (0.14 mmol)/kg/d would be adequate for all[14].

23.4.2 *Infants* Human milk contains about 2.8 mg (0.12 mmol)/100 ml (range 2.6–3.0 mg; 0.11–0.12 mmol)[15] so the newborn ingest about 25 mg (1 mmol)/d or about 7.2 mg (0.3 mmol)/kg. At 3 months the intake is 6 mg (0.25 mmol)/kg, and at 6 months 5 mg (0.21 mmol)/kg.

23.4.3 *Pregnancy* The fetus accumulates about 8.0 mg (0.33 mmol)/d over 40 weeks[16]. Assuming 50 per cent absorption, the extra maternal requirement for the fetus is 16 mg (0.66 mmol)/d. The mother also needs an extra 10 mg (0.41 mmol)/d for the accumulation of placental and other tissues[17]. However, physiological adaptation in pregnancy and release from maternal stores ensure an adequate supply.

23.4.4 *Lactation* As the Mg content of breast milk is about 2.8 mg (0.12 mmol)/100 ml[15] so the average secretion of Mg in breast milk is about 25 mg/d. Assuming 50 per cent absorption from the maternal diet the lactational increment is 50 mg (2.1 mmol)/d.

23.4.5 Using the above and the balance data for adults from Jones *et al*[14], the RNIs and LRNIs for Mg given in table 23.1 are therefore calculated from the EARs per kg body weight:

		Estimated Average Requirement
Infants	0–3 months	7 mg/kg/d
	4–6 months	6 mg/kg/d
Children	6 months–18 years	4.5 mg/kg/d (interpolated from 6.0 to 3.4 mg/kg/d)
Adults	18 years and over	3.4 mg/kg/d
Lactation—increment		50 mg/d

Table 23.1 *Dietary Reference Values for Magnesium mg/d (mmol/d*)*

Age	Lower Reference Nutrient Intake	Estimated Average Requirement	Reference Nutrient Intake
0–3 months	30 (1.2)	40 (1.7)	55 (2.2)
4–6 months	40 (1.7)	50 (2.1)	60 (2.5)
7–9 months	45 (1.9)	60 (2.5)	75 (3.2)
10–12 months	45 (1.9)	60 (2.5)	80 (3.3
1–3 years	50 (2.1)	65 (2.7)	85 (3.5)
4–6 years	70 (2.9)	90 (3.7)	120 (4.8)
7–10 years	115 (4.7)	150 (6.7)	200 (8.0)
11–14 years	180 (7.4)	230 (9.5)	280 (11.5)
15–18 years	190 (7.8)	250 (10.3)	300 (12.3)
19–50 years men	190 (7.8)	250 (10.3)	300 (12.3)
19–50 years women	150 (6.2)	200 (8.2)	270 (10.9)
50+ years men	190 (7.8)	250 (10.3)	300 (12.3)
50+ years women	150 (6.2)	200 (8.2)	270 (10.9)
Pregnancy	no increment		
Lactation			+50 (+2.1)

*1 mmol = 24.3 mg

23.5 **Intakes** Magnesium is present in the chloroplasts of green plants and the main sources of Mg in the diet are cereals and green vegetables. The household diet provides on average 294 (12.1 mmol)/d, 33 per cent derived from cereals and 18 per cent from green vegetables[18]. Mean intakes from the Dietary and Nutritional Survey of British Adults were 323 and 237 mg/d (13.3 and 9.8 mmol/d) for men and women respectively[19]. Meat and animal products are rich in Mg but the simultaneous intake of calcium, phosphate and protein from these sources reduces its bioavailability[20].

23.6 **Guidance on high intakes** There is no evidence that large dietary intakes of Mg are harmful to humans with normal renal function. Excessive circulating levels of Mg are almost impossible to achieve by ingestion from foods but high levels induced by intravenous administration interfere with nerve transmission causing paralysis and eventually death[21]. When taken in doses of 3–5 g (123–206 mmol) Mg salts have a cathartic effect[22] and if taken often enough for this reason can lead to high blood Mg levels that can be toxic or even fatal[23].

23.7 References

[1] Aikawa J K. Effect of specific nutrient deficiencies in man: Magnesium In: Rechcigl M, ed. *CRC Handbook Series in Nutrition and Food, Section E: Nutritional Disorders, volume III, Effect of Nutrient Deficiencies in Man*. West Palm Beach, Florida: CRC Press Inc, 1978; 169–178.

[2] Harper H A. *Review of Physiological Chemistry* 11th ed. Los Altos: Lange Medical Publications, 1967; 392–000.

[3] Foy A. Magnesium, the neglected cation. *Med J Aust*, 1980; **1**: 305–306.

[4] Widdowson E M, McCance R A, Spray C M. The chemical composition of the human body. *Clin Sci* 1951; **10**: 113–125.

[5] Schroeder H A, Nason A P, Tipton I H. Essential metals in man: magnesium. *J Chronic Dis* 1969; **21**: 815–841.

[6] Flink E B. Magnesium deficiency and magnesium toxicity in Man. In: Prasad A, ed. *Trace Elements in Human Health and Disease Vol II*. New York: Academic Press, 1976; 1–21.

[7] Iseri L T. Magnesium in coronary heart disease. *Drugs* 1984; **28**: (Suppl) 151–160.

[8] Meyers D. Ischaemic heart disease and the water factor: a variable relationship. *Br J Prev Soc Med* 1975; **29**: 98–102.

[9] Roth P, Werner E. Intestinal absorption of magnesium in man. *Int J Appl Rad Isot* 1979; **30**: 523–526.

[10] Department of National Health and Welfare. *Recommended Nutrient Intakes for Canadians*. Ottawa: Canadian Govt Pub Centre, Canada, 1983.

[11] Schwartz R, Spencer H, Welsh J J. Magnesium absorption in human subjects from leafy vegetables intrinsically labelled with stable 26 Mg. *Am J Clin Nutr* 1984; **39**: 571–576.

[12] Seelig M S. Magnesium requirements in human nutrition *J Med Soc New Jersey* 1982; **70**: 849–854.

[13] Marshall D H, Nordin B E C, Speed R. Calcium, phosphorus and magnesium requirement. *Proc Nutr Soc* 1976; **35**: 163–173.

[14] Jones J E, Manalo R, Flink E B. Magnesium requirements in adults. *Am J Clin Nutr* 1967; **20**: 632–635.

[15] Department of Health and Social Security. *Artificial Feeds for the Young Infant*. London: HMSO, 1980. (Reports on health and social subjects; 18)

[16] Ziegler E E, O'Donnell A M, Nelson S E, Fomon S J. Body composition of the reference foetus. *Growth* 1976; **40**: 329–341.

[17] Widdowson E M. Chemical composition and nutritional needs of the fetus at different stages of gestation. In: Aerbi H, Whitehead R, eds *Maternal Nutrition during Pregnancy and Lactation*. Bern: Hans Huber, 1980; 39–48.

[18] Lewis J, Buss D H. Trace nutrients, 5 Minerals and vitamins in the British household food supply. *Br J Nutr* 1988; **60**: 414–424.

[19] Gregory J, Foster K, Tyler H, Wiseman M. *The Dietary and Nutritional Survey of British Adults*. London: HMSO, 1990.

[20] Dyckner T, Webster P O. *Magnesium: A Short Review*. Malmo, Sweden: E D Searle AB, 1983.

[21] Lipsitz P J. Nutrient toxicities in animals and man: Magnesium, In: *CRC Handbook Series in Nutrition and Food, Section E: Nutritional Disorders, Volume 1. Effect of Nutrient Excesses and Toxicities in Animals and Man*. West Palm Beach, Florida: CRC Press Inc 1978; 113–117.

[22] Goodman L S, Gilman A Z. *The Pharmacological Basis of Therapeutics* 3rd ed. New York: MacMillan, 1965; 1785–1791.

[23] Outerbridge E W, Papageorgiou A, Stern L. Magnesium sulphate enema in the newborn. *J Am Med Ass* 1973; **224**: 1392–1393.

24. Phosphorus

24.1 **Function and essentiality** About 80 per cent of the phosphorus (P) in the human body ie 600–900 g (19–29 mol) is present in bones as a calcium salt that gives rigidity to the skeleton. The rest is in soft tissues as inorganic phosphate and as a constituent of all the major classes of biochemical compounds. The energy that drives most metabolic processes is derived from the phosphate bonds of Adenosine triphosphate (ATP) and other high energy phosphate compounds. Phosphorylation-dephosphorylation reactions are crucial to many aspects of metabolic control.

24.2 **Metabolism** Absorption of P is about 60 per cent of intake[1]. Plasma concentrations fall within the range 24.7–43.3 mg/L (0.8–1.4 mmol/L) and are regulated by excretion. At low P intakes, plasma P falls and urinary excretion is reduced. To maintain a plasma phosphate concentration of 23.9 mg (0.8 mmol)/L an intake of 400 mg (12.9 mmol)/d with a bioavailability of 60 per cent is needed[1]. This is well below usual intakes.

24.3 **Requirements** Phosphorus requirements are conventionally set as equal to calcium in mass terms, ie 1 mg P: 1 mg Ca. However these elements are present in the body in nearly equimolar amounts and the Panel took the view that it was more rational to set the ratio in the diet as 1 mmol P: 1 mmol Ca and recommended that as a matter of prudence the RNI for P be set equal to the calcium RNI in mmol* (see Table 22.3 and paras 1.3.16 and 22.11.1). For Ca intakes different from the RNI, P intake should be equivalent to *actual* Ca intakes.

24.4 **Intakes** As phosphate is a major constituent of all plant and animal cells, P is present in all natural foods. It is also present in many food additives. Household food purchases in Britain provide 1.2–1.3 g (39–42 mmol)/person/d[2] of which about 10 per cent is added in manufacture[3].

24.5 **Guidance on high intakes** As discussed in para 22.8 a varying Ca:P ratio can be tolerated by adult populations with no effect on Ca balance[4], although for infants the ratio remains extremely important and should not be outside the range of 1.2:1 to 2.2:1 mg/mg or 0.9:1 to 1.7:1 mmol/mmol[5]. Nevertheless the maximum tolerable daily intake is set at 70 mg/kg body weight[6] which is about 4.5 g/d for a 65 kg man and well above any level likely to be obtained from dietary sources.

*1 mmol Ca = 40 mg, 1 mmol P = 30.9 mg

24.6 References

[1] Marshall D H, Nordin B E C, Speed R. Calcium, phosphorus and magnesium requirement. *Proc Nutr Soc* 1976; **35**, 163–173.

[2] Gilbert L, Wenlock R W, Buss D H. Phosphorus in the British household food supply. *Hum Nutr: Appl Nutr* 1985; **39A**: 208–212.

[3] Davidson L S P, Passmore R. *Human Nutrition and Dietetics*. 7th ed. London: Churchill Livingstone, 1980.

[4] Spencer M, Cramer L, Osis D, Worris C. Effect of phosphorus on the absorption of calcium and on the calcium balance in man. *J Nutr* 1978; **108**: 447–457.

[5] Department of Health and Social Security. *Artificial feeds for the Young Infant*. London: HMSO, 1980. (Reports on health and social subjects; 18).

[6] World Health Organization. *Evaluation of Certain Food Additives and Contaminants* Geneva: World Health Organization, 1982. (WHO Technical Report Series; 683).

25. Sodium

25.1 **Function and Essentiality** Sodium (Na) is the principal cation in extracellular fluid where it exists in its ionised state. Its physiological roles include the maintenance of (i) extracellular fluid (ECF) volume which is closely related to total body Na content, (ii) extracellular fluid oncotic pressure, (iii) acid base balance, (iv) electrophysiological phenomena in muscle and nerves and (v) the generation of transmembrane gradients which enable the energy dependent uptake of nutrients (eg amino acids and hexoses) by cells including those of the intestinal mucosa and renal tubules.

25.2 **Metabolism**

25.2.1 An adult male weighing 65 to 70 kg has a total body Na of 4 mol (92 g); of this 500 mmol (11.5 g) is in the intracellular fluid at an activity concentration of 2 mmol/L (46 mg/L), 1500 mmol (34.5 g) is sequestered in bone and 2,000 mmol (46 g) is in the ECF. Intestinal Na absorption is virtually complete and occurs in the distal small intestine and colon. Its concentration in the ECF of 135–145 mmol/L (3.1–3.3 g/L) is maintained by renal excretion and conservation (See Annex 8). The kidneys filter 25 mol (575 g) of Na daily; since daily dietary intakes (50–200 mmol; 1.15–4.6 g) approximate only 0.2–0.8 per cent of this amount, almost all of this filtered Na needs to be reabsorbed. Renal Na reabsorption is highly efficient and adaptable. In pregnancy the glomerular filtration rate and the corresponding filtered load of Na can be doubled.

25.2.2 Regulation of the Na content of ECF is closely related to the systemic control of ECF volume. If the body Na burden is increased, water is also retained and the ECF volume increases; conversely, if the body Na burden falls the ECF volume decreases. Regulation of these changes in ECF volume is mediated by sensors of pressure and distension which are located in the cardiac atria and right ventricle, the pulmonary vasculature, the carotid arteries and the aortic arch. The nerve pathways from these sensors end in the medulla and hypothalamus of the brain. When ECF or blood volume falls retention is stimulated, sympathetic activity increases, stimulation of nerves supplying the afferent renal arterioles induces vasoconstriction, and a redistribution of renal blood flow which by reducing gomerular filtration increases Na and water retention. Additionally stimulation of nerves to the juxtaglomerular apparatus increases renin production leading to an increase in circulating angiotensin II, adrenal medullary secretion of noradrenalin and adrenalin, and pituitary release of adrenocorticotrophin (ACTH) and antidiuretic hormone (ADH). ACTH and angiotension II induce adrenal cortical secretion of aldosterone and other mineralocorticoids which stimulate Na retention and potassium loss by the kidneys and distal bowel. Increased secretion of ADH promotes water reabsorption from the renal distal tubules.

25.2.3 Several factors increase renal Na excretion. These natriuretic factors include a specific natriuretic hormone, and vasodilators, parathormone, prostaglandins and kinins. Some of these may act on the renal vasculature, others may have direct effects on renal tubular reabsorption; atrial natriuretic polypeptide may affect both processes.

25.2.4 In infants and old people Na and fluid homeostasis are less efficient. Neonates are less able to conserve Na than are adults, and the ECF volume does not reach the adult proportion of body weight until about one year of age. Glomerular filtration in children is less variable then in adults, but tubular Na reabsorption is as efficient. Thus although children's ability to excrete excessive Na loads is limited, they are able to respond to deprivation by reducing urinary Na loss almost to zero. In the elderly the onset of renal responses to altered Na intakes, in particular reduced intakes, is slow although such adaptation is ultimately achieved. Since the elderly may be on inadvertently or therapeutically restricted Na intakes they may become Na depleted, and thus susceptible to anorexia and confusion which could further compromise their general nutrient intake thereby creating a disadvantageous cycle.

25.3 **Requirements**

25.3.1 Healthy adults maintain balance on intakes as low as 3–20 mmol/d (69–460 mg/d)[1,2], and some healthy populations have daily intakes of less than 40 mmol (920 mg)[3, 4]. The role of higher Na intakes in the pathogenesis of hypertension has generated much interest, but the evidence supporting this or indicating the relative importance of Na intakes is unclear[5]. High body mass index (BMI) (obesity), alcohol and smoking are important contributory factors to the development of hypertension[4]. In adolescents obesity may increase the sensitivity of blood pressure to dietary Na intake[6]. The lower Na intakes of 'less developed communities' with lower blood pressure than those seen in developed societies with increased incidences of hypertension may reflect different lifestyles rather than a causal relationship between Na intake and increased blood pressure, although more recent evidence is in favour of the latter[7].

25.3.2 After BMI and alcohol consumption have been allowed for, a relationship does exist between urinary Na excretion (assumed to be a marker of intake) and increasing blood pressure with age[4]. However this correlation was not as strong as that found either between urinary potassium (K) excretion or urinary Na: K excretion ratios with increasing blood pressure. Although restricted Na intakes reduce blood pressure in individuals with established hypertension, they do not do so reliably in those with normal blood pressure. It has been calculated that a reduction of daily Na intake from 170 mmol to 70 mmol (3.9 to 1.6 g) might reduce systolic blood pressure by 2.2 mm Hg and diastolic pressure by 0.1 mm Hg, but recent evidence suggests this may be a considerable underestimate[7]. The Panel accepted the possibility that public health benefits such as reduced cardiovascular disease mortality might arise from such a change, but other interventions such as reduction of obesity, increased potassium, reduced energy intakes, altered quantity and quality of fat intake and reduced alcohol consumption may also have at least as great an impact on such diseases. The

Panel cautioned against any trend towards increased Na intakes. The Panel further agreed that current Na intakes were needlessly high, and decided to set DRVs on the basis of the balance of risks and benefits which might practically be expected to occur, given the prevailing socio-cultural environment.

25.3.3 The determination of a potentially toxic threshold for Na intake is also difficult. The possibility of a genetic susceptibility to Na related hypertension in perhaps 10 per cent of the population is of some concern. This association with elevated diastolic and systolic blood pressures may be apparent at intakes of 140–205 mmol/d (3.2–4.7 g/d).

25.3.4 *Adults* On these bases it is not possible to derive an EAR for Na but the Panel suggests that the LRNI for adults is set at 25 mmol/d (575 mg/d) with an RNI of 70 mmol/d (1600 mg) (Table 25.1). The Panel were unable to offer guidance on high consumption though noted that usual intakes are in excess of 140 mmol/d (3.22 g/d). The Panel saw no physiological advantage in exceeding this intake and considered that it would not be appropriate to increase these intakes further.

25.3.5 *Infants and children* The LRNIs have been estimated by calculating the daily increments in total body Na content (140 mmol/L of ECF and 2 mmol/L of intracellular fluid) allowing for the declining proportion with age of ECF in body mass[8] with an allowance for dermal, faecal and some urinary losses. The LRNI in infants up to 6 months approximates to calculated intakes for breastfed infants in whom, on the basis of 850 ml milk consumed daily and a Na content of 7 mmol/L, intakes up to 3 months of age are 1.4 mmol/kg/d and 0.9 mmol/kg/d at 4–6 months of age (Table 25.1).

25.3.6 *Environmental effects* Sodium requirements may be increased with unaccustomed hard exercise or exposure to high ambient temperatures. In such

Table 25.1 *Dietary Reference Values* for Sodium mmol/d** (mg/d)*

Age	Lower Reference Nutrient Intake	Reference Nutrient Intake
0–3 months	6 (140)	9 (210)
4–6 months	6 (140)	12 (280)
7–9 months	9 (200)	14 (320)
10–12 months	9 (200)	15 (350)
1–3 years	9 (200)	22 (500)
4–6 years	12 (280)	30 (700)
7–10 years	15 (350)	50 (1,200)
11–14 years	20 (460)	70 (1,600)
15–18 years	25 (575)	70 (1,600)
19–50 years	25 (575)	70 (1,600)
50+ years	25 (575)	70 (1,600)

*No Estimated Average Requirements have been derived for sodium.
**1 mmol = 23 mg Na: 1 g salt (NaCl) contains 17.1 mmol Na.

circumstances daily sweat losses may increase acutely from 2-4 mmol (46-92 mg) to 350 mmol (8.0 g). However adaptation provides a more dilute sweat resulting in a daily loss of 30 mmol (690 mg), and a need for a continuing intake above the range proposed is not established, although in the short term additional Na (salt) may be required.

25.4 **Intakes** Daily Na intakes are 2–10 g (90–440 mmol). In the UK mean daily urinary Na excretion has been estimated as 187 mmol (4.3 g) and 131 mmol (3.0 g) in men and women respectively with a urinary Na/K ratio of more than two[9]. In the Dietary and Nutritional Survey of British Adults mean Na intakes, excluding discretionary salt, were 3,376 and 2,351 mg/d (147 and 102 mmol/d) in men and women respectively, while mean 24 hour urinary excretion was 173 mmol (3979 mg) and 132 mmol (3036 mg) respectively[10]. A wide range of daily urinary Na excretion of 18–150 mg (0.8–6.6 mmol) has been noted in normal children.

25.5 References

[1] Simpson F O. Sodium intake, body sodium and sodium excretion. *Lancet* 1988; **2**: 25–28.

[2] Luft F C. Sodium, chloride and potassium. In: Brown M, ed. *Present Knowledge in Nutrition* 6th Ed. Washington DC: International Life Sciences Institute Nutrition Foundation, 1990; 233–240.

[3] Glieberman L. Blood pressure and dietary salt in human populations. *Ecol Fd Nutr* 1973; **2**: 143–156.

[4] Intersalt Cooperative Research Group. Intersalt: an international study of electrolyte excretion and blood pressure. Results for 24 hour urinary sodium and potassium excretion. *Br Med J* 1988; **297**: 319–328.

[5] Swales J D. Salt saga continued. *Br Med J* 1988; **297**: 307–308.

[6] Rocchini A P, Key J, Bondie D *et al.* The effect of weight loss on the sensitivity of blood pressure to sodium in obese adolescents. *New Engl J Med* 1989; **321**: 580–585.

[7] Law M R, Frost C D, Wald N J. By how much does dietary salt reduction lower blood pressure? *Br Med J* 1991; **302:** 811–815, 815–818, 819–824.

[8] Friis-Hanson B. Body weight compartments in children: changes during growth and related changes in body composition. *Pediat* 1961; **28**: 169–181.

[9] Sanchez-Castillo C P, Warrender S, Whitehead T P, James W P T. An assessment of the sources of dietary salt in a British population. *Clin Sci* 1987; **72**: 95–102.

[10] Gregory J, Foster K, Tyler H, Wiseman M. *The Dietary and Nutritional Survey of British Adults*. London: HMSO, 1990.

26. Potassium

26.1 **Function and essentiality** Potassium (K) is predominantly an intracellular cation. This compartmentalisation of K is maintained by the energy dependent cellular uptake of the element and simultaneous extrusion of sodium by the cell membrane bound enzyme Na: K adenosine triphosphatase. This process is fundamental to the cellular uptake of molecules against electrochemical and concentration gradients, to the electrophysiology of nerves and muscle, and to acid-base regulation[1, 2].

26.2 **Metabolism** An adult male is estimated to contain 40–50 mmol (1.6–2.0 g)/kg body weight, on which basis a 70 kg adult would contain 2800–3500 mmol (110–137 g). At least 95 per cent of this is intracellular at an activity concentration of 150 mmol/L (5.9 g/L); the residue is present in the ECF at a concentration of 3.5–5.5 mmol/L (137–215 mg/L). The total body K reflects lean tissue mass and consequently varies with muscularity.

26.3 **Homeostasis** The homeostasis of K is imperfectly understood and many factors are involved (see Annex 8). Over 90 per cent of dietary K is absorbed in the proximal small intestine. The body content is regulated by renal glomerular filtration and tubular secretion but up to 10 per cent of the daily loss can occur via the distal ileum and the colon and a small amount is lost in sweat. The glomerular filtration of K is approximately 3 per cent of the value for sodium, and amounts to only about 680 mmol/d (26.5 g/d). However, renal tubular secretion of the element, which is regulated predominantly by aldosterone, is highly efficient and the kidney is able to excrete K considerably in excess of this filtered load. As long as renal function is normal it is almost impossible to induce K excess on habitual dietary intakes. An additional, but usually less important, regulation of ECF and plasma K excess is achieved by the capacity of cells induced by glucose and insulin to take up K.

26.4 **Deficiency**

26.4.1 Potassium deficiency alters the electrophysiological characteristics of cell membranes causing weakness of skeletal muscles. The effect on cardiac muscle is reflected by electrocardiographic changes characteristic of impaired polarisation which may lead to arrhythmias and cardiac arrest. Similar changes in intestinal muscle cause intestinal ileus (loss of motility). Mental depression and confusion can also develop. Potassium is needed for lean tissue synthesis and an adequate K intake is needed to achieve effective homeostasis of sodium and renal function. Potassium deficiency arising from an inadequate dietary intake is unlikely because of the ubiquity of K in foodstuffs.

26.4.2 Young normotensive men on a K intake of 10 mmol/d (390 mg/d) were less able to excrete an imposed sodium excess than when they had a K intake of 90 mmol/d (3.5 g/d)[3]; simultaneously their blood pressure increased. In an international study K excretion, an assumed indicator of K intake, was negatively related to blood pressure and there was a positive relationship between urinary Na:K excretion and increasing blood pressure[4]. Potassium intakes of 65 and 100 mmol/d (2.5 and 3.9 g/d) reduce blood pressure in normotensive and hypertensive individuals and increase urinary sodium loss[5, 6]. Although some studies contradict these findings it seems reasonable to ensure that habitual daily K intakes are maintained at suitable levels to ensure optimal metabolism of sodium. It has been calculated that an increase in K intakes of 60–80 mmol/d (2.3–3.1 g/d) might induce a fall of 4 mm Hg systolic blood pressure with a possible 25 per cent reduction in deaths related to hypertension[5].

26.5 **Requirements** These are difficult to determine precisely but they can be gauged from the amount accumulated with growth and from reported urinary and faecal excretion, although the latter, of course, may represent homeostatic excretion of excessive intakes or losses incurred in maintaining sodium homeostasis. An additional allowance can be made for amounts lost via the skin and hair. The basal K losses of children have not been clearly defined; observed urinary excretion range from 0.7–2.3 mmol/kg/d (27–90 mg/kg/d). The amount needed for growth and lean tissue synthesis has been taken as 50 mmol (2.0 g)/kg body weight, and the Panel has used these factors with an allowance for integuemental and faecal losses in estimating DRVs for K factorially up to 18 years of age (Table 26.1).

26.6 **Intakes** In the Dietary and Nutritional Survey of British Adults mean K intakes were 3187 and 2434 mg/d (82 and 62 mmol/d) in men and women respectively and mean 24 urinary K excretions were 3000 mg (77 mmol) and 2420 mg (62 mmol) respectively[7]. Potassium is particularly abundant in vegetables, potatoes, fruit (especially bananas) and juices. Dietary trends with decreased consumption of vegetables and fruit and increased consumption of

Table 26.1 *Dietary Reference Values* for Potassium mmol/d** (mg/d)*

Age	Lower Reference Nutrient Intake	Reference Nutrient Intake
0–3 months	10 (400)	20 (800)
4–6 months	10 (400)	22 (850)
7–9 months	10 (400)	18 (700)
10–12 months	12 (450)	18 (700)
1–3 years	12 (450)	20 (800)
4–6 years	16 (600)	28 (1,100)
7–10 years	24 (950)	50 (2,000)
11–14 years	40 (1,600)	80 (3,100)
15–18 years	50 (2,000)	90 (3,500)
19–50 years	50 (2,000)	90 (3,500)
50+ years	50 (2,000)	90 (3,500)

*No Estimated Average Requirements have been derived for Potassium.
**1 mmol = 39.1 mg.

foods with sodium based preservatives and other additives favour reduced K and increased sodium intakes.

26.7 **Guidance on high intakes** Reported K intakes by Western populations are in the range of 40–150 mmol/d (1.6–5.9 g/d). Intakes above 450 mmol (17.6 g) may induce symptomatic hyperkalaemia in some individuals and would represent a threshold for acute toxicity but such amounts would only be achieved by supplementation and on usual dietary intakes toxicity is unlikely[8].

26.8 References

1 Pitts R F. *Physiology of the Kidney and Body Fluids* 2nd Ed. Chicago: Year Book Medical Publishers 1968.

2 Patrick J. Assessment of body potassium stores. *Kidney Int* 1977; **11**: 476–490.

3 Krishna G G, Miller E, Kapoor S. Increased blood pressure during potassium depletion in normotensive men. *New Engl J Med* 1989; **320**: 1177–1182.

4 Intersalt Cooperative Research Group. Intersalt: an international study of electrolyte excretion and blood pressure. Results for 24 hour urinary sodium and potassium excretion. *Br Med J* 1988; **297**: 319–328.

5 Rose G. Desirability of changing Potassium intake in the community. In: Whalton P *et al*, eds. *Potassium in Cardiovascular and Renal Disease*. New York: Marcel Dekker, 1986; 411–416.

6 Matlou S M, Isles C G, Higgs A *et al*. Potassium supplementation in Blacks with mild to moderate essential hypertension. *J Hyperten* 1986; **4**: 61–64.

7 Gregory J, Foster K, Tyler H, Wiseman M. *The Dietary and Nutritional Survey of British Adults*. London: HMSO, 1990.

8 National Academy of Sciences. *Recommended Dietary Allowances* 9th Ed. Washington DC: National Academy of Sciences, 1980.

27. Chloride

27.1 **Function and Essentiality** Chloride (Cl) is the major extracellular and intracellular counter anion to sodium and potassium, with 70 per cent of the body burden in the ECF, and the remainder in the intracellular space, connective tissue and bone[1]. Plasma Cl is maintained at 95–106 mmol/L* (3.4–3.8 g/L). Its concentration in interstitial fluid is slightly higher whereas the intracellular concentration of chloride has been varyingly reported between 4–25 mmol/L (142–890 mg/L). The total body Cl in adult men is about 33 mmol (1.2 g)/kg body weight and the accumulation of Cl by children has been calculated on this basis.

27.2 **Metabolism** Chloride is absorbed passively in the proximal small intestine where it follows the electrochemical gradient created by the transport of the major cationic electrolytes. Active Cl uptake in exchange for bicarbonate occurs in the distal small intestine and colon and electrogenic Cl secretion occurs in the intestinal crypt enterocytes. Dietary Cl deficiency has only been described in healthy infants who were fed an infant formula which provided less than 2 mmol (71 mg)/L[2].

27.3 **Requirements** It has been argued that Cl and Na interact in inducing hypertension in man[3,4]. Since the dietary intake and systemic metabolism of Cl matches closely and is interdependent with that of sodium, the Panel concluded that in the absence of more definitive information intakes of Cl from the diet should equal sodium intakes in molar terms and DRVs for Cl should therefore correspond to those of sodium (see table 25.1).

27.4 **Intakes** Daily Cl intake in the UK is 85–145 mmol/d (3.0–5.1 g/d) and is derived principally from sodium chloride. In a United Kingdom study daily urinary Cl excretion was 182 and 127 mmol/d (6.5 and 4.5 g/d) in men and women respectively[5]. In the Dietary and Nutritional Survey of British Adults mean Cl intakes were 5,179 and 3,573 mg/d (150 and 100 mmol/d) in men and women respectively[6]. Daily urinary Cl excretion in children aged 3–18 years was 3.8 g (110 mmol)[1].

27.5 **References**

[1] Pitts R F. *Physiology of the Kidney and Body Fluids*. 2nd ed. Chicago: Year Book Medical Publishers, 1968.

[2] Rodriguez-Soriano J, Vallo A, Castillo G, Oliveros R, Cea J M, Balzategui M J. Biochemical features of dietary chloride deficiency syndrome: a comparative study of 30 cases. *J Pediatr* 1983; **103**: 209-214.

*1 mmol = 35.5 mg

[3] Kurtz T W, Al-Bander H A, Morris R C. 'Salt-Sensitive' essential hypertension in men. Is the sodium ion alone important? *New Eng J Med* 1987; **317**: 1043–1048.

[4] Weinberger M H. Sodium chloride and blood pressure. *New Engl J Med* 1987; **317**: 1084–1086.

[5] Sanchez-Castillo C P, Branch W J, James W P T. A test of the validity of the lithium marker technique for monitoring dietary sources of salt in men. *Clin Sci* 1987: **72**: 87–94.

[6] Gregory J, Foster K, Tyler H, Wiseman M. *The Dietary and Nutritional Survey of British Adults*. London: HMSO, 1990.

28. Iron

28.1 **Function and essentiality**

28.1.1 Iron (Fe) is a component of haemoglobin (Hb), myoglobin and many enzymes and is stored in the reticulo-endothelial system as ferritin and haemosiderin. Iron stores are influenced by long-term nutrition, and can account for up to 30 per cent of total body Fe. A plasma ferritin concentration of 1 μg/L represents 8–10 mg (140–180 μmol) of stored Fe[1]. When requirements exceed the quantity absorbed from the diet, Fe stores are mobilised. Plasma ferritin of 12 μg/L or less suggests that Fe stores have become depleted.

28.1.2 Iron deficiency ultimately results in defective erythropoeisis leading to a normocytic or microcytic hypochromic anaemia[2]. However, functional consequences of Fe deficiency may occur in the absence of anaemia[3]. These include adverse effects on work capacity[4], intellectual performance[5] and behaviour[6]. Resistance to infection[7], and to thermoregulation[8] have been demonstrated in Fe deficient states

28.2 **Metabolism** Certain groups of the UK population are more vulnerable to Fe deficiency, either due to high physiological requirements to meet tissue growth (infants and toddlers, adolescents, pregnant women), high losses (menstruating women) or poor absorption (the elderly, and people consuming foods high in inhibitors of absorption eg polyphenols such as tannin in tea). Iron status is most accurately determined from combined measures of serum ferritin, transferrin saturation and erythrocyte protoporphyrin[9], although more recently the use of circulating transferrin receptor measurements as an index of tissue Fe status has been undergoing evaluation[10]. Deficiency is common among children where late weaning and inappropriate foods may precipitate problems, as demonstrated, for example, in London among infants of Bangladeshi parents[11], and children in Bradford where Ehrhardt found anaemia (Hb less than 11 g/dl) in 12 per cent of white and 28 per cent of Asian preschool children[12]. Similar results were obtained in Birmingham where 26 per cent of 470 screened children aged 6 months to 6 years, were anaemic (27 per cent of Asians, and 18 per cent of other, mainly European, children).

28.3 **Requirements**

28.3.1 Iron homeostasis is regulated by both uptake and transfer at the intestinal mucosa and although there are preliminary reports describing prolonged intestinal Fe losses there are no major excretory pathways for endogenous Fe. Other daily losses of endogenous Fe include that in desquamated gastrointestinal cells (0.14 mg), Hb (0.38 mg), bile (0.24 mg), and urine (0.1 mg)[13]. Losses through skin and sweat are so small, when skin contamination is eliminated[14], that the Panel considered them to be negligible. Blood loss depletes the body of Fe (haemoglobin is 0.347 per cent Fe).

28.3.2 The degree to which physiological requirements vary from person to person is not known precisely but basal Fe losses appear to have a coefficient of variation of about 15 per cent among normal healthy individuals. In infants, children and adolescents, Fe is also required for expanding red cell mass and growing body tissues and in women of child-bearing age menstrual losses must be added to basal losses. The dietary requirement also depends on the bioavailability of Fe from the diet. According to FAO a diet typical for most segments of the population in industrialized countries comprises generous quantities of meat, poultry, fish, and/or foods containing high amounts of ascorbic acid[15]. The Panel accepted that Fe absorption from a diverse diet can be assumed to be 15 per cent[15]. However, the Panel cautioned that Fe in diets containing little or no meat is less well absorbed and that people habitually consuming such diets may need a higher Fe intake. Unfortunately, data do not exist to quantify this precisely. As discussed in Annex 8, many factors influence absorption and utilisation of nutrients and those affecting Fe are shown in Table 28.1. For example, high intakes of ascorbic acid increase absorption and hence lower the required intake, whereas inhibitors of absorption such as tannin in tea raise the required intake.

28.3.3 *Infants* Although breast-fed infants can absorb approximately 50 per cent of the Fe in milk, infants up to the age of 3 months fed on formulated milks are assumed to absorb only 10 per cent of the Fe in milk[16]. Using these estimated losses and an absorption of 15 per cent the Panel has calculated DRVs for Fe as given in Table 28.2.

28.3.4 *Menstruating women* There are few systematic data on menstrual blood loss in the UK. Studies in Sweden show marked variation of menstrual losses between women but relatively constant losses from period to period for individual women[17]. Overall, blood losses in women have a skewed distribution (Table 28.2); 95 per cent lose 118 ml per period or less, whereas the median and

Table 28.1 *Factors affecting iron absorption**

Enhancers	Inhibitors
Dietary	
Organic acids: ascorbic, citric, lactic, malic, tartaric	Tannins, polyphenols,
	Phosphates, phytate
	Bran, lignin
Fructose, sorbitol	Proteins: egg albumen, egg yolk, legume protein
Alcohol	
Amino acids: cysteine, lysine, histidine	Inorganic elements: Ca, Mn, Cu, Cd, Co
Physiological	
Iron deficient and anaemic states	Iron overload
Fasting	Achlorhydria
Pregnancy	Copper deficiency

*See also Annex 8

Table 28.2 *Dietary Reference Values for Iron mg/d (μmol/d*)*

Age	Lower Reference Nutrient Intake	Estimated Average Requirement	Reference Nutrient Intake
0–3 months	0.9 (15)	1.3 (20)	1.7 (30)
4–6 months	2.3 (40)	3.3 (60)	4.3 (80)
7–9 months	4.2 (75)	6.0 (110)	7.8 (140)
10–12 months	4.2 (75)	6.0 (110)	7.8 (140)
1–3 years	3.7 (65)	5.3 (95)	6.9 (120)
4–6 years	3.3 (60)	4.7 (80)	6.1 (110)
7–10 years	4.7 (80)	6.7 (120)	8.7 (160)
11–14 years (males)	6.1 (110)	8.7 (160)	11.3 (200)
(females)	8.0 (140)**	11.4 (200)**	14.8 (260)**
15–18 years (males)	6.1 (110)	8.7 (160)	11.3 (200)
(females)	8.0 (140)**	11.4 (200)**	14.8 (260)**
19–50 years (males)	4.7 (80)	6.7 (120)	8.7 (160)
(females)	8.0 (140)**	11.4 (200)**	14.8 (260)**
50+ years	4.7 (80)	6.7 (120)	8.7 (160)

*1 μmol = 55.9 μg

**The distribution of iron requirements in women of childbearing age is skewed as shown below and these DRVs exclude those with high menstrual losses resulting in iron requirement above point a, 2 sd above the EAR which is set at the 75th centile. For those women iron intakes should be increased and the most practical way of achieving this would be to take iron supplements.

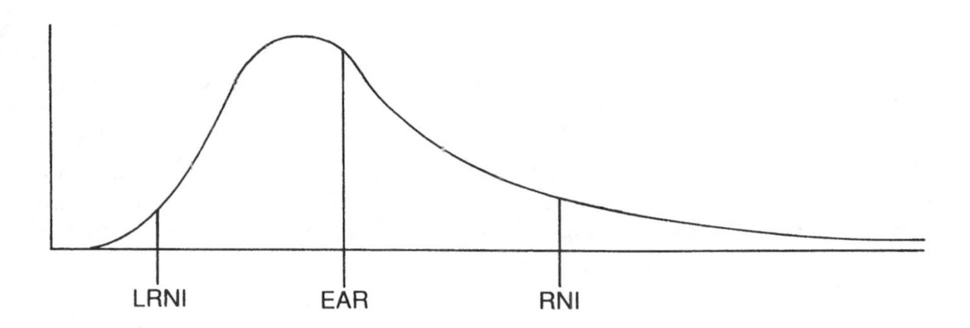

mean losses are 30 ml and 44 ml respectively. Assuming a Hb concentration of 13 g/100 ml, with the mean blood loss of 44 ml, the calculated loss of endogenous Fe is about 19.8 mg which on a 28 day cycle averages 0.7 mg/d. This is additional to Fe losses of 0.86 mg/d from other routes (see para 28.3.1). Assuming 15 per cent absorption gives a mean requirement of 10.4 mg (190 μmol)/d. Similarly the 95th centile of blood loss of 118 ml represents 1.90 mg Fe/d giving a dietary requirement of 18.4 mg (330 μmol)/d. However, these calculations do not take into account the possibility of higher efficiency of absorption and lower Hb concentrations which may offset Fe losses among women with high menstrual losses. In the UK the average Fe intake among women aged 18–49 years is 12.1 mg/d of whom 5 per cent had Hb levels of less than 110 g/L and 17 per cent had serum ferritin levels of less than 13 μg/L[18].

The DRVs assume a Gaussian distribution (see para 1.3.8) but menstrual blood losses are highly skewed (see Table 28.2). Therefore the Panel decided that the 75th centile of blood losses of 52.4 ml per period was appropriate for calculating the EAR. Using the above calculation procedure gives an EAR of 11.4 mg (200 μmol)/d. Allowing 2 sd each side of the EAR gives an LRNI of 8.0 mg (140 μmol)/d and an RNI of 14.8 mg (260 μmol)/d. The Panel acknowledged that this RNI might not meet the requirements of approximately 10 per cent of the women with the highest menstrual losses and for these women the most practical way of meeting their high Fe requirements would be to take iron supplements.

28.3.5 *Pregnancy* The requirement of Fe for the products of conception have been estimated to be 680 mg (12 mmol)[19]. Ideally all women of child-bearing age should have sufficient stores to cope with the metabolic demands made by pregnancy which can be met without further increase because of cessation of menstrual losses and by the mobilisation of maternal stores and increased intestinal absorption[20]. However, when iron stores are inappropriately low at the start of pregnancy, supplementation with Fe may be necessary.

28.3.6 *Lactation* Reported Fe concentrations in breast milk are 0.4 mg (7 μmol)/L during weeks 6–8 post-partum, falling to 0.29 mg (5 μmol)/L during weeks 17–22[21]. Assuming that the volume of milk produced per day is 850 ml, this amounts to 0.25–0.34 mg/d (5–6 μmol/d). This Fe secretion may be offset by lactational amenorrhoea.

28.3.7 *Blood donors* Information supplied by the National Blood Transfusion Service indicates that regular blood donors, who give blood at intervals of not less than 6 months, are able to replenish their own Fe stores. This is probably achieved by an increased efficiency of absorption and therefore higher Fe intakes are probably not necessary. However, more frequent donations, particularly by women of child-bearing age, may warrant a higher Fe intake to maintain adequate Fe status.

28.4 **Intakes** The most recent figures from the National Food Survey indicate that the Fe content of food obtained for consumption at home in 1988 averaged 10.9 mg (0.2 mmol)/person/d[22]. Adult Fe intakes in Great Britain averaged 14.0 mg (250 μmol)/d and 12.3 mg (220 μmol)/d among men and women respectively[18]. For women intakes from foods only averaged 11.6 mg (200 μmol)/d while for those taking Fe supplements intakes from these supplements averaged 7.5 mg (130 μmol)/d[23].

28.5 **Guidance on high intakes** Most cases of Fe poisoning occur in children. The acute toxic dose in infants has been estimated to be approximately 20 mg (0.4 mmol)/kg, and the lethal dose about 200–300 mg (3.6–5.4 mmol)/kg body weight[24]. Individual case reports on poisoning in adults indicate that a 100 g (1,800 mmol) dose of Fe is lethal[25] although survival may be possible with treatment[26]. The inherited disorder, haemochromatosis, estimated to cause disease in 0.3–0.8 per cent of white people[27], is associated with inappropriately high Fe absorption, resulting in a gradual accumulation of Fe in the tissues. However, it cannot be prevented by dietary treatment alone.

28.6 **Research needs** More information is needed on the Fe status of different groups of the UK population, including infants, children and the elderly. This should be coupled with reliable measures of intake. Particular attention should be given to the measurement of losses of body Fe, the determination of physiological requirements for infants, the optimal Fe fortification to be added to infant formulas and other foods, and the possibility of undesirable nutritional effects of high Fe concentration due to interactions with other micronutrients which could result in reduced bioavailability, and the formation of free radicals. Short and long-term adaptive responses to diets of differing Fe levels and absorbabilities need to be demonstrated along with the health and socio-economic consequences of Fe deficiency, including psychomotor development and behaviour in children. The role of Fe in modifying immune function requires further evaluation.

28.7 References

[1] Walters G O, Miller F M, Worwood M. Serum ferritin concentration and iron stores in normal subjects. *J Clin Pathol* 1973; **26**: 770–772.

[2] Expert Scientific Working Group. Summary of a report on assessment of the iron nutritional status of the United States population. *Am J Clin Nutr* 1985; **42**: 1318–1330.

[3] Scrimshaw N S. Functional consequences of iron deficiency in human populations. *J Nutr Sci Vitaminol* 1984; **30**: 47–63.

[4] Gardner G W, Edgerton V R, Senewiratne B, Barnard R J, Ohira Y. Physical work capacity and metabolic stress in subjects with iron deficiency anaemia. *Am J Clin Nutr* 1977; **30**: 910–917.

[5] Soemantri A G, Pollitt E, Kim I. Iron deficiency anaemia and educational achievement. *Am J Clin Nutr* 1985; **42**: 1221–1228.

[6] Oski F A, Honig A S, Helu B, Howanitz P. Effect of iron therapy on behaviour performance in nonanaemic, iron-deficient infants. *Pediatrics* 1983; **71**: 877–880.

[7] Srikantia S G, Bhaskaram C, Prasad J S, Krishnamachari K A V R. Anaemia and immune response. *Lancet* 1976; **1**: 1307–1309.

[8] Martinez-Torres C, Cubeddu L, Dillman E *et al.* Effect of exposure to low temperature on normal and iron-deficient subjects. *Am J Physiol* 1984; **246**: 380–383.

[9] Cook J D, Finch C A, Smith N J. Evaluation of the iron status of a population. *Blood* 1976; **48**: 449–455.

[10] Flowers C H, Skikne B S, Covell A M, Cook J D. The clinical measurement of serum transferrin receptor. *J Lab Clin Med* 1989; **114** 368–377.

[11] Harris R J, Armstrong D, Ali R, Loynes A. Nutritional survey of Bangladeshi children aged under 5 years in the London Borough of Tower Hamlets. *Arch Dis Child* 1983; **58**: 428–432.

[12] Erhardt P. Iron deficiency in young Bradford children from different ethnic groups. *Br Med J* 1986; **292**: 90–93.

[13] Green R, Chalton R, Seftel H, Bothwell T H, Mayet F, Adams B, Finch C A, Layrisse M. Body iron excretion in man. A collaborative study. *Am J Med* 1968; **45**: 336–353.

[14] Brune M, Magnussen B, Persson H, Hallberg L. Iron losses in sweat. *Am J Clin Nutr* 1986; **43**: 438–443.

[15] Food and Agriculture Organization. *Requirements of Vitamin A, Iron, Folate and B12. Report of a Joint FAO/WHO consultation. Rome: FAO, 1988. (Food and Nutrition Series No 23).*

[16] *Flanagan P R, Mechanisms and regulation of intestinal uptake and transfer of iron. Acta Paediatr Scand* 1989; **361** (suppl); 21–30.

[17] Hallberg L, Hogdahl A-M, Nilsson L, Rybo G. Menstrual blood loss—a population study. *Acta Obstet Gynaecol Scand* 1966; **45**: 320–351.

[18] Gregory J, Foster K, Tyler H, Wiseman M. *The Dietary and Nutritional Survey of British Adults*. London: HMSO, 1990.

[19] Committee on Iron Deficiency. Iron deficiency in the United States. *J Am Med Ass* 1968; **203**: 407–412.

[20] Svanberg B, Arvidsson B, Bjorn-Rasmussen E, Hallberg L, Rossander L, Swolin B. Dietary iron absorption in pregnancy—a longitudinal study with repeated measurements of non-haem iron absorption from whole diet. *Acta Obstet Gynecol Scandinav* 1975; **48** (suppl): 43–68.

[21] Vuori E. Intake of copper, iron, manganese and zinc by healthy, exclusively breast-fed infants during the first 3 months of life. *Br J Nutr* 1979; **42**: 407–411.

[22] Ministry of Agriculture, Fisheries and Food. *Household Food Consumption and Expenditure, 1988*. London: HMSO, 1989.

[23] Ministry of Agriculture, Fisheries and Food. *Report of the Working Group on Dietary Supplements and Health Foods*. London: MAFF, 1991.

[24] Pierron H, Sauzay F, Bellon-Serre V, Sepulcre J, Perrimond H, David J M. Intoxication martiala orale aigui accidentelle d'origine medicamenteuse en pediatrie. *Ann Ped* 1987; **34**: 333–335.

[25] Cernelc M, Kusar V, Jeretin S. Fatal peroral iron poisoning in a young woman. *Acta Haemat* 1968; **40**: 90–94.

[26] Eriksson F, Johnsson S V, Mellstedt H, Strandberg O, Wester P O. Iron intoxication in two adult patients. *Acta Med Scand* 1984; **196**: 231–236.

[27] Edwards C Q. Early detection of hereditary hemochromatosis. *Ann Intern Med* 1984; **101**: 707–708.

29. Zinc

29.1 **Function and Essentiality** Zinc (Zn) is present in all tissues. It is an essential component of a number of enzymes in which it has structural, regulatory, or catalytic roles[1]. Additionally, it has a structural role in a number of non-enzymic proteins for example in maintaining the aggregation of the presecretory insulin granules and, possibly, in maintaining the configuration of mammalian gene transcription proteins, and the integrity of biomembranes. Thus, either directly or indirectly, Zn is involved in the major metabolic pathways contributing to the metabolism of proteins, carbohydrates, energy, nucleic acids and lipids. Early features of deficiency include growth retardation, and defects of rapidly dividing tissues such as skin, intestinal mucosa, and the immune system.

29.2 **Metabolism** The adult human contains approximately 2 g (31 mmol) Zn, of which about 60 and 30 per cent respectively are in skeletal muscle (30–50 mg/kg) and bone (100–200 mg/kg), and 4–6 per cent is present in skin[2]. Since Zn turnover in these tissues is slow, these depots do not provide a reliable source of the element at times of deprivation, unless there is an increased turnover of the tissue, such as during catabolism, when Zn is released adventitiously and is available for use in other tissues. Conversely, since Zn is essential for the synthesis of lean tissue, it is when this is occurring, rather than when tissue is being broken down, that it may become a limiting nutrient. As a general rule it is assumed that the body has no specific Zn reserve and that it is dependent on a regular dietary supply of the element. The best dietary Zn sources are red meats. The amount from plant sources varies. Unrefined cereals contain Zn in sufficient amounts to offset the limited bioavailability of the metal. White flour is a poor Zn source[3].

29.3 **Homeostasis** Zinc is absorbed throughout the gut but, since there is a large enteropancreatic circulation of the element, net intestinal absorption occurs in the distal small intestine. Many factors affect bioavailability (see Annex 8) but regulation of faecal losses is important in systemic Zn homeostasis[2,4]. With inappropriately high Zn intakes homeostasis of the element is achieved by sequestation in the mucosal cells by metallothionein, a cysteine rich protein.

29.4 **Requirements**

29.4.1 *Adults* The assessment of Zn requirements in adults has been approached on the basis of determining basal losses during metabolic studies of deprivation, the turnover time of radiolabelled endogenous Zn pools, deduction from metabolic studies of patients receiving total parenteral nutrition, and factorial analyses. None are ideal but all indicate that in order to avoid disturbed metabolism of other nutrients the systemic needs are 2–3 mg/d

(30–46 μmol/d). On a factorial basis, using assorted data on basal faecal and urinary losses, and on losses via skin, hair and, where appropriate, semen or menstruation, it has been estimated that minimal losses are in the order of 2.2 and 1.6 mg/d (30 and 20 μmol/d) in men and women respectively[3,5]. Assuming a 30 per cent absorptive efficiency these figures translate to EARs of 7.3 and 5.5 mg/d (110 and 85 μmol/d). Assuming a normal distribution RNIs are 9.5 and 7.0 mg/d (145 and 110 μmol/d) and LRNIs are 5.5 and 4.0 mg/d (85 and 60 μmol/d) respectively (Table 29.1).

29.4.2 *Infants* In the absence of better information, daily Zn requirements for infants and children have been calculated factorially[6]. Growth increments have been estimated on the basis of growth progressing along the 50th centile and on a lean tissue Zn content of 30 mg (0.5 mmol)/kg. Urine and sweat losses were taken as 10 and 20 μg (0.15 and 0.30 μmol)/kg/d respectively and faecal losses as 77 μg (1.2 μmol)/kg/d. This gives a daily requirement of 1.0 mg (15 μmol/d) which, when adjusted to allow for 30 per cent efficiency of absorption from formulas, represents an EAR of 3.3 mg (50 μmol)/d. Allowing for a notional 2 sd the RNI is 4 mg (60 μmol)/d. The LRNI has been based on an absorptive efficiency of 50 per cent.

Table 29.1 *Dietary Reference Values for Zinc mg/d (μmol/d*)*

Age	Lower Reference Nutrient Intake	Estimated Average Requirement	Reference Nutrient Intake
0–3 months	2.6 (40)	3.3 (50)	4.0 (60)
4–6 months	2.6 (40)	3.3 (50)	4.0 (60)
7–9 months	3.0 (45)	3.8 (60)	5.0 (75)
10–12 months	3.0 (45)	3.8 (60)	5.0 (75)
1–3 years	3.0 (45)	3.8 (60)	5.0 (75)
4–6 years	4.0 (60)	5.0 (75)	6.5 (100)
7–10 years	4.0 (60)	5.4 (80)	7.0 (110)
Males			
11–14 years	5.3 (80)	7.0 (110)	9.0 (140)
15–18 years	5.5 (85)	7.3 (110)	9.5 (145)
19–50 years	5.5 (85)	7.3 (110)	9.5 (145)
50+ years	5.5 (85)	7.3 (110)	9.5 (145)
Females			
11–14 years	5.3 (80)	7.0 (110)	9.0 (140)
15–18 years	4.0 (60)	5.5 (85)	7.0 (110)
19–50 years	4.0 (60)	5.5 (85)	7.0 (110)
50+ years	4.0 (60)	5.5 (85)	7.0 (110)
Pregnancy	No increment		
Lactation:			
0–4 months			+6.0 (+90)
4+ months			+2.5 (+40)

1 μmol = 65.4 μg

29.4.3 *Children* For children over one year of age RNIs have been based on interpolated basal losses from adults and calculated increments for growth. The values were calculated on the basis of a 30 per cent absorption. Future research will probably show that these estimates are generous.

29.4.4 *Pregnancy* There is evidence that extra Zn is required during pregnancy. The additional Zn accumulated during the last trimester of gestation is 0.78 mg (12 μmol)[7], so given a physiological and systemic need of 2.0 mg (31 μmol) and absorptive efficiencies of 20–50 per cent, the dietary requirements of late pregnancy would be 5.6–14.0 mg/d (85–210 μmol/d). Since studies have shown no increase in customary daily Zn intake by pregnant women and no benefit from Zn supplements[8], it is considered probable that in healthy women metabolic adaptation ensures an adequate transfer of Zn to the fetus.

29.4.5 *Lactation* Additional Zn requirements for lactation have been computed on the basis of a daily milk volume of 850 ml and on a total daily milk Zn secretion of 2.13 mg (33 μmol) in the initial 4 months of lactation and 0.94 mg (14 μmol) thereafter; as yet insufficient data are available to enable any allowance for maternal adaptation increasing the bioavailability of dietary Zn during lactation.

29.5 **Intakes** Many studies of Zn intake show a wide range which probably reflect daily variations in intake and the short periods over which the intakes were assessed. Nonetheless most studies indicate average intakes of 9–12 mg/d. In the Dietary and Nutritional Survey of British adults, mean Zn intakes were 11.4 and 8.4 mg/d by men and women respectively[9]. Daily intakes of pregnant women in the UK are similar to those of non-pregnant women estimated at 9.1 mg/d in women on mixed diets and 7.5 mg/d in North East London Asians and 10.2 mg/d in vegetarians and non-vegetarians[7].

29.6 **Guidance on high intakes** Gross Zn toxicity may arise from acute ingestion of water which has been stored in galvanised containers, or the use of such water for renal dialysis. Symptoms such as nausea, vomiting and fever develop after acute ingestion of 2 g (31 mmol) Zn or more. However, of greater concern is the effect of chronic ingestion of high Zn levels. Prolonged exposure to large amounts 75–300 mg/d (1.15–4.59 mmol/d) have been associated with features of copper deficiency such as microcytic anaemia, and neutropenia. In short term studies 50 mg (0.76 mmol) of Zn daily interfered with metabolism of both iron and copper[10]. The development of these effects probably depends on both the relative molar ratios of the elements involved and on their absolute amounts. It is not known at present whether or not long term adaptation in the metabolism of metals will compensate for the interactions.

29.7 **Research needs** There is a need to understand further the metabolism and function of Zn and to develop more reliable means of assessing status, determining physiological requirements and consequently the required dietary intakes needed to meet these.

29.8 References

[1] Vallee B, Galdes A. The metalobiochemistry of zinc enzymes. In: Meister A, ed. *Advances in Enzymology*. Chichester, New York: John Wiley, 1984; 283–430.

[2] Jackson M J, Physiology of zinc: general aspects. In: Mills C, ed. *Zinc in Human Biology*. London: Springer Verlag, 1989; 1–4.

[3] Hambidge K M, Casey C E, Krebs N F. Zinc. In: Mertz W, ed. *Human and Animal Nutrition*. Vol 2. New York: Academic Press, 1986; 1-137.

[4] Taylor C M, Bacon J R, Aggett P J, Bremner I. The homeostatic regulation of zinc absorption and endogenous zinc losses in zinc deprived man. *Am J Clin Nutr* 1991; **53**: 755–763.

[5] King J C, Turnland J R, Human zinc requirements. In: Mills C, ed. *Zinc in Human Biology*. London: Springer Verlag, 1989; 335-350.

[6] Hambidge K M. Zinc in the nutrition of children. In: Chandra R, ed. *Trace Elements in Children*. New York: Raven Press, 1991: 65–77.

[7] Aggett P J. Extra zinc in pregnancy. *Contemp Rev Obstet Gynaecol* 1989; **1**: 181–189.

[8] Mahomed K, James D K, Golding J, McCabe R. Zinc supplementation during pregnancy: a double blind randomised controlled trial. *Br Med J* 1989; **299**: 826–830.

[9] Gregory J, Foster K, Tyler H, Wiseman M. *The Dietary and Nutritional Survey of British Adults*. London: HMSO, 1990.

[10] Yadrick M K, Kenney M A, Winterfeldt E A. Iron, copper and zinc status: response to supplementation with zinc or zinc and iron in adult females. *Am J Clin Nutr* 1989; **49**: 145–150.

30. Copper

30.1 **Function and essentiality** Copper (Cu) is a component of many enzymes, including cytochrome oxidase, and superoxide dismutase (Cu/Zn SOD)[1]. Synthesis of a range of neuroactive amines and peptides (eg catecholamines and enkephalins) also involves Cu enzymes. Features of Cu deficiency in infants and the young include leucopenia and skeletal fragility[2] and increased susceptibility to respiratory tract and other infections[3]. Anaemia may develop if deficiency is prolonged and severe. Apart from neutropenia, such signs are seen rarely. Studies with adults suggest that early features of Cu deficiency can include defects in cardiovascular function[4–6].

30.2 **Bioavailability** The factors affecting Cu bioavailability are not understood (see Annex 8), but it ranges between 35 and 70 per cent and appears to be lower in the elderly than in the young. The bioavailability of Cu from milk-based formulas is approximately 50 per cent[7].

30.3 **Requirements** There are no adequate data on human Cu requirements and the Panel were unable to derive EARs or LRNIs with sufficient confidence. Nevertheless sufficient data for infants and from biochemical changes in adults associated with varying Cu intakes were available on which to base RNIs (table 30.1).

30.3.1 *Infants* The full-term infant has larger Cu stores than at other stages of development, the liver typically containing 8 mg (130 μmol). Copper status of the term infant probably begins to be influenced by dietary intake at 4–8 weeks. Requirements have been calculated factorially on the basis of a tissue Cu content of 1.38 μg (0.02 μmol)[8], and an adjustment to allow for a possible loss of endogenous Cu[9]. Assuming an absorptive efficiency of 50 per cent[7] infant RNIs approximate to 47, 39 and 36 μg/kg/d (0.7, 0.6 and 0.6 μmol/μg/d) in successive 3 months periods of infancy.

30.3.2 *Children* The RNIs were interpolated from 36 μg (0.6 μmol)/kg/d at 9 months to 27 μg (0.4 μmol)/kg/d at 3 years, 25 μg (0.4 μmol)/kg/d at 4 years, 19 μg (0.3 μmol)/kg/d at 14 years, and 17 μg (0.3 μmol)/kg at 15 years.

30.3.4 *Adults* Review of published balance data suggested that balance can be achieved on intakes of 1.2 mg (19 μmol)/d (Mills C F, personal communication). Features concomitant with Cu deprivation such as declines in SOD and cytochrome oxidase activities, and altered metabolism of enkephalins have been detected at intakes of 0.8–1.0 mg/d (13–16 μmol)/d. An RNI of 1.2 mg (19 μmol)/d was therefore proposed for adults which is approximately 17 μg (0.3 μmol)/kg/d (Table 30.1).

Table 30.1 *Dietary Reference Values* for Copper mg/d (μmol/d**)*

Age	Reference Nutrient Intake
0–3 months	0.3 (5)
4–6 months	0.3 (5)
7–9 months	0.3 (5)
10–12 months	0.3 (5)
1–3 years	0.4 (6)
4–6 years	0.6 (9)
7–10 years	0.7 (11)
11–14 years	0.8 (13)
15–16 years	1.0 (16)
18–50 years	1.2 (19)
50+ years	1.2 (19)
Pregnancy	No increment
Lactation	+0.3 (+5)

*No Estimated Average Requirements or Lower Reference Nutrient Intakes have been derived for Copper.
**1 μmol = 63.5 μg

30.3.5 *Pregnancy* The estimated requirements for the products of conception amount to 0.033, 0.063 and 0.148 mg/d (0.5, 1.0 and 2.3 μmol/d) for first, second and third trimesters respectively[10], which can probably be met by the mother's adaptive responses.

30.3.6 *Lactation* Assuming a milk secretion of 850 ml milk/d with a Cu content of 0.22 mg (3.5 μmol)/L[11] and 50 per cent absorption, the increment required for lactation is 0.38 mg (6 μmol)/d.

30.4 **Intakes** Estimated Cu intakes by infants were 0.3, 0.45 and 0.59 mg/d (5, 7 and 9 μmol/d) at 3, 6 and 9 months of age respectively[12]. The average household Cu intake estimated from the NFS by Lewis and Buss was 1.25 mg/person/d plus 0.26 mg/person/d available in some instances from alcoholic drinks and confectionery[13]. Scottish pregnant women consumed 1.5 mg/d[14]. Mean Cu intakes of men and women in the Dietary and Nutritional Survey of British Adults were 1.63 and 1.23 mg/d respectively[15].

30.5 **Guidance on high intakes** High intakes of copper are toxic but chronic Cu intoxication has not been reported in the UK. However in the USA and West Germany Cu toxicity has been associated with water contaminated with over 1.6 mg (25 μmol)/L[16].

30.6 **Research needs** The Panel recommended further research on the significance of Cu deficiency in the UK in relation to cardiovascular disease, blood pressure and metabolism of neuroactive catecholamines and peptides. Further work on the functions of copper in humans is necessary and the development of diagnostic indices of Cu status.

30.7 References

[1] Prohaska J R. Biochemical functions of copper in animals. In: Prasad A, ed. *Essential and Toxic Trace Elements in Human Health and Disease*. New York: Alan R Liss, 1988; 105–124.

[2] Danks D M, Copper deficiency in humans. *Ann Rev Nutr* 1988; **8**: 235–257.

[3] Castillo-Duran C, Fisberg M, Valzuela A *et al*. Controlled trial of copper supplementation during the recovery from marasmus *Am J Clin Nutr* 1983; **37**: 898–903.

[4] Reiser S, Smith J C, Mertz W *et al*. Indices of copper status in humans consuming a typical American diet containing either fructose or starch. *Am J Clin Nutr* 1985; **42**: 242–251.

[5] Bhathena S J, Recant L, Voyles N R *et al*. Decreased plasma enkephalins in copper deficiency in man. *Am J Clin Nutr* 1986; **43**: 42–45.

[6] Klevay L M, Inman L, Johnson L K *et al*. Increased cholesterol in plasma in a young man during experimental copper depletion. *Metabolism* 1984; **33**: 1112–1118.

[7] Miller C A. Study of the influences on mineral homeostasis in infants fed synthetic milk formulae. CNAA, 1987. Phd Thesis.

[8] Widdowson E M, Dickerson J W T. Chemical composition of the body. In: Comar C, Bronner F, eds. *Mineral Metabolism: an Advanced Treatise*. Vol 2, New York: Academic Press, 1964; 1–247.

[9] Zlotkin S H, Buchanan B E. Meeting copper intake requirements in the parenterally fed preterm and full-term infant. *J Pediatr* 1983; **103**: 441–446.

[10] Shaw J C L. Trace elements in the foetus and young infant. *Am J Dis Child* 1980; **134**: 74–81.

[11] Casey C E, Neville M C, Hambidge K M. Studies in human lactation. The secretion of zinc, copper and manganese in human milk. *Am J Clin Nutr* 1989; **49**: 773–785.

[12] Purvis G A, Bartholomay S. Commercially prepared baby foods. In: Tsang R, Nichols B, eds. *Nutrition During Infancy*. Philadelphia: Hanley and Belfus, 1988; 399–417.

[13] Lewis J, Buss D H. Trace nutrients; 5. Minerals and vitamins in the British household food supply. *Brit J Nutr* 1988; **60**: 413–424.

[14] Tuttle S, Aggett P J, Campbell D, Macgillivary I. Zinc and copper nutrition in human pregnancy: a longitudinal study in normal primagravidae and in primagravidae at time of delivery of a growth retarded baby. *Am J Clin Nutr* 1985; **41**: 1032–1041.

[15] Gregory J, Foster K, Tyler H, Wiseman M. *The Dietary and Nutritional Survey of British Adults*. London: HMSO, 1990.

[16] Spitalny K C, Brondum J, Vogt R L, Sargent H E, Kappel S. Drinking-water-induced copper intoxication in a Vermont family. *Pediatrics* 1984; **74**: 1103–1106.

31. Selenium

31.1 **Functions and essentiality** Selenium (Se) is an integral part of the enzyme glutathione peroxidase (GSHPx), one of the mechanisms whereby intracellular structures are protected against oxidative damage[1]. Selenium deficiency results both in a decrease in GSHPx activity and in GSHPx protein[2]. GSHPx activity in blood and other tissues is linearly related to Se concentrations up to a level of 100 ng/ml in whole blood[3]. Other selenoproteins have been isolated from mammalian tissues and of particular interest is the role of Se in the hepatic microsomal deiodination of thyroxine[4]. Between 55 and 65 per cent of dietary Se is absorbed and the major route of excretion is in the urine, which reflects dietary intakes, as do levels in tissues and blood. Thus the Se 'status' of people correlates with the amount and availability of Se in their diet and the local geochemical environment[1–3].

31.2 **Requirements**

31.2.1 *Adults* Blood Se levels in the UK are just above the value (100 ng/ml) at which GSHPx activity reaches a plateau[5,6] suggesting that current levels of Se in diets are adequate. No adverse consequences arise from somewhat lower blood levels of Se or GSHPx which are below saturation[7]. However, since intakes that permit functional saturation appear to be the norm in the UK, the RNI has been established at a level to maintain this, at 1.0 μg (13 nmol)/kg (table 31.1). Supplementation studies using DL selenomethionine show that in Chinese males saturation of GSHPx can be acheived on an intake of about 41 μg/d[8]. On a body weight basis this would correspond to 50 μg/d in a UK male. However, no evidence of deficiency is seen in populations with intakes of 40 μg/d[7]. Since the Se responsive cardiomyopathy, Keshan Disease, is not seen in populations with mean intakes of 19 μg/d (equivalent to 23 μg/d in a UK male)[9], and given the considerable functional reserve at low GSHPx saturations[7], the Panel considered 40 μg/d a suitable LNRI. There is insufficient evidence to suggest that smoking or the use of oral contraceptive agents increase the requirement for Se. Neither is there any convincing evidence that high intakes protect against cancer or cardiovascular disease[3].

31.2.2 *Pregnancy and Lactation* Women should have an adequate Se intake prior to becoming pregnant and since adaptive changes in the metabolism of Se occur during pregnancy[10], no advantage is seen in recommending extra Se at this time. Concentrations of Se in colostrum vary from 15 to 80 ng/ml and fall during the first month of lactation to about 8–30 ng/ml, remaining relatively constant thereafter. To maintain infant serum at about 70 ng/ml (whole blood of about 80 ng/ml) a daily intake from breast milk of about 8–10 ng/g is necessary[11]. Human milk from the UK has been reported to contain 10–20 ng/ml[12]. In the absence of more specific data, a possible extra requirement during lactation has been calculated on the basis of milk with a Se content

Table 31.1 *Dietary Reference Values* for Selenium $\mu g/d$* (μmol/d**)

Age	Lower Reference Nutrient Intake	Reference Nutrient Intake
0–3 months	4 (0.1)	10 (0.1)
4–6 months	5 (0.1)	13 (0.2)
7–9 months	5 (0.1)	10 (0.1)
10–12 months	6 (0.1)	10 (0.1)
1–3 years	7 (0.1)	15 (0.2)
4–6 years	10 (0.1)	20 (0.3)
7–10 years	16 (0.2)	30 (0.4)
11–14 years	25 (0.3)	45 (0.6)
Men		
15–18 years	40 (0.5)	70 (0.9)
19–50 years	40 (0.5)	75 (0.9)
50+ years	40 (0.5)	75 (0.9)
Women		
15–18 years	40 (0.5)	60 (0.8)
19–50 years	40 (0.5)	60 (0.8)
50+ years	40 (0.5)	60 (0.8)
Pregnancy No increment	—	—
Lactation:	+15 (+0.2)	+15 (+0.2)

*No Estimated Average Requirements have been derived for Selenium.
**1 μmol = 79 μg

of about 12 ng/ml and 60 per cent absorption. This gives an increment in intake of about 15 μg (0.2 μmol)/d.

31.2.3 *Infants* At birth, blood Se levels resemble those in adults but then fall to a minimum by about 3 months before increasing to reach adult levels at 1–3 years. Breast-fed infants receive 5–13 μg/d (60–160 nmol/d). Intakes from formula are generally low, only 2–4 μg/d and the trend in blood concentrations reflects methods of infant feeding[13,14]. In models Se appears to be less well absorbed from infant formulas than from human milk[15]. For non-breast fed infants the RNI has been set at 1.5 μg/kg at 4–6 months and 1.0 μg/kg at 7–12 months with an allowance for growth of 0.2 μg/kg weight gain.

31.2.4 *Children* Selenium nutrition has not been extensively investigated in children. In the UK, blood Se levels were found to be about 80 per cent of UK adult levels at 1 year, increasing to adult values by 3 years and remaining relatively constant thereafter[14]. Similar trends have been reported in New Zealand and West Germany. The RNI has been calculated on a body weight basis from the adult figure, with an additional requirement for growth set at 0.2 ng/g weight gain.

31.3 **Intakes** Selenium is present in foods mainly as the amino acids selenomethionine and selenocysteine and derivatives. Estimation of adequate Se intake is helped by the recognition of clinical disease with the extremes of naturally occurring dietary intakes of Se. In China, intakes of Se less than 12 μg (0.15 μmol)/d are associated with an increased incidence of an endemic Se responsive cardiopathy (Keshan Disease). However in New Zealand and Finland where habitual intakes are 15–40 μg/d (0.2–0.5 μmol/d) no Se responsive disease has been identified[1–3]. In Southern England Se intakes approximate 65 μg (0.8 μmol)/d[16]. Cereals, meat and fish contribute the bulk of Se to the diet with cereals providing about 50 per cent of this[12,16].

31.4 **Guidance on high intakes** Evidence of disturbed Se homeostasis occurs at intakes above 750 μg (9.5 μmol)/d[17], and early nail dystrophy has been observed in adults ingesting 900 μg (11.4 μmol)/d. Thus, given the absence of any demonstrable benefit from exceeding intakes much lower than these[3], the Panel recommended that the maximum safe Se intake from all sources should be 450 μg (5.7 μmol)/d for adult males, corresponding to 6 μg/kg/d.

31.5 References

1 Levander O A. Selenium. In: Mertz W, ed. *Trace Elements in Human and Animal Nutrition*. 5th ed, vol 2. Orlando, Florida: Academic Press, 1986; 209–279.

2 Levander O A. A global view of human selenium nutrition. *An Rev Nutr* 1987; **7:** 227–250.

3 Casey C E. Selenophillia. *Proc Nutr Soc* 1988; **47:** 55–62.

4 Arthur J R, Nicol F, Beckett F J. Hepatic iodothyronine deiodinase: the role of selenium. *Biochem J* 1990; **272:** 537–540.

5 Thomson C D, Rea H M, Doesburg V M, Robinson M F. Selenium concentrations and glutathione peroxidase activities in whole blood of New Zealand residents. *Br J Nutr* 1977; **37:** 457–460.

6 Diplock A T, Chaudhry F A. The relationship of selenium biochemistry to selenium-responsive disease in man. In: Prasad A, ed. *Essential and Toxic Trace Elements in Human Health and Disease*. New York: Alan R Liss, 1988; 211–226.

7 Robinson M F. The New Zealand selenium experience. *Am J Clin Nutr* 1988; **48:** 521–534.

8 Yang G A, Zhu L Z, Liu S J *et al*. Human selenium requirements in China. In: Combs G, *et al* eds. *Selenium in Biology and Medicine*. New York: Nostrand Rheinhold/AVJ, 1987; 589–607.

9 Yang G, Ge K, Chen J, Chen X. Selenium-related endemic diseases and the daily requirement of humans. *Wld Rev Nutr Dietet* 1988; **55:** 98–152.

10 Swanson C A, Reaner D C, Veillon C, King J C, Levander O A. Quantitative and qualitative aspects of selenium utilisation in pregnant and non pregnant women: an application of stable isotope methodology. *Am J Clin Nutr* 1983; **38;** 169–180.

11 Smith A M, Picciano M F, Milner J A. Selenium intakes and status of human milk and formula fed infants. *Am J Clin Nutr* 1982; **35:** 521–526.

12 Thorn J, Robertson J, Buss D H, Bunton N G. Trace nutrients. Selenium in British food. *Br J Nutr* 1978; **39**: 391–396.

13 Lombeck I, Kasperek K, Harbisch H D, Feinendegen L E, Bremer H J. The selenium state of healthy children. *Europ J Pediatr* 1977; **125**: 81–88.

[14] Ward K P, Arthur J R, Russell G, Aggett P J. Blood selenium content and glutathione peroxidase activity in children with cystic fibrosis, coeliac disease, asthma and epilepsy. *Eur J Pediatr* 1984; **142:** 21–24.

[15] Raghib M H, Chan W Y, Rennert O M. Comparative studies of selenium-75 (selenite and selenomethionine) absorption from various milk diets in suckling rats. *J Nutr* 1986; **116:** 1456–1463.

[16] Bunker V W, Lawson M S, Stranfield M F, Clayton B E. Selenium balance studies in apparently healthy and housebound elderly people eating self-selected diets. *Br J Nutr* 1988; **59:** 171–180.

[17] Yang G, Yin S, Zhou L *et al*. Studies of safe maximal daily dietary Se intake in a seleniferous area in China. Part II Relation between Se intake and the manifestation of clinical signs and certain biochemical alterations in blood and urine. *J Trace Elem Electrolytes Health Dis* 1989; **3:** 123–130.

32. Molybdenum

32.1 **Function and essentiality** Molybdenum (Mo) is essential for the enzymes xanthine oxidase/dehydrogenase, aldehyde oxidase and sulphite oxidase which are involved in the metabolism of DNA and sulphites[1].

32.2 **Requirements** Functional defects that were responsive to Mo developed in adults fed 25 μg (0.3 μmol*)/d[2]. Hamilton and Minski (1972) reported a mean intake of 128 μg/d from typical UK diets[3]. For other countries intakes of ostensibly healthy subjects have been reported to be 44–460 μg/d for USA adults, 48–96 μg/d for New Zealand, 44–260 μg/d for Sweden[1] and 120 μg/d for Finland[4]. Therefore the Panel set no RNIs but safe intakes are believed to lie between 50 and 400 μg/d (0.5 and 4 μmol/d) for adults. On evidence from infants who were breastfed intakes between 0.5 and 1.5 μg/kg/d should be appropriate[5]. In the absence of other evidence the Panel suggested similar safe intakes for children up to 18 years of age.

32.3 **Guidance on high intakes** High dietary Mo intakes (10–15 mg/d: 142–214 ng/kg/d) may be associated with altered metabolism of nucleotides[6], and with impaired copper bioavailability[1].

32.4 **References**

[1] Mills C F, Davis G K. Molybdenum. In: Mertz W, ed. *Trace elements in Human and Animal Nutrition*. Fifth Edition, Vol 2. New York: Academic Press, 1986; 429–461.

[2] Chiang G, Swenseid M E, Turnlund J. Studies of biochemical markers indicating molybdenum status in humans. *FASEB J* 1989; **3**: Abstr No 4922.

[3] Hamilton E I, Minksi M J. Abundance of the chemical elements in man's diet and possible reactions with environmental factors. *Sci Total Envir* 1972, **1**: 341–375.

[4] Varo P, Koivistoinen P. Mineral element composition of Finnish foods. *Acta Agric Scand* 1980; **22** (Suppl): 165–171.

[5] Casey C E, Neville M C. Studies in human lactation. 3 Molybdenum and nickel in human milk during the first month of lactation. *Am J Clin Nutr* 1987; **45**, 921–926.

[6] Kovalskii V V, Iarovaia G A, Shmavonjan D M. Modification of human and animal purine metabolism in conditions of various molybdenum bio-geochemical areas. *Zh Obshch Biol* 1961; **22**: 179–191.

*1 μmol = 95.9 μg

33. Manganese

33.1 **Function and Essentiality** Manganese (Mn) is a component of enzymes such as pyruvate carboxylase, mitochondrial superoxide dismutase and arginase, and it also activates many other enzymes eg hydrolases, glycosyl transferases, kinases, prolinase and phosphotransferases[1]. The body contains 12–20 mg (0.2–0.4 mmol*) of Mn, most of which is intracellular. About 25 per cent of this is in the skeleton and is relatively immobile. Highest concentrations are found in the pancreas and liver Absorption occurs throughout the length of the small intestine but the efficiency is reportedly low, and there is as yet no evidence on how it alters with Mn deprivation or excess. Systemic Mn homeostatis is achieved principally through hepato-biliary and intestinal secretion. Studies in animal models, and preliminary studies in human infants, suggest that in the early postnatal period intestinal uptake and whole body retention is increased. This appears to be a consequence of an efficient intestinal uptake and transfer of the element and reduced hepato-biliary secretion[2].

33.2 **Requirements** Human Mn deficiency has not been observed other than in two experimental studies only one of which was part of a systematic study of Mn metabolism. It would seem therefore that current population intakes are adequate[3]. Recourse to this pragmatic approach of determining DRVs is further enforced because the lack of adequate data on body composition data and of detailed studies of turnover and metabolism. The Panel therefore set no RNIs but safe intakes are believed to lie above 1.4 mg (26 μmol)/d for adults and above 16 μg (0.3 μmol)/kg/d for infants and children.

33.3 **Intakes** Total Mn intakes in Britain were estimated at 4.6 mg (84 μmol)/person/d of which half was derived from tea[4]. Observed mean dietary Mn intakes in the UK include 5.5 mg and 3.3 mg/d in pregnant and non-pregnant women[5] and 60 μg/kg/d in children aged 3 months to 8 years[6]. The calculated total Mn output in human breast milk during the first three months postpartum is 1.9 μg/d and 1.6 μg/d in the ensuing three months[7]. Healthy term infants fed a formula based on cow's milk had intakes of 28–42, 16–24 and 18–32 μg/kg/d at 1, 2 and 3 months of age with respective mean maximum retentions of 7.7, 6.1 and 8.0 μg[8]. Older infants on mixed weaning diets have intakes of 71 μg (1.3 μmol)/kg/d and 8 μg (0.2 μmol)/kg/d at 6 and 12 months[9].

33.4 **Guidance on high intakes** Manganese is one of the least toxic of all elements because when excess is consumed absorption is very low and that which is absorbed is efficiently excreted via the bile and kidneys[10]. Toxic

*1 mmol = 55 mg

reactions in man have only been reported in miners exposed to Mn ores, but these were attributed to continuous absorption from dust in the lungs rather than from the intestine[11,12].

33.5 References

[1] Keen C L, Lonnerdal B, Hurley L S. Manganese. In: Frieden E, ed. *Biochemistry of the Essential Ultratrace Elements*. New York: Plenum Press, 1984; 89–132.

[2] Kies C. *Nutritional Bioavailability of Manganese*. Washington DC: American Chemical Society, 1987.

[3] Anonymous. Manganese deficiency in humans: fact or fiction. *Nutr Rev* 1988; **46:** 348–352.

[4] Wenlock R W, Buss D H, Dixon E J. Trace nutrients 2. Manganese in British foods. *Br J Nutr* 1979; **41:** 253-261.

[5] Armstrong J. *Trace Element Metabolism in Human Pregnancy*. M. Phil. Thesis. Aberdeen: Robert Gordon's Institute of Technology, 1985.

[6] Alexander F W, Clayton B E, Delves H T. Mineral and trace metal balances in children receiving normal and synthetic diets. *Quart J Med* 1974; **43:** 89–111.

[7] Casey C E, Neville M C, Hambidge K M. Studies in human lactation: secretion of zinc, copper and manganese in human milk. *Am J Clin Nutr* 1989; **49:** 773–785.

[8] Miller C. *A study of the Influences on Mineral Homeostatis in Infants fed synthetic Milk Formulae* Ph.D. Thesis. Aberdeen: Robert Gordons Institute of Technology, 1987.

[9] Gibson R S, DeWolfe M S. The dietary trace metal intake of some Canadian full-term and low birthweight infants during the first twelve months of infancy. *J Can Diet Assoc* 1980; **41:** 206–215.

[10] Underwood E J. *Trace elements in Human and Animal Nutrition*. 4th ed. New York: Academic Press, 1977; 170–181.

[11] Borg D C, Cotzias G C. Incorporation of manganese into erythrocytes as evidence for a manganese porphyrin in man. *Nature* 1958; **182:** 1677–1678.

[12] Cotzias G C. Manganese and heart disease. *Physiol Rev* 1958; **38:** 503–532.

34. Chromium

34.1 **Function and essentiality** Chromium (Cr) appears to function biologically in an organic complex which potentiates the action of insulin[1,2]. It may also participate in lipoprotein metabolism and in maintaining the structure of nucleic acids, and in gene expression[3]. The cationic trivalent form (Cr III) is biochemically active, whereas anionic hexavalent Cr VI is metabolised differently and is more toxic. The two forms are inter-convertible and both are found in tissues[4]. Gross Cr deficiency has not been seen in humans except for some patients on long term parenteral nutrition[5].

34.2 **Sources of chromium** Because of inadequate analytical techniques and possible Cr contamination, values published prior to 1980 should be viewed with caution. Foods with a high Cr content include brewers' yeast, meat, whole grains, legumes and nuts. Highly refined foods are reported as being low in Cr and sugars may stimulate urinary Cr excretion[6].

34.3 **Requirements** There are no reliable objective measures of Cr deficiency but deficiency symptoms have been reported on intakes of 6 μg (0.12 μmol*)/d which can be prevented by an intravenous supplement of 20 μg (0.38 μmol)/d[7]. Using regression equations, the theoretical requirement from balance studies for adults is 23 μg (0.38 μmol) and range from 25 to 30 μg/d (0.5–0.6 μmol/d). The Cr content of breast milk ranges from 0.06–1.56 ng/ml[8]. On an intake of breast milk of 850 ml/d, the estimated Cr intake for infants would be 51–1326 ng/d. In adults observed intakes vary from 13 to 49 μg/d[9-11], and in the elderly from 27 to 61 μg/d[12,13]. The Panel set no RNIs but a safe and adequate level of intake is believed to lie above 25 μg (0.5 μmol)/d for adults and between 0.1 and 1.0 μg/kg/d (2 and 19 nmol/kg/d) for children and adolescents.

34.4 **Guidance on high intakes** No adverse effects have been noted from Cr III but intakes of 19.2–38.5 mmol/d (1–2 g/d) of the hexavalent form can cause renal and hepatic necrosis[14,15].

34.5 **References**

[1] Campbell W J, Mertz W. Interaction of insulin and chromium (III) on mitochondrial swelling. *Am J Physiol* 1963; **204** (Suppl 2): 1028–1030.

[2] Mertz W. Chromium occurrence and functions in biological systems. *Physiol Rev* 1969; **49:** 163–239.

[3] Okada S. Ohba H, Taniyama M. Alterations in ribonucleic acid synthesis by chromium (III). *J Inorg Biochem* 1981; **15:** 223-231.

*1 μmol = 52 μg

[4] Underwood E J. *Trace Elements in Human and Animal Nutrition*. 4th Ed. New York: Academic Press, 1977; 263–270.

[5] Freund H F, Atamian S, Fischer J E. Chromium deficiency during total parenteral nutrition. *J Am Med Ass* 1979; **241:** 496–498.

[6] Schroeder H A, Nason A P, Tipton H I. Chromium deficiency as a factor in atherosclerosis. *J Chron Dis* 1970; **23:** 123–142.

[7] Offenbacher E G, Pi-Sunyer F X. Chromium in human nutrition, *Ann Rev Nutr* 1988; **8:** 543–563.

[8] Casey C E, Hambidge K M. Chromium in human milk from American mothers. *Br J Nutr* 1984; **52:** 73–77.

[9] Kumpulainen J, Vuori E, Makinen S, Kara R. Dietary chromium intake of lactating Finnish mothers: effect on the Cr content of their breast milk. *Br J Nutr* 1980; **44:** 257–263.

[10] Gibson R S, Scythes C A. Chromium, selenium, and other trace element intakes of a selected sample of Canadian premenopausal women. *Biol Trace El Res* 1984; **6:** 105–116.

[11] Anderson R A, Kozlovsky A S. Chromium intake, absorption and excretion of subjects consuming self selected diets. *Am J Clin Nutr* 1985; **41:** 1177–1183.

[12] Bunker V W, Lawson M S, Delves H T, Clayton B E. The uptake and excretion of chromium by the elderly. *Am J Clin Nutr* 1984; **39:** 792–802.

[13] Gibson R S, MacDonald A C, Martinez O B. Dietary chromium and manganese intakes of a selected sample of Canadian elderly women. *Hum Nutr: App Nutr* 1985; **39A:** 43–52.

[14] Frisdedt B, Lindqvist B, Schutz A, Ovrum P. Survival in a case of acute oral chronic acid poisoning with acute renal failure treated with dialysis. *Acta Med Scand* 1965; **177:** 153–159.

[15] Kaufman D B, Di Nicola W, McIntosh R. Acute potassium dichromate poisoning. *Am J Dis Child* 1970; **119:** 374–376.

35. Iodine

35.1 **Function and essentiality** Iodine (I) forms part of the hormones thyroxine (T_4) and triiodothyronine (T_3), which are necessary for the maintenance of metabolic rate, cellular metabolism and integrity of connective tissue. In the fetus I is necessary for the development of the nervous system during the first three months of gestation; infants born to severely deficient mothers are likely to suffer from cretinism[1,2]. Iodine deficiency is now rare in the UK, but is still common in many areas in the world, including some parts of Europe[3].

35.2 **Metabolism** Inorganic I is efficiently absorbed from normal diets. Excretion is mainly via the urine[4]. Iodide ions are concentrated by the thyroid and to a lesser extent by the salivary and gastric glands. Apart from these glands iodide ions are equally distributed throughout body tissues and form the "iodide pool". About 20 per cent of I in blood is in the form of iodide, and levels do not vary significantly with different thyroid states. Goitrogens such as thiocyanates and perchlorates interfere with I uptake by the thyroid. The quantities of Ca, F, Mg, and Mn ions in hard water may be goitrogenic. Brassicas, cassava, maize, bamboo shoots, sweet potato and lima beans contain goitrogenic cyanoglucosides, but in the UK these foods are only likely to be important where they are consumed in conjunction with a diet low in I[5].

35.3 **Sources of iodine** Iodine occurs in foods largely as inorganic iodides or iodates. Milk has become a major source of I in the UK as the I content of cow milk has risen during recent years from 23 to 104 μg/kg (0.2–0.8 μmol/kg) in 1965 to between 30 and 280 μg/kg (0.2–23 μmol/kg) in 1985[6]. The reasons for this rise are the increase in I in the environment from adventitious sources such as I-supplemented cattle feed, particularly during the winter months, the use of iodinated casein as a lactation promoter in cows, and the contamination of milk from teat dips containing iodophors as sterilising agents[7]. The amount of I in human milk has also increased over the last 50 years and correlates with increases in intake. Seafoods are rich sources, with some dried seaweed preparations containing up to 5,000 μg (40 μmol)/kg. Sea fish may contain up to 1,200 μg (10 μmol)/kg. Foods containing the red dye erythrosine also contain large amounts of I, but this is in a bound form and the bioavailability from this source is reported to be between 1 and 5 per cent[6].

35.4 **Requirements**

35.4.1 *Adults* A urinary I excretion of less than 50 μg/g creatinine is usually associated with a high incidence of goitre in a population[8,9]. There are no data on I requirements and the Panel did not calculate an EAR. Nevertheless in adults an intake of 70 μg/d appears to be the minimum necessary to avoid signs of goitre in a population[10,11]. Increasing I intake from 100 to 500 μg/d made no difference to the incidence of goitre in one study[9]. The level of I in the thyroid gland has been shown to be normal at I intakes of 100 μg/d, and showed no further increase at intakes of up to 300 μg/d[12]. The minimum I requirement is therefore about 70 μg (0.6 μmol)/d for adults and the Panel made this the LRNI. In order to provide a margin of safety and to allow for the possible effects of different dietary patterns the Panel has set the RNI at 140 μg (1.1 μmol)/d (Table 35.1).

35.4.2 *Infants and children* Some children have been reported as receiving human milk containing 30–40 μg/L without signs of I deficiency[13] and, in order to allow a margin of safety, a value of 50 μg/d has been taken as the RNI for the young infant. It is not possible to extrapolate RNIs for older infants and children from those estimated for adults on a weight basis, since this would result in values similar to those estimated in areas with a high incidence of goitre. RNIs and LRNIs have therefore been extrapolated from adult values using EARs for energy, which being based on BMR have a weight component.

35.5 **Intakes** In most European countries dietary intakes of I are in excess of requirements. Average intake in the UK was calculated from the Total Diet Study as 255 μg (2 μmol)/person/d[6]. In the Dietary and Nutritional of Survey of British Adults mean I intakes were 243 and 176 μg/d for men and women respectively[14]. In the United States daily intakes of infants were assessed in 1982 and 1984 at 200 μg and 140 μg respectively; for small children the values were 460 and 160 μg and for teenagers 470–710 μg and 210–360 μg/d[15].

35.6 **Guidance on high intakes** High I intakes can cause toxic modular goitre and hyperthyroidism. Few cases of toxicity have been reported in people with

Table 35.1 *Dietary Reference Values* for Iodine μg/d* (μmol/d**)

Age	Lower Reference Nutrient Intake	Reference Nutrient Intake
0–3 months (formula fed)	40 (0.3)	50 (0.4)
4–6 months	40 (0.3)	60 (0.5)
7–9 months	40 (0.3)	60 (0.5)
10–12 months	40 (0.3)	60 (0.5)
1–3 years	40 (0.3)	70 (0.6)
4–6 years	50 (0.4)	100 (0.8)
7–10 years	55 (0.4)	110 (0.9)
11–14 years	65 (0.5)	130 (1.0)
15–18 years	70 (0.6)	140 (1.1)
19–50 years	70 (0.6)	140 (1.1)
50+ years	70 (0.6)	140 (1.1)
Pregnancy—No increment		
Lactation—No increment		

*No Estimated Average Requirements have been derived for Iodine.
**1 μmol = 127 μg

intakes of less than 5,000 μg (40 μmol)/d although transient mild effects have been demonstrated in previously deficient individuals receiving only 150–200 μg/d[16]. Normal subjects with an intake of 1,000–2,000 μg/d showed an increased I concentration in the thyroid gland, but no other changes[17]. An intake of 10–20 mg/d in Japanese fisherman resulted in an incidence of iodine goitre of 6–12 per cent[18]. There appears to be a weak relationship between consistently high I intakes and thyroid cancer. The placenta is permeable to I and the foetus is more susceptible to I-induced hyperthyroidism than the adult. Transient hyperthroidism has been reported in neonates following high I exposure in the mother, particularly in areas of I deficiency[19]. Because there remains a small number of elderly people in the UK who may be sensitive to high intakes[20], the Panel recommended that the safe upper limit on intakes 17 μg (0.1 μmol)/kg be retained[21], or not more than 1,000 μg (8 μmol)/d[22].

35.7 References

1 Delange F M. Relation of thyroid hormones to human brain development. In: Hetzel B, Smith R, eds. *Fetal Brain Disorders: Recent Approaches to the Problem of Mental Deficiency.* Amsterdam: Elsevier, 1981; 285–296.

2 Hetzel B S, Mano M T, A review of experimental studies of iodine deficiency during fetal development. *J Nutr* 1989; **119:** 145–151.

3 Anonymous, Goitre and iodine deficiency in Europe. *Lancet* 1985; **i:** 1289–1292.

4 Vought R L, London W T, Lutwak L, Dublin T D. Reliability of estimates of serum inorganic iodine and daily fecal and urinary iodine excretion from single casual specimens. *J Clin Edocrinol Metab* 1963; **23:** 1218–1228.

5 Gaitan E. Goitrogens. *J Clin Endocrinol Metab* 1988; **2:** 683–702.

6 Wenlock R W, Buss D H, Moxon R E, Bunton N G. Trace elements 4: Iodine in British Foods. *Br J Nutr* 1982; **7:** 381–390.

7 Wenlock R W, Changing patterns of dietary iodine intake in Britain. In: *Dietary Iodine and Other Aetiological Factors in Hyperthyroidism.* Conference Report, Southampton: MRC Environmental Epidemiology Unit, 1987; 1–6. (MRC Scientific Report No 9).

8 Committee on Nutrition for National Defence. *Manual for Nutrition Surveys.* Washington DC: Committee on Nutrition for National Defence, 1963.

9 Moulopoulu D S, Koutras D A, Mantzos J *et al.* Iodine intake and thyroid function in normal individuals. In Nagataki S, Torizuka K, eds. *The Thyroid.* New York: Elsevier, 1988; 283–286.

10 Stanbury J B, Ermans A M, Hetzel B S, Pretell E A, Querido A. Endemic goitre and cretinism: public health significance and prevention. *WHO Chronicle* 1974; **28:** 220–228.

11 Lamberg B A. Endemic goitre in Finland and changes during 30 years of iodine prophylaxis. *Endocrinol Exp* 1986; **20:** 35–47.

12 Ermans A M, Kinthaert J, Camus M. Defective intrathyroidal iodine metabolism in nontoxic goiter; inadequate iodination of thyroglobulin. *J Clin Endocrinol Metab* 1968; **28:** 1307–1316.

13 Gushurst C A, Mueller J A, Green J A, Sedor F. Breast milk iodide: reassessment in the 1980's. *Pediatrics* 1984; **73:** 354–357.

14 Gregory J, Foster K, Tyler H, Wiseman M. *The Dietary and Nutritional Survey of British Adults.* London: HMSO, 1990.

15 Pennington J A, Young B E, Wilson D B, Johnson R D, Vanderveen J E. Mineral content of foods and total diets: the selected minerals in Foods Survey 1982 to 1984. *J Am Dietet Assoc* 1986; **86:** 876–891.

[16] Livadas D P, Koutras D A. The toxic effects of small iodine supplements in patients with autonomous thyroid nodules. *Clin Endocrinol* 1977; **7:** 121–127.

[17] Freund G, Thomas W C, Bird E D *et al*. Effect of iodinated water supplies on thyroid function. *J Clin Endocrinol Metab* 1966; **26:** 619–624.

[18] Suzuki H, Higuchi T, Saura K *et al*. Endemic coast goitre in Hokkaido, Japan. *Acta Endocrinol* 1965; **50:** 161–176.

[19] Braverman L E. Iodine excess and thyroid function. In: *Dietary Iodine and Other Aetiological Factors in Hyperthyroidism* Conference Report, Southampton: MRC Environmental Epidemiology Unit, 1987; 29–37. (MRC Scientific Report No 9).

[20] Phillips D I, Nelson M, Barker D J P, Morris J A, Wood T J. Iodine in milk and incidence of thyrotoxicosis in England. *Clin Endocrinol* 1988; **28:** 61–66.

[21] JECFA *WHO/FAO Joint Expert Committee on Food Additives*. Geneva: World Health Organization, 1988.

[22] Pennington J A T. A review of iodine toxicity reports. *J Am Dietet Assoc* 1990; **90:** 1571–1581.

This chapter and the safe intake level have been revised to take account of some inconsistencies within the previous chapter.

36. Fluoride

36.1 **Function and Essentiality** No essential function for fluoride (F) has been proven in humans. However, it forms calcium fluorapatite (3Ca3[PO4]2CaF2) in tooth and bone and may have a role in bone mineralisation. It protects against dental caries and assists remineralisation of bone and teeth in pathological demineralising conditions. An inverse relationship between the prevalence of dental caries and the fluoride concentration of the drinking water was observed in the 1940s and the addition of fluoride to the drinking water to a level of 1ppm (1mg/l) leads to a decrease in the prevalence of caries (for review see [1,2]). A compilation of 113 water fluoridation studies, from all over the world, found that artificial water fluoridation is effective in reducing caries experience by approximately 50%, regardless of climate, race or social conditions[2].

36.2 **Requirements** Ionic fluoride is rapidly and nearly completely absorbed passively from the stomach but protein-bound organic fluoride is less bioavailable[3]. As there does not appear to be a physiological requirement for fluoride, the Panel set no RNI. Nevertheless, because of its role in the prevention of dental caries, the Panel endorses the recommendation for the continued fluoridation of water supplies to achieve levels of 1ppm.

36.3 **Intakes** Total fluoride intakes depend on the concentration of fluoride in the water supplies. However, only about 10% of the UK population receives a water supply which has either been fluoridated or has a naturally occurring fluoride content at or around 1 ppm. The MAFF Total Diet Study has estimated that adults had a mean intake of 1.82mgF/d in non-fluoridated water areas or 2.90mgF/d in fluoridated water areas, assuming an average consumption of 1.1L water daily[4]. Tea contains high concentrations of fluoride and provides 70% of the average fluoride intake. Extreme tea consumers drinking tea made from fluoridated water may reach intakes of 12mg/day[5]. A study of adolescents in the UK estimated from dietary records that the intake of fluoride from drinks (water, soft drinks and tea) was 0.96mg/d[6].

36.4 The concentration of fluoride in breast milk is low and ranges from 5–25μg/L[1] (0.26–1.3μmol/L)[7]. The consumption of fluoride by infants aged six months to one year and fed with a British milk formula reconstituted with unfluoridated water has been estimated to be 0.010–0.012mg/kg body weight/d[8]. Consumption of drinking-water fluoridated to a concentration of 1ppm results in a daily oral fluoride intake of 0.22mg/kg body weight in a 1 month-old bottle-fed baby (daily fluid intake 200ml/kg body weight, contributing 0.2mg/kg body weight, and

[1] 1μmol = 19μg

fluoride from reconstituted feed contributing 0.02mg/kg body weight). The daily intake per kg body weight falls with increasing age. A child aged 3–4 years, weighing 15kg, drinking 1 litre of water daily, and ingesting 0.3mg fluoride daily from food (4) and 0.5mg fluoride daily from toothpaste[9], would consume 0.12mg/kg body weight daily.

36.5 *Supplements* The British Dental Association recommends fluoride supplements as a protection against dental caries for infants and young children in areas where the water supply contains less than 0.7 ppm F. The dosage depends on the age of the child and the level of fluoride in the local water supply (see Table 1)[9].

Table 1 *Recommended fluoride supplement level (mg/day) depending on age and fluoride concentration in the drinking water.*

	Concentration of Fluoride in drinking water		
Age	<0.3 ppm	0.3–0.7 ppm	>0.7 ppm
6 months to 2 years	0.25	0.00	0.00
2–4 years	0.50	0.25	0.00
4–16 years	1.00	0.50	0.00

(From [9])

36.6 **Guidance on high intakes** Excessive fluoride intakes can cause dental fluorosis and very high intakes can lead to skeletal fluorosis. Dental fluorosis affects the enamel during the formation of the teeth before they erupt, and can range from very mild mottling, which is only detectable by close examination of dried teeth in good light, to severe fluorosis with pitting of the enamel and widespread brown staining of the teeth. In areas where the water contains 1ppm fluoride, about 10% of children show some tooth mottling indicative of very mild dental fluorosis[10]. More pronounced mottling is seen in children living in areas where the fluoride concentration is higher. Two surveys have shown that bottle fed infants have a higher prevalence of mottling and a higher fluorosis index than do breast-fed infants but they were within the aesthetically acceptable level[11,12]. The prevalence of very mild and mild fluorosis has increased in the USA since the 1940s when water fluoridation was introduced but the largest increases have been in non-fluoridated areas[7].

36.7 Excessive intakes of fluoride over a prolonged period of time (20–80 mg/d for 10–20 years) can lead to skeletal fluorosis, resulting in ossification of the ligaments and fusion of the spine (for review, see [1]). Occupational skeletal fluorosis was most commonly seen in people working in aluminium production, magnesium foundries, fluorspar processing and superphosphate manufacture, prior to the introduction of adequate controls. Endemic, as opposed to occupational, skeletal fluorosis occurs in parts of the Indian sub-continent, China and Africa but has not been observed in temperate countries (where the quantity of water drunk is generally lower) with drinking water concentrations less than 4ppm[13]. In an area of the USA where the water naturally contained 8ppm, radiological and clinical examination of residents found no evidence of deleterious bone changes from fluoride exposure although bone thickening was seen in 10–15% of the population[14]. Acute toxic doses range from 1 to 5 mg/kg body weight; doses exceeding 15 to 30 mg/kg body weight may be fatal[15].

36.8 **Safe Intakes** A water fluoride concentration of 1ppm contributes substantially to protection against dental caries, without causing cosmetically significant dental mottling. Therefore fluoride intakes, expressed as mg/kg body weight/day, associated with this level of water fluoride concentration can be considered safe. Fluoride intakes in infants and children in unfluoridated areas without supplementation are below that required for optimal dental health[8].

36.8.1 *Infants up to 6 months* Fluoride intakes of about 0.22mg/kg body weight/day (0.9mg/day) are found in the first month of life in formula-fed infants in areas with fluoridated water. This falls to about 0.13mg/kg body weight/day (1.0mg/day) in 6 month old infants. Intakes of fluoride up to **0.22mg/kg body weight/day** in infants up to 6 months are safe.

36.8.2 *Infants and children up to 6 years* Fluoride intake per kg body weight falls with increasing age. Up to 6 years, which is the period of mineralisation of the crowns of the anterior permanent teeth (ie those that are vulnerable to cosmetically significant dental mottling), fluoride intakes of up to 0.12mg/kg body weight/day (1.8mg/day for a child aged 3–4 years; 2.3mg/day for a child aged 5–6 years) are found in areas with fluoridated water and are not associated with cosmetically significant dental mottling. Intakes of fluoride of **0.12mg/kg body weight/day** in infants and children between 6 months and 6 years of age are safe.

36.8.3 *Children over 6 years and adults* After 6 years of age it is no longer possible for further exposure to fluoride to give rise to cosmetically significant mottling but the dental benefit from continued exposure persists. An adult weighing 60kg, drinking 1.1 litres of fluoridated water daily, and ingesting 2mg fluoride from food[4] would have a daily fluoride intake of 0.05mg/kg body weight (3mg/day). This exposure is less than those associated with skeletal fluorosis and has not been shown to be associated with adverse effects. Intakes of fluoride of **0.05 mg/kg body weight** daily in children aged over 6 years and in adults are therefore safe. Consumers of exceptionally large quantities of tea, in areas with fluoridated water, may have fluoride intakes several times greater (estimated as up to 12mg/day in a 60kg adult or 0.2mg/kg/day). Fluoride may be less readily absorbed from tea than from water, but nevertheless the absence of any reports of adverse effects from such exposures in the UK indicates that there is a further wide safety margin above the more usual intakes in fluoridated areas.

36.9 **References**

1 World Health Organisation. **Fluorine and fluorides. Environmental Health Criteria 36**. World Health Organisation: Geneva, 1984.

2 Murray J J, Rugg-Gunn A J and Jenkins G N. Fluorides in caries prevention. Third Edition. Butterworth-Heinemann Ltd, Oxford, 1991.

3 Rao G S. Dietary intake and bioavailability of fluoride. **Ann Rev Nutr** 1984;**4**:115–136.

4 Sherlock J C. Fluorides in foodstuffs and the diet. **J Roy Soc Health** 1984;**1**:34–36.

[5] Walters C B, Sherlock J C, Evans W H, Read J I. Dietary intake of fluoride in the United Kingdom and fluoride content of some foodstuffs. **J Sci Food Agric**, 1983;**34**:523–528.

[6] Rugg-Gunn A J, Hackett A F, Appleton D R, Eastcote J E, Dowthwaite L, Wright, W G. The water intake of 405 Northumbrian adolescents aged 12–14 years. **Brit Dent J** 1987;**162**:335–340.

[7] Department of Health and Human Services. **Review of fluoride: Benefits and risks**. Report of the ad hoc subcommittee of the committee to coordinate environmental health and related programs public health service. Centres for Disease Control: Atlanta, 1991.

[8] Vlachou A, Drummond B K, Curzon, M E J. Fluoride concentrations of infant foods and drinks in the UK. **Caries Res** 1992;**26**:29–32.

[9] Dowell T B, Joyston-Bechal S. Fluoride supplements—age related dosages. **Brit Dent J** 1981; **150**: 273–275.

[10] Dean H T, Arnold F A, Elvove E. Domestic water and dental caries, V, additional studies of the relation of fluoride domestic waters to dental caries experience in 4425 white children aged 12–14 years, of 13 cities in 4 states. **Public Health Rep**, 1942;**52**:1443–1452.

[11] Forsman B. Dental fluorosis and caries in high fluoride districts in Sweden. **Comm Dent Oral Epidemiol**, 1974;**2**:132–148.

[12] Forsman B. Early supply of fluoride and enamel fluorosis. **Scand J Dent Res**, 1977;**85**:22–30.

[13] Victoria Committee. **Report of the committee of inquiry into the fluoridation of victorian water supplies.** Melbourne: FD Atkinson, Government Printer, 1980; 278pp.

[14] Leone N C, Stevenson C A, Hilbish T F, Sosman M C. A roentgenologic study of human population exposed to high fluoride domestic water. **Am J Roentgenol radium Ther Nucl Med** 1955;74:874–855.

[15] Kaminsky L S, Mahoney M C, Leach J, Melius J, Miller M J. Fluoride: Benefits and risks of exposure. **Critical Reviews in Oral Biology and Medicine**, 1990;**1**: 261–281.

37. Other Minerals

37.1 **Aluminium** Aluminium (Al) comprises approximately 8 per cent of the earth's crust, making it the third most common element and the most abundant metal. It is found in all plants and animals, and levels vary with the amount of Al available in the environment. Although a number of roles have been described for the Al^{+++} ion in physiological processes, such as an involvement in the succinic dehydrogenase-cytochrome C system *in vitro*[1], there is no conclusive evidence that Al performs an essential function in any living species. Attempts to induce deficiency by providing an aluminium-free environment in species such as the rat have been unsuccessful.

37.2 **Arsenic** Arsenic (As) essentiality in humans has yet to be demonstrated. Although As intake is usually positively related to the quantity of seafoods in the total diet, much of the element in seafoods is present in the form of arsenobetaine—a compound which, although readily absorbed, is rapidly excreted unchanged. Soluble inorganic forms of penta- and trivalent As are rapidly methylated both within the digestive tract and in tissues but whether such modification modifies their bioavailability is not known. Typical estimates of total intake for Europe and USA range from 10 to 30 μg/d (0.1–0.4 μmol)/d*. Arsenic is highly toxic and the WHO/FAO Joint Expert Committee on Food Additives suggests a provisional maximum tolerable daily intake of inorganic As of 2 μg/kg body weight. Although no limit was derived for the consumption of organic As the need for further study of the toxicity of such forms was emphasised[2].

37.3 **Antimony** There is no evidence that antimony (Sb) is an essential element. Intakes of 0.25 to 1.25 mg/d (2–10 μmol/d†) have been reported for children in the USA. About 15 per cent of ingested Sb is absorbed, much of which accumulates in the liver, kidneys, skin and adrenals. Toxic effects include gastrointestinal symptoms and irregular respiration. Most instances of dietary Sb poisoning stem from the consumption of soft drinks stored in enamelled containers[3].

37.4 **Boron** (B) shows binding and structural characteristics intermediate between metals and non-metals and, like carbon, has a tendency to form double bonds and macromolecules including complexes with vicinal hydroxyl groups in organic compounds, many of which are of biological interest (eg sugars, polysaccharides, adenosine-5-phosphate, pyridoxine, riboflavin, dehydroascorbic acid, pyridine nucleotides and steroid hormones). Two fungal

---

*1 μmol = 75 μg
†1 μmol = 51 μg

antibiotics have been identified as containing B[4]. Nielsen has reported that B-deprivation depressed growth and elevated plasma alkaline phosphatase activity in chicks fed inadequate cholecalciferol[3]. However, the role of B in humans is unknown and the essentiality of B for humans remains to be demonstrated. There do not appear to be any published studies relating to the question of B toxicity.

37.5 **Bromine** The physiological function of bromine (Br) is unclear. Bromide appears to be able to substitute for the chloride ion in some reactions in a number of species[5]. There is conflicting evidence as to whether Br is concentrated by the thyroid gland in animals and in humans[6]. There is one reported study suggesting that deficiency occurs in humans: low serum and brain Br concentrations were found in haemodialysis patients, due to removal of the bromide ion by dialysis. Patients complaining of insomnia found that quality of sleep improved when Br was added to the dialysate[7]. The evidence for essentiality in man is very weak, and there are no recommendations for optimum dietary intakes in any species. Bromine is ubiquitous in the environment and it is unlikely that any deficiency would occur in humans.

37.6 **Cadmium** Although animals reared on diets virtually free of cadmium (Cd) exhibit poor reproductive efficiency and growth, there are no adequate data to support the essentiality of Cd for humans, and its potential toxicity is of more concern[8,9]. Human Cd exposure is in evolutionary terms a relatively recent phenomenon arising from industrial activity and smoking in the past two centuries. There is no effective homeostatic mechanism for the metal and relative body content increases steadily throughout life as the element is sequestered by the cysteine rich protein metallothione in tissues such as the liver and renal cortex. Systemic Cd deposits have a biological half-life of 15-30 years[8]. Cadmium reacts both in the intestinal mucosa and systemically with zinc, copper, manganese and iron. The intestinal transfer of Cd is increased in models deprived of zinc, iron, Cd and copper[10]. However it is not known how important these interactions are at customary dietary Cd intakes. On the other hand inhalational Cd exposure by smoking cigarettes during pregnancy is associated with an increased placental accumulation of Cd and zinc and with evidence consistent with a reduced delivery of zinc to the fetus and reduced birth weight[11].

37.7 **Caesium** There is no evidence that caesium (Cs) is an essential element. However, it can be present in the environment mainly as the radioisotope caesium-137 (half-life 30 years). The body deals with Cs in the same way as potassium, concentrating it in the muscle[3]. Thus, as the result of radioactive fallout meat from animals fed on pastures with Cs^{137} from this source may be contaminated.

37.8 **Cobalt** Cobalt (Co) is an essential trace element but is utilised by man only in the form of vitamin B_{12}. Requirements for this nutrient are discussed in section 13. Average intakes of Co are about 0.3 mg (5 μmol*)/d and the total

*1 μmol = 59 μg

body content about 1.5 mg. When Co salts have been used as a non-specific bone marrow stimulus in the treatment of certain refractory anaemias, doses of 29.5 mg (500 μmol)/d produced serious toxic effects including goitre, hypothyroidism and heart failure[12].

37.9 **Germanium** Germanium (Ge) is not an essential element. It is a relatively abundant element naturally present in the diet at trace levels of about 1 mg/d which are excreted rapidly and are not harmful. There is no evidence that Ge has any nutritional value or is otherwise beneficial to health. However, there is evidence that consumption of Ge at doses of the order of 50 to 250 mg/d (0.7–3.4 mmol*/d) over periods of 4–18 months can cause serious harm to health[13] and even death. There are not adequate data to define a safe maximum intake.

37.10 **Lead** There have been a small number of studies suggesting that lead (Pb) may be an essential element in the rat. Deprivation of Pb appeared to result in poor growth, disturbance of iron metabolism and altered levels of some metabolites[5]. The evidence is far from conclusive for the rat and there is no evidence that Pb is essential for humans.

37.11 **Lithium** Lithium (Li) is not of proven essentiality for humans[14]. However, goats deprived of Li develop reproductive inefficiency. The main focus on Li has been on its pharmacological role in the management of psychoses and affective disorders. Lithium is absorbed efficiently by the intestine and is excreted predominantly in the urine. Assessments of dietary Li intake vary considerably. This may reflect difficulties with analysis of the element. High Li doses in humans cause interference with metabolism of glucose, teratogenecity, and hypothyroidism with goitre development. No pharmacological basis for its therapeutic efficacy in psychoses has as yet been established other than the concept that Li may alter the distribution of electrolytes within the brain.

37.12 **Mercury** Mercury (Hg) is not an essential element. Metallic and organic Hg are trace contaminants of food. Methyl mercury, entering the food chain via marine sediments, is a potential problem. It is readily absorbed in the intestine, and accumulates in the brain. Most foods contain less than 5 μg (0.02 μmol†)/kg, giving average intakes of Hg of about 2–3 μg/d, but fish such as tuna may contain up to 1,000 mg (5 mmol)/kg. Toxic effects of Hg appear as Minamata disease after a pollution incident in Japan in the 1950's when fish and shellfish were found to have levels of methyl mercury up to 29 mg (145 μmol)/kg, resulting in a methyl mercury intake by the local population of 3 mg (15 μmol)/d or higher.

37.13 **Nickel** The biochemical function of nickel (Ni) has not been clearly defined, but it has been recognised as essential in animals and birds. Deficiency

---

*1 μmol = 72.6 μg
†1 μmol = 200.6 μg

results in depressed growth and haemopoesis. The human requirement for Ni is unknown and could be as low as 5 μg/d[15]. Intakes in the UK are estimated to lie between 140 and 150 μg/d (2.4 and 2.5 μmol/d*)[16] and there is no indication of deficiency. Nickel is relatively non-toxic and it has been estimated that the level of toxicity in humans lies around 250 mg (4.3 mmol)/d[15].

37.14 **Silicon** Studies with rats and chicks indicate that silicon (Si) is essential for the normal development of connective tissues and the skeleton. The Si content of the human aorta, trachea, lungs and tendons is particularly high. Aorta Si has been claimed to decline with age and the concentration in arterial wall decreases with the development of atherosclerosis[17]. It has been estimated that humans assimilate 9–14 mg (0.3–0.5 mmol†)/d, but most dietary Si in the form of silica remains unabsorbed. In contrast, silicic acid in foods and beverages is absorbed readily. Cereal grains are rich Si sources. Human requirements for Si are not known and estimates of intake differ widely. Hamilton and Minski (1972–1973) suggest that the UK diet provides 1.2 g/d[18]; a Finnish study suggested that 29 mg/d was typical[19].

37.15 **Silver** Silver (Ag) occurs naturally in very low concentrations in soils, plant and animal tissues. Although it has been shown to interact with copper and selenium *in vivo*[20], it has not been shown to perform any essential function in humans.

37.16 **Strontium** There is no evidence that strontium (Sr) is an essential element for man, but it is widely distributed in the environment and is present in foods particularly of plant origin, concentrated in the bran rather than the endosperm of grains and in the peel of root vegetables[21]. The Sr content of drinking water varies usually between 0.02 and 0.06 mg/L[22], although values as high as 1.6 mg (18 μmol**)/L have been reported[23]. Estimates of Sr intakes from dietary surveys and from national food supply statistics are generally in the range of 1–3 mg/d although one study in Britain showed an intake of 0.86 μg/d[18]. The total body content is only about 323 mg (3.7 mmol) of which 99 per cent is present in the bones[22]. Absorption of Sr in adults has been reported to be 19 per cent with losses in the urine, sweat, hair and other fluids. There is little evidence of Sr toxicity but it appears that a wide margin of safety exists between dietary levels of stable Sr likely to be ingested from ordinary foods and water supplies and those that induce toxic effects. However the longlived isotope of strontium, Sr^{90}, produced in atomic explosions, is hazardous when deposited in the human skeleton.

37.17 **Sulphur** Sulphur (S) occurs in tissues as the sulphate anion (SO_4^{--}), a constituent of the high molecular weight proteoglycans which are fundamental components of the extracellular matrices. Dermatan sulphate, chondroitin sulphate and keratan sulphate are typical proteoglycans of tissues such as

---

*1 μmol = 58.7 mg
†1 mmol = 28.1 mg
**1 μmol = 87.6 μg

cartilage and the vascular and reproductive systems[25]. In a different role, sulphate is involved in the detoxification of phenols, alcohols, amines and thiols in which their derivatives are excreted in the form of sulphate conjugates[26]. The "active" sulphate (phosphoadenosine phosphosulphate) required for the above purposes is probably derived from the oxidation of S derived from the amino acids cysteine and methionine. This process proceeds via the generation of sulphite and the highly active molybdenum-dependent sulphite oxidase system and there is no obligatory requirement for dietary sulphate[27]. Intakes in excess of approximately 0.7 mg (22 μmol*)/d probably exceed the sulphate-absorptive capacity of the small intestine and facilitate the bacterial reduction of sulphate to sulphide in the colon.[28].

37.18 **Tin** It is doubtful whether tin (Sn) is an essential element. Average intakes in the UK have been estimated to be 187 μg/d for an adult. Between 90 and 99 per cent of Sn in food is excreted in the faeces, depending on the chemical form, since Sn (II) is four times better absorbed than Sn (IV). Most retained Sn accumulates in the skeleton. The toxic dose of inorganic Sn is 5–7 mg (40–60 μmol†)/kg body weight, but organic Sn is far more toxic. Very high intakes of inorganic Sn of 250 mg/kg from food cause gastrointestinal symptoms. Chronic exposure to high levels results in growth depression and altered immune function, possibly due to interactions between Sn and Zn or Se[3].

37.19 **Vanadium** In vitro and animal studies led to the proposal that vanadium (V) has a specific physiological role in humans as a regulator of (Na,K)-ATPase, and therefore regulates the Na+ pump by means of a redox mechanism[29]. This has yet to be proven. It may also have a role in methyl and/ or labile methyl metabolism[30], and expression of some endocrine function[15]. Urinary output in man is estimated to be 10 μg/d[31]. Unlike cadmium and lead, V does not accumulate in body tissues with age[29]. Reported concentrations in serum measured by neutron activation analysis range from 0.016–0.139 ng/ml in women and 0.024–0.939 ng/ml in men[31]. The absolute requirement, for example as needed in total parental nutrition, is possibly only about 1–2 μg (20–40 nmol**)/d.

37.20 References

1 Martin R B. The chemistry of aluminium as related to biology and medicine. *Clin Chem* 1986; **32**: 1797–1806.

2 World Health Organization. Toxicological evaluation of certain food additives and contaminants. *WHO Food Additives Series* 1990; **26**: 156–160.

3 Nielsen F H. In: Mertz W, ed. *Trace Elements in Human and Animal Nutrition* vol II. New York: Academic Press, 1986; 415–463.

4 Nielsen F H. Boron: An over looked element of potential nutritional significance. *Nutrition Today* 1988; **2**: 4–7.

---

*1 mmol = 32 mg
†1 μmol = 118.7 μg
**1 μmol = 50.9 μg

[5] Nielsen F H. Ultra-trace elements in nutrition. *Ann Rev Nutr* 1984; **4**: 21–41.

[6] Van Leeuwen F X, Sangster B. The toxicology of bromide ion. *CRC Crit Rev Toxicol* 1987; **18**: 189–203.

[7] Oe P L C, Vis R D, Meijer J H G, Van Langevelde F, Allon W, Vandermeer L, Verheul H. Bromine deficiency and insomnia in patients on dialysis. In: McHowell J *et al.* eds. *Trace Element Metabolism in Man and Animals. Acad Sci Australia* 1981; **4**: 391–404.

[8] Kostial K. Cadmium. In: Mertz W, ed. *Trace Elements in Human and Animal Nutrition* vol 2, London: Academic Press, 1986; 319–345.

[9] Friberg L, Elinder C G. Cadmium toxicity in humans. In: Prasad A, ed. *Essential and Toxic Trace Elements in Human Health and Disease* New York: Alan R Liss, 1988; 559–587.

[10] Flanagan P B, McLellan J S, Haist J, Cherian M, Chamberlain M J, Valberg L S. Increased dietary cadmium absorption in mice and human subjects with iron deficiency. *Gastroenterology* 1978; **74**: 841–846.

[11] Kuhnert B R, Kuhnert P M, Debanne S, Williams T G. The relationship between cadmium, zinc and birth weight in pregnant women who smoke. *Am J Obstet Gynecol* 1987; **157**: 1247–1251.

[12] Smith R M, Cobalt. In: Mertz W, ed. *Trace Elements in Human and Animal Nutrition* Vol I London: Academic Press, 1987; 143–183.

[13] Matsusaka T, Fujii M, Nakano T, *et al.* Germanium-induced nephropathy: report of two cases and review of the literature. *Clinical Nephrology* 1988; **30**: 341–345.

[14] Mertz W. Lithium. In: Mertz W, ed. *Trace Elements in Human and Animal Nutrition* Vol 2. London: Academic Press, 1986; 391–397.

[15] Nielsen F H, Fluoride, vanadium, nickel, arsenic and silcon in total parenteral nutrition. *Bull NY Acad Med* 1984; **60**: 177–195.

[16] Smart G A, Sherlock J C. Nickel in foods and the diet. *Fd Add Contam* 1987; **4**: 61–71.

[17] Carlisle E M. Silicon. In: Mertz W, ed. *Trace Elements in Human and Animal Nutrition* 5th ed, Vol 2. New York: Academic Press, 1986; 373–390.

[18] Hamilton E I, Minski M J. Abundance of the chemical elements in man's diet and possible relations with environmental factors. *Sci Total Environ* 1972/73; **1**: 375–394.

[19] Varo P, Koivistoinen P. Mineral element composition of Finnish foods. *Acta Agric Scand* 1980; **22** (suppl): 161–171.

[20] Underwood E J. *Trace Elements in Human and Animal Nutrition*. 4th ed. New York: Academic Press, 1977; 444–445.

[21] Duckworth R B, Hawthorn J. Uptake and distribution of strontium in vegetables and cereals. *J Sci Food Agric* 1960; **11**: 218–225.

[22] Schroeder H A, Tipton I H, Nason A P. Trace metals in man: strontium and barium. *J Chron Dis* 1972; **25**: 491–517.

[23] Wolf N, Gedaila I, Yariv S, Zuckerman H. The strontium content of bones and teeth of human foetuses. *Arch Oral Biol* 1973; **18**: 233–238.

[24] Spencer H, Li M, Samachson J, Laszlo D. Metabolism of strontium-85 and calcium-45 in man. *Metab* 1960; **9**: 916–925.

[25] Muir H. The coming of age of proteoglycans. *Trans Biochem Soc* 1990; **18**: 787–789.

[26] Williams R T. *Detoxification Mechanisms*. London: Chapman and Hall, 1959.

[27] Stipanuk M H. Metabolism of Sulfur-containing amino acids. *Ann Rev Nutr* 1986; **6**: 179–209.

[28] Florin T, Neale G, Gibso G R, Cristl S A, Cummings J H. Metabolism of dietary sulphate: absorption and excretion in humans. *Gut* 1991; **32**: (in press).

[29] Golden M H N, Golden B E. Trace elements. Potential importance in human nutrition with particular reference to zinc and vanadium. *Br Med Bull* 1981; **37**: 31–36.

[30] Nielsen F H, Myron D R, Uthus E O. Newer trace elements—vanadium and arsenic. Deficiency signs and possible metabolic roles. In: Kirchgessner M, ed. *Trace Element Metabolism in Man and Animals* 1978; **3**: 244–247.

[31] Nechay B R. Mechanisms of action of vanadium. *Ann Rev Pharmacol Toxicol* 1984; **24**: 501–524.

Annex 1. Weights and Heights of the UK Population

1. **Introduction** As many DRVs, including those for energy, are related to body weight, it is essential to have standard weights for use in calculations which are representative of various age and sex groups of the UK population. In the past the appropriate reference standards for younger people have been those of Tanner *et al*[1]. These standards were based on measurements of normal British children which were made in 1959, and they were adjusted to take account of secular anthropometric trends in 1965. These standards have become increasingly out of date and the Panel, at the request of its Working Group on Energy and Protein, has sought acceptable data for use in its calculations. The 50th centiles are given in Tables A1–A4, where possible, along with 3rd and 97th or 5th and 95th centiles. Although corresponding heights have not been used in calculations by the Panel, these are given in the Tables for information.

2. **Children aged 3 months to 5.0 years** Data were obtained by Mrs E Hoinville from the records of the Pre-school Child Growth Surveys carried out on behalf of the Department of Health and Social Security (DHSS) by the Department of Human Nutrition of the London School of Hygiene and Tropical Medicine. A total of 12 271 children were measured in 4 surveys carried out between 1973 and 1982. All measurements were taken within 1 week of the age point given in the tables. Because the 4 surveys had a degree of overlap there were larger numbers in the 1 to 3 year age groups. In addition children who were measured longitudinally from 3 months to 5 years were measured twice at age 5.

3 **Children aged 5.5 to 11.5 years** Data were obtained by Dr S Chinn of the Department of Community Medicine, St Thomas's Hospital, London, from the records of the National Study of Health and Growth (NSHG) of 14,584 children measured in 1985 and 1986. The NSHG included a nationally representative sample in 1986 and a sample weighted towards inner city children and children from ethnic minorities in 1985. In order to make the combined sample more nationally representative the Caucasian children studied in 1985 and the non-Caucasian children studied in 1986 were omitted. The 1986 Caucasian children have been taken as representative of England and Wales; the 1985 ethnic minority children taken as representative of their appropriate groups; and the 1985 plus the 1986 Scottish children as representative of Scotland. Taller heights and heavier weights were reported on a nationally representative sample of schoolchildren aged 10/11 years measured in 1983[2]. However these children were weighed clothed and their exact ages were unrecorded as they were recruited to the survey as 10 year olds. Hence, with fieldwork lasting a year, their actual ages varied between 10 years and 11 years 11 months.

4 **Children aged 12.5 to 15.5 years** Data were made available to the Panel by Dr N G Norgan from the British Schoolchildren's Size Survey of the HUMAG Research Group, Loughborough University of Technology. This study was sponsored by the Syndicate of British Retailers and Garment Manufacturers

and covered 3500 boys aged 5 to 15.9 years who were measured in 1978 and 4500 girls aged 5 to 16.9 years who were measured in 1986. Details of the sample methodologies were made available to the Panel and confirmed that the samples were representative of Caucasian children only, and were designed to yield about 300 children in each age and sex group. The weight and height centiles for children aged 12.5 to 15.5 years only have been utilised as the two studies in paras 2 and 3 above had larger and more nationally representative samples of younger children.

5 **Adults aged 16 to 64 years** Data from the OPCS Survey of Adult Heights and Weights have been taken. This survey studied a nationally representative sample of 10 018 people aged 16–64 years in 1980. Median values for weights and heights in each 5 year range have been taken from the Report of the Survey[3]. A further 2197 British adults were measured in 1986/87 by OPCS in the Dietary and Nutritional Survey of British Adults. This showed that there had been a significant increase in the prevalence of obesity and overweight defined as Body Mass Index (BMI) greater than 30 or 25 respectively. The median weights of women had not changed between 16 and 34 years but had risen slightly between 35 and 64 years. However, the median weights of men had increased by about 1 kg between 16 and 49 years and by about 3 kg between 50 and 64 years[4]. Although the sample in this survey was nationally representative, the numbers in each age group were small compared with the 1980 survey. The results of the 1980 survey[3] have therefore been used while acknowledging that adult men, particularly over 50 years of age, may be heavier.

6 **The elderly aged 65 years and over** Data from the Nottingham Activity and Ageing Survey were made available to the Panel by Dr A B Lehmann of the Department of Health Care of the Elderly of the University of Nottingham Medical School. Full details of the sampling and methodology have been published[5]. Briefly, an effective sample of 406 men and 636 women aged 65 and over was obtained from a sample of 1,599 elderly people randomly selected from the Nottinghamshire Family Practitioner Records between May and September 1985. Those included were weighed in light clothes, without shoes. The composition of this sample was similar to the 1981 national census data in terms of age, sex and social class, so the demographic composition was close enough for the Nottingham data to be regarded as representative. The sample excluded the 3 per cent from that age group in residential accommodation. There is accumulating evidence that the institutionalised elderly may not be representative, in nutritional terms, of their age groups as a whole[6]. For this reason the Nottingham weights used were limited to those living in the community.

7 **References**

[1] Tanner J M, Whitehouse R H, Takaishi M. Standards from birth to maturity for height, weight, height velocity and weight velocity: British children, 1965. *Arch Dis Child* 1966; **41**: 454–471, 613–635.

[2] Department of Health. *The Diets of British Schoolchildren*. London: HMSO, 1989. (Reports on health and social subjects; 36).

[3] Knight I, Eldridge J. *The Heights and Weights of Adults in Great Britain*. London: HMSO, 1984.

[4] Gregory H, Foster K, Tyler H, Wiseman M. *The Dietary and Nutritional Survey of British Adults*. London: HMSO, 1990.

[5] Dalloso H M, Morgan K, Bassey E J, Ebrahim S B J, Fentem P H, Arie T H D. Levels of customary physical activity among the old and very old living at home. *J Epidemiol Comm Health* 1988; **42**: 121–127.

[6] Evans J G. Ageing and nutrition: questions needing answers. *Age Ageing* 1989; **18**: 145–147.

Table A.1 *Weights (kg)—Males*

Age	No of Observations	Centiles				
		3rd	5th	50th	95th	97th
3 m	590	4.65	—	6.12	—	7.70
6 m	794	6.29	—	8.00	—	10.00
9 m	883	7.45	—	9.20	—	11.55
12 m	1,037	8.10	—	10.04	—	12.48
1.5 y	1,089	9.13	—	11.30	—	14.03
2.0 y	1,030	10.00	—	12.39	—	15.11
2.5 y	1,033	10.85	—	13.42	—	16.30
3.0 y	1,012	11.53	—	14.40	—	17.83
3.5 y	967	12.25	—	15.32	—	19.10
4.0 y	968	13.00	—	16.22	—	20.49
4.5 y	912	13.72	—	17.00	—	21.90
5.0 y	1,832	14.25	—	18.25	—	22.75
5.5 y	1,134	15.3	—	19.3	—	25.1
6.5 y	1,175	17.1	—	21.7	—	29.0
7.5 y	1,125	18.8	—	24.2	—	33.0
8.5 y	994	20.6	—	26.8	—	37.1
9.5 y	1,013	22.5	—	29.7	—	41.5
10.5 y	1,104	24.5	—	32.7	—	46.6
11.5 y	648	27.0	—	35.9	—	53.0
12.5 y	335	—	30.9	39.0	54.1	—
13.5 y	229	—	33.0	45.5	61.6	—
14.5 y	269	—	37.5	52.0	68.8	—
15.5 y	277	—	41.4	56.5	74.5	—
16–19 y	481	—	—	64.5	—	—
20–24 y	518	—	—	70.0	—	—
25–29 y	539	—	—	73.0	—	—
30–34 y	523	—	—	74.5	—	—
35–39 y	459	—	—	74.5	—	—
40–44 y	438	—	—	75.5	—	—
45–49 y	401	—	—	74.5	—	—
50–54 y	424	—	—	74.5	—	—
55–59 y	441	—	—	73.0	—	—
60–64 y	326	—	—	74.0	—	—
65–74 y	211	50.0	53.0	71.0	93.4	99.3
75+ y	162	46.9	49.0	69.0	87.7	92.1

Table A.2 *Weights (kg)—Females*

Age	No of Observations	Centiles				
		3rd	5th	50th	95th	97th
3 m	552	4.50	—	5.70	—	7.10
6 m	814	5.93	—	7.44	—	9.35
9 m	833	6.94	—	8.55	—	10.55
12 m	976	7.52	—	9.50	—	11.76
1.5 y	1,023	8.60	—	10.65	—	13.30
2.0 y	1,019	9.50	—	11.80	—	14.82
2.5 y	1,009	10.39	—	12.84	—	16.31
3.0 y	1,007	11.20	—	13.85	—	17.85
3.5 y	940	11.70	—	14.90	—	19.90
4.0 y	936	12.25	—	15.75	—	20.50
4.5 y	907	13.25	—	16.75	—	22.00
5.0 y	1,779	14.00	—	17.75	—	23.41
5.5 y	1,049	15.0	—	18.9	—	24.8
6.5 y	1,070	16.8	—	21.3	—	29.0
7.5 y	1,024	18.5	—	23.8	—	33.4
8.5 y	947	20.2	—	26.6	—	37.8
9.5 y	974	21.0	—	29.7	—	42.7
10.5 y	1,053	23.9	—	33.0	—	48.7
11.5 y	645	26.6	—	36.7	—	57.3
12.5 y	373	—	30.5	41.0	55.5	—
13.5 y	376	—	35.5	47.0	63.1	—
14.5 y	389	—	40.2	50.5	65.0	—
15.5 y	393	—	42.5	52.5	64.2	—
16–19 y	499	—	—	55.5	—	—
20–24 y	548	—	—	58.5	—	—
25–29 y	560	—	—	58.0	—	—
30–34 y	561	—	—	60.0	—	—
35–39 y	495	—	—	60.0	—	—
40–44 y	486	—	—	61.5	—	—
45–49 y	419	—	—	62.5	—	—
50–54 y	498	—	—	62.5	—	—
55–59 y	497	—	—	63.0	—	—
60–64 y	414	—	—	63.5	—	—
65–74 y	272	52.2	46.7	63.0	90.0	94.8
75+ y	313	40.0	41.7	60.0	81.3	84.6

Table A.3 *Heights (cm)—Males*

Age	No of Observations	Centiles				
		3rd	5th	50th	95th	97th
3 m	589	56.2	—	61.1	—	65.6
6 m	793	63.4	—	67.9	—	72.1
9 m	827	68.0	—	72.1	—	77.2
12 m	1,034	70.5	—	75.8	—	80.7
1.5 y	1,078	76.6	—	82.0	—	87.7
2.0 y	1,039	81.0	—	86.9	—	93.1
2.5 y	1,024	84.5	—	91.4	—	98.1
3.0 y	—	—	—	—	—	—
3.5 y	1,649	90.9	—	98.6	—	106.1
4.0 y	—	—	—	—	—	—
4.5 y	—	—	—	—	—	—
5.0 y	1,830	99.6	—	107.9	—	116.5
5.5 y	1,134	103.4	—	112.4	—	121.3
6.5 y	1,175	109.3	—	118.6	—	127.9
7.5 y	1,125	114.5	—	124.5	—	134.4
8.5 y	994	119.4	—	130.0	—	140.6
9.5 y	1,013	124.1	—	135.3	—	146.5
10.5 y	1,104	128.9	—	140.5	—	152.1
11.5 y	648	134.0	—	145.5	—	157.1
12.5 y	335	—	139.1	149.6	162.0	—
13.5 y	299	—	142.2	156.6	172.0	—
14.5 y	269	—	147.9	164.7	178.9	—
15.5 y	277	—	154.1	170.3	184.8	—
16–19 y	500	—	—	175.3	—	—
20–24 y	537	—	—	176.3	—	—
25–29 y	557	—	—	175.3	—	—
30–34 y	541	—	—	175.3	—	—
35–39 y	481	—	—	175.3	—	
40–44 y	453	—	—	173.3	—	—
45–49 y	415	—	—	173.8	—	—
50–54 y	441	—	—	172.8	—	—
55–59 y	446	—	—	171.3	—	—
60–64 y	338	—	—	170.3	—	—

Table A.4 *Heights (cm)—Females*

Age	No of Observations	Centiles				
		3rd	5th	50th	95th	97th
3 m	547	55.5	—	60.0	—	64.0
6 m	812	61.6	—	66.3	—	70.3
9 m	830	65.9	—	70.4	—	75.2
12 m	975	69.0	—	74.2	—	79.5
1.5 y	1,021	74.8	—	80.6	—	86.4
2.0 y	1,023	79.7	—	85.7	—	91.9
2.5 y	1,005	83.5	—	90.2	—	96.9
3.0 y	—	—	—	—	—	—
3.5 y	1,600	90.2	—	97.6	—	105.5
4.0 y	—	—	—	—	—	—
4.5 y	—	—	—	—	—	—
5.0 y	1,778	99.1	—	107.3	—	115.7
5.5 y	1,049	103.0	—	111.6	—	120.2
6.5 y	1,070	108.5	—	117.8	—	127.2
7.5 y	1,024	113.6	—	123.6	—	133.6
8.5 y	949	118.6	—	129.2	—	139.7
9.5 y	973	123.5	—	134.6	—	145.8
10.5 y	1,056	128.4	—	140.2	—	152.0
11.5 y	643	133.2	—	145.9	—	158.6
12.5 y	373	—	139.0	151.3	163.6	—
13.5 y	376	—	146.8	156.8	168.1	—
14.5 y	389	—	150.6	160.3	170.6	—
15.5 y	394	—	151.5	161.9	171.4	—
16–19 y	523	—	—	161.3	—	—
20–24 y	582	—	—	161.8	—	—
25–29 y	516	—	—	161.8	—	—
30–34 y	583	—	—	162.3	—	—
35–39 y	516	—	—	161.3	—	—
40–44 y	498	—	—	160.8	—	—
45–49 y	439	—	—	160.3	—	—
50–54 y	519	—	—	159.8	—	—
55–59 y	503	—	—	159.3	—	—
60–64 y	420	—	—	158.8	—	—

Annex 2. Equations for estimating the basal metabolic rate (BMR) for older children, adolescents, adults and the elderly

BMR (MJ/d)			
Males	10–17 y	BMR = 0.074W + 2.754	SEE = 0.44
	18–29 y	BMR = 0.063W + 2.896	SEE = 0.64
	30–59 y	BMR = 0.048W + 3.653	SEE = 0.70
Females	10–17 y	BMR = 0.056W + 2.898	SEE = 0.47
	18–29 y	BMR = 0.062W + 2.036	SEE = 0.50
	30–59 y	BMR = 0.034W + 3.538	SEE = 0.47
Males	60–74 y	BMR = 0.0499W + 2.930 (n = 189)	
	75+ y	BMR = 0.0350W + 3.434 (n = 112)	
Schofield equations for all men over 60 years:		BMR = 0.049W + 2.459 (n = 50)	
Females	60–74 y	BMR = 0.0386W + 2.875 (n = 109)	
	75+ y	BMR = 0.0410W + 2.610 (n = 96)	
Schofield equations for all women over 60 years:		BMR = 0.038W + 2.755 (n = 38)	
BMR (kcal/d)			
Males	10–17 y	BMR = 17.7W + 657	SEE = 105
	18–29 y	BMR = 15.1W + 692	SEE = 156
	30–59 y	BMR = 11.5W + 873	SEE = 167
Females	10–17 y	BMR = 13.4W + 692	SEE = 112
	18–29 y	BMR = 14.8W + 487	SEE = 120
	30–59 y	BMR = 8.3W + 846	SEE = 112

W = body weight (kg), SEE = Standard error of estimate.

The equations for the elderly incorporate some of the original data collated by Schofield *et al* (1985) together with data on 101 men aged 60–70 years studied by Durnin and unpublished Italian data on 170 men and 180 women kindly supplied by Professor Anna Ferro-Luzzi. Those data collected in the tropics and used by Schofield proved to be appreciably lower than the European data and have been excluded.

Annex 3. Energy expenditure of various activities of moderate duration grouped according to Physical Activity Ratio (PAR*)

PAR 1.2 (1.0 to 1.4)	
Lying at rest:	reading.
Sitting at rest:	watching TV; reading; writing; calculating; playing cards; listening to radio; eating.
Standing at rest.	
PAR 1.6 (1.5 to 1.8)	
Sitting:	sewing; knitting; playing piano; driving.
Standing:	preparing vegetables; washing dishes; ironing; general office and laboratory work.
PAR 2.1 (1.9 to 2.4)	
Standing:	mixed household chores (dusting and cleaning); washing small clothes; cooking activities; hairdressing; playing snooker; bowling.
PAR 2.8 (2.5 to 3.3)	
Standing:	dressing and undressing; showering; 'hoovering'; making beds:
Walking:	3–4 km/h; playing cricket;
Industrial:	tailoring; shoemaking; electrical; machine tool; painting and decorating.
PAR 3.7 (3.4 to 4.4)	
Standing:	mopping floor; gardening; cleaning windows; playing table tennis; sailing.
Walking:	4–6 km/h; golf;
Industrial:	motor vehicle repairs; carpentry, chemical; joinery; bricklaying.
PAR 4.8 (4.5 to 5.9)	
Standing:	polishing furniture; chopping wood; heavy gardening; volley ball.
Walking:	6–7 km/h:
Exercise:	Dancing; moderate swimming; gentle cycling; slow jogging;
Occupational:	labouring; hoeing; road construction; digging and shovelling; felling trees
PAR 6.9 (6.0 to 7.9)	
Walking:	uphill with load or cross-country; climbing stairs.
Exercise:	average jogging; cycling.
Sports:	football; more energetic swimming; tennis; skiing.

*for discussion and definition of PAR see paras 2.3.3 and 2.3.4.

Annex 4. Classification of occupational work as light, moderate and moderate–heavy

Light PAR* = 1.7	Moderate PAR* = 2.7 in men = 2.2 in women	Moderate–heavy PAR* = 3.0 in men = 2.3 in women
Professional and technical workers; Administrative and managerial; Sales Representatives, Clerical and related workers; Housewives; Unemployed.	Sales workers; Service workers; Domestic helpers. Students; Transport workers; Some construction workers eg joiners, roofing workers.	Equipment operators; Labourers; Agricultural, eg animal husbandry, forestry and fishing; Some construction workers, eg bricklayers, masons.

*PAR = Physical Activity Ratio integrated over the period of the working day.

Annex 5. Examples of calculations of estimated daily energy expenditures of men and women aged 25 years and of median weight in light activity occupations and three categories of non-occupational activities

		Category of non-occupational activity					
		Inactive		Moderately active		Very active	
	Time hours	PAR	MJ(kcal)/d	PAR	MJ(kcal)/d	PAR	MJ(kcal)/d
Men							
Bed	8.0	1.0	2.44 (580)	1.0	2.44 (580)	1.0	2.44 (580)
Occupational	5.5	1.7	2.85 (680)	1.7	2.85 (680)	1.7	2.85 (680)
Non-occupational	10.5	1.5	4.79 (1,140)	1.7	5.43 (1,300)	1.9	6.07 (1,450)
Total energy expenditure			10.08 (2,400)		10.72 (2,560)		11.36 (2,710)
PAL (TEE)/(BMR)			1.4		1.5		1.6
Women							
Bed	8.0	1.0	1.88 (450)	1.0	1.88 (450)	1.0	1.88 (450)
Occupational	5.5	1.7	2.19 (520)	1.7	2.19 (520)	1.7	2.19 (520)
Non-occupational	10.5	1.5	3.70 (880)	1.7	4.18 (1,000)	1.9	4.68 (1,120)
Total energy expenditure			7.77 (1,850)		8.25 (1,970)		8.75 (2,090)
PAL (TEE)/(BMR)			1.4		1.5		1.6

PAR = Physical Activity Ratio (see para 2.3.3)
PAL = Physical Activity Level (see para 2.3.9)
TEE = Total Energy Expenditure (see para 2.3.1.3)
BMR = Basal Metabolic Rate (see para 2.3.2)

Annex 6. Examples of calculated energy expenditure from typical time use, energy cost of activity (PAR) in a group of young women office workers of median body weight

Activity		Time (h)	PAR	MJ(kcal)
In bed		8.00	1.0	1.88 (450)
Office work,	sitting	4.50	1.2	1.27 (300)
	standing	1.00	1.6	0.38 (90)
	walking slow	0.25	3.7	0.22 (50)
Sitting,	eating	1.50	1.2	0.42 (100)
	driving	0.50	1.2	0.14 (30)
	watching TV	3.00	1.2	0.85 (200)
	miscellaneous	1.00	1.2	0.28 (70)
Standing,	cooking	0.75	1.8	0.32 (80)
	personal	0.50	2.1	0.25 (60)
	shopping	0.75	2.1	0.37 (90)
	miscellaneous	1.00	2.1	0.49 (120)
	housework	0.50	2.8	0.33 (80)
Walking,	slow	0.25	2.8	0.16 (40)
	normal	0.50	3.7	0.43 (100)
TOTAL		24.00		7.80 (1,860)

Annex 7 Calculation of basal metabolic rate (BMR), total daily energy expenditure and Estimated Average Requirements (EARs) of energy for older children and adolescents

	Age (years)							
	10.5	11.5	12.5	13.5	14.5	15.5	16.5	17.5
Boys								
Weight kg	33	36	39	46	52	57	60	65
BMR MJ/d	5.12	5.35	5.58	6.05	6.53	6.86	7.13	7.45
TEE MJ/d	8.00	8.37	8.73	9.47	10.21	10.74	11.16	11.65
Growth MJ/d	0.25	0.29	0.33	0.38	0.42	0.21	0.13	0.13
Estimated Average Requirement MJ/d	8.25	8.66	9.06	9.85	10.63	10.95	11.29	11.78
Girls								
Weight kg	33	37	41	47	51	53	54	56
BMR MJ/d	4.81	5.00	5.21	5.52	5.70	5.80	5.88	5.95
TEE MJ/d	7.11	7.39	7.71	8.16	8.43	8.58	8.69	8.80
Growth MJ/d	0.27	0.31	0.36	0.40	0.42	0.21	0.10	0.10
Estimated Average Requirement MJ/d	7.38	7.70	8.07	8.56	8.85	8.79	8.79	8.90
Boys								
Weight kg	33	36	39	46	52	57	60	65
BMR kcal/d	1,223	1,279	1,334	1,447	1,561	1,640	1,705	1,780
TEE kcal/d	1,912	2,000	2,086	2,264	2,442	2,566	2,668	2,785
Growth kcal/d	60	70	80	90	100	50	30	30
Estimated Average Requirement kcal/d	1,972	2,070	2,166	2,354	2,542	2,616	2,698	2,815
Girls								
Weight kg	33	37	41	47	51	53	54	56
BMR kcal/d	1,149	1,194	1,246	1,319	1,362	1,387	1,405	1,423
TEE kcal/d	1,700	1,766	1,842	1,951	2,014	2,051	2,078	2,104
Growth kcal/d	65	75	85	95	100	50	25	25
Estimated Average Requirement kcal/d	1,765	1,841	1,927	2,046	2,114	2,101	2,103	2,129

BMR = basal metabolic rate
TEE = total energy expenditure

Annex 8. The efficiency of absorption and utilisation of nutrients—bioavailability

1 The efficiency (usually expressed as a percentage) with which any dietary nutrient is used in the body is known as its *bioavailability*. For some nutrients (amino acids, lipids, available polysaccharides) this is high (90 per cent or more), but for others, especially some vitamins and inorganic minerals, and non-starch polysaccharides, it is low and poorly predictable. Bioavailability is an important concept in the nutritional evaluation of foodstuffs and composite diets, and must be taken into account when calculating the DRVs for nutrients, especially those with variable bioavailabilities, so that they meet estimated needs[1-3].

2 Examples of factors which influence bioavailability are listed in Table A8. These arise from (i) the nature of the diet and of the nutrient itself; (ii) intestinal factors which influence luminal and mucosal digestion and absorption; and (iii) systemic factors which control the intestinal absorption and systemic distribution of a nutrient, its metabolism, and its ultimate fate. Whereas the bioavailability of all nutrients is influenced both by intestinal and by systemic factors it can be seen from Table A8 that the metabolism of minerals and vitamins is particularly influenced by the physico-chemical properties of the nutrients themselves, acting either independently or with those of other dietary components.

3 Because the absorption and utilisation of a nutrient may vary not only with the nutrient itself but also with the food in which it is eaten and the rest of the diet, as well as with host factors, it is not possible to apply a single figure which will define the 'bioavailability' of any nutrient. However, it is possible to give some guidance based on usual dietary patterns eaten by particular groups, and on evidence of host influences.

4 When needs for a nutrient are low then either the intestinal absorption may be reduced or the mechanisms for its clearance can be increased, or both. Conversely when requirements are high increased acquisition and conservation of the nutrient may occur. The time scale of such homeostatic mechanisms is not known, but by these means the body has an appreciable capacity to adapt to a low dietary intake or a reduced availability arising from the nature of the diet. Thus the measured bioavailability of several nutrients from a meal would be lower when needs for that nutrient are low than it would be from an identical meal if the body's requirements were high. In the former circumstances the reduced bioavailability may be independent of the dietary source.

5 The difficulty of selecting appropriate functional endpoints with which to measure the utilisation of many nutrients has led to an ambiguity in which the term *bioavailability* is sometimes equated with the efficiency of a nutrient's net or true absorption, or both. For example, whereas in the case of iron the relative incorporation of an ingested isotope into erythrocyte haemoglobin is a useful measure of bioavailability, with most other minerals crucial functional indices have either not been identified or would not be ethically or practically feasible

Table A8 *Examples of factors which influence the absorption and utilisation of nutrients*

Diet

Chemical form of the nutrient:
eg haem iron v inorganic iron, pyridoxine v pyridoxine glucosides, amino-acid and hexose complexes (condensation interactions), monoglutamyl v polyglutamyl folate, isomeric form (amino acids, hexoses), physical form (starches), oxidation state.

Antagonistic ligands:
phosphates, phytate, carbonates, polyphenols, oxalates (minerals), nitrates, avidin, factors in wheat bran (some B vitamins)

Facilitatory ligands:
Ascorbate, carboxylic acids, some sugars, amino acids.

Ligands which may facilitate absorption but increase renal excretion:
EDTA, picolinate.

Competitive interactions:
Fe v Cu v Zn v Cd

Inhibitors of proteolysis impair release of amino acids, complexed vitamins and metals, and facilitatory ligands.

Breakdown of nutrient:
Thiaminase in fish and some cereals.

Luminal

pH and redox state.
Efficiency of dietary hydrolysis.
Bacterial fermentation (non-starch polysaccharides).

Mucosal

Entrainment of uptake and transfer mechanisms (influenced by systemic factors listed below).
Changes in mucosal structure and function.
Proteolytic inhibitor of folate conjugase.

Systemic factors

Anabolic requirements:
growth in infancy and childhood, pregnancy and lactation.
Post-catabolic states.
Endocrine influences.
Hepatic and renal function.
Infection and stress.
Homeostatic setting for nutrient determined by previous dietary supply, supply and metabolism of other nutrients.

in human studies. In practice the closest estimate of bioavailability is the proportion of intake that is absorbed or retained in the body. As a consequence estimates of bioavailability for some nutrients, such as iron, zinc and copper, have focussed on the luminal factors which limit their bioavailability; this places undue emphasis on dietary characteristics which do not allow for the host's ability to compensate. Similarly this approach would not measure the bioavailability of nutrients which are absorbed efficiently but which for some reason are not then utilised.

6 Studies in animal models, in which host factors may be more easily standardised, provide some information about the metabolism of a nutrient and the effect on this of factors which influence bioavailability. They may also enable the stratification of bioavailability of nutrients from human diets; but this information cannot necessarily be extrapolated quantitatively to humans.

7 It is clear that any measurement of bioavailability can be interpreted reliably only in the context of the circumstances in which it was assessed[1-3]. Even if the studies are well characterised with respect to the factors which influence bioavailability the extrapolation of such data to the derivation of DRVs has to be done in the light of current knowledge of the metabolism of the nutrient concerned. The judgements involved for any nutrient and the limited information on which they can be based[3] are explained in the appropriate sections. Differences in these judgements of bioavailability are one of the principal sources of discrepancy between different sets of recommendations.

8 References

1 O'Dell B L. Bioavailability of trace elements. *Nutrition Reviews* 1984; **42**: 301–308.

2 Bender A E. Nutritional significance of bioavailability. In: Southgate D *et al* eds. *Nutrient Availability: Chemical and Biological Aspects*. London: Royal Society of Chemistry, 1989; 3–9.

3 Southgate D A T. Conceptual issues concerning the assessment of nutrient bioavailability. In: Southgate D *et al*, eds. *Nutrient Availability: Chemical and Biological Aspects*. London: Royal Society of Chemistry, 1989; 10–12.